Can **Adventu**re **Prev**ent Dementia?

A guide to outwitting Alzheimer's

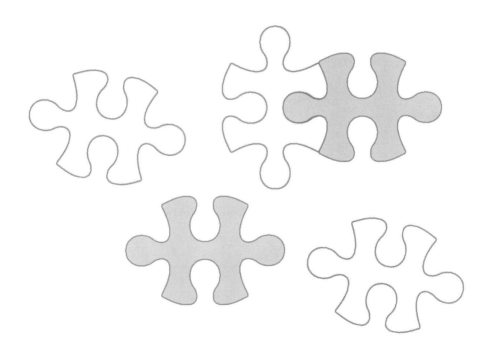

Dr Helena Popovic MBBS

Published by Choose Health, Australasia

First published in Australia and New Zealand in 2023

Liability Disclaimer

The material contained in this book is general in nature and does not constitute medical advice. It is not intended to provide specific guidance for any particular circumstances and it should not be relied on as a basis for any decision to take action on any matter it covers. Readers should obtain medical advice before acting on any information in this book. The author disclaims all responsibility and liability to any person, arising directly or indirectly, from any person taking or not taking action based upon the information in this publication.

 A catalogue record for this book is available from the National Library of Australia

Title: Can Adventure Prevent Dementia? — A guide to outwitting Alzheimer's
Author: Dr Helena Popovic MBBS
Edition: First
ISBN: 9780994335791 (pbk)
Notes: Includes bibliographical references
Subjects: Dementia | Alzheimer's | Longevity | Health | Nutrition |
          Exercise | Care | Fathers and daughters
Editor: Rosemary Peers
Proofreader: Camilla Cripps
Cover design, internal design, formatting and artwork: Sue Finlay Graphics
Libraries Australia ID 71978442. Contributed by Libraries Australia

Proudly printed in Australia

Dedication

This book is dedicated to four extraordinary individuals with an unshakeable commitment to improving the lives of everyone touched by dementia: Lori La Bey, Lauren Miller Rogen, Seth Rogen and Dr Richard S Isaacson MD.

* * * * *

Lori La Bey became a passionate advocate for people with dementia when her mother was diagnosed with early-onset Alzheimer's in her 50s. Lori gave up her career to care for her mother for the next 30 years and was shocked at the lack of information, support and hope for patients and their families. In response, she established **Alzheimer's Speaks** (alzheimersspeaks.com) to provide free education, tools and resources for patients, friends, caregivers and health professionals.

Lori's mission is to raise dementia awareness and connect people around the globe in order to shift the dementia journey **from crisis to comfort**. In 2011 she launched **Alzheimer's Speaks Radio:** (blogtalkradio.com/alzheimersspeaks), the first radio show and podcast dedicated to dementia. Her podcast remains the most informative, insightful and uplifting program for people with all forms of dementia and their caregivers. Above all, Lori's empathy and wisdom are a wellspring of strength, encouragement and optimism. Her far-sighted motto is **'What's good for dementia is good for the world'**.

* * * * *

Lauren Miller Rogen is a screenwriter, director, producer and philanthropist who lost her mother and grandmother to Alzheimer's. When her mother was diagnosed, Lauren was only in her 20s but she wasted no time in co-founding the nonprofit **HFC (Hilarity for Charity)** (wearehfc.org) with her writer, actor and entrepreneur husband **Seth Rogen**.

The goals of HFC (which would also qualify as an acronym for Help For Caregivers) are to assist people with in-home care and support TODAY, while offering brain health education and promoting research for TOMORROW. To date, the HFC team has raised over

US$12 million and awarded 300 000 hours of in-home care to families. HFC also has virtual support groups that pair people who are in similar situations.

One of HFC's unique innovations is **HFCUniverse** (hfcuniverse.learnworlds.com), a digital brain health education program for high school and college students. Blending scientific rigour, humour and age-specific classroom learning, HFCUniverse is North America's only national Alzheimer's prevention program for teens and young adults.

In October 2022 HFC celebrated their 10th anniversary with a gala fundraising celebrity event and a pledge that heartfelt **care can lead to cure**.

* * * * *

Dr Richard Isaacson MD is a world-renowned neurologist, researcher and director of the Florida Atlantic University Center for Brain Health within the Schmidt College of Medicine. He also runs the university's **Alzheimer's Prevention Clinic** and leads a research program aimed at reducing the risk of Alzheimer's, Parkinson's and Lewy body dementia in people with a family history of these diseases.

Dr Isaacson is a **genuine pioneer** in dementia prevention. When he established the first-ever Alzheimer's Prevention Clinic in the USA at Weill Cornell Medicine and New York-Presbyterian in 2013, he encountered skepticism and disdain from many of his academic colleagues. At the time, the words 'Alzheimer's' and 'prevention' were deemed incompatible. Despite ongoing reproval, he held his ground and has gone on to show that a personalised, comprehensive medical and lifestyle strategy can delay — and in many cases prevent — the onset of Alzheimer's. His **courage and conviction** continue to spearhead breakthroughs in dementia research. Dr Isaacson is also instrumental in creating **free online courses** on brain health (faumedicine.org/alz/course) and Alzheimer's prevention — (alzu.org) for anyone, anywhere in the world.

* * * * *

I extend my profound gratitude to all four of you.

Contents

PART ONE – Our decisions are more powerful than our DNA

PART TWO – Obstacles or opportunities?

PART THREE – Let movement be your medicine

PART FOUR – Let food be your medicine

PART FIVE – Slow ageing despite fast living

PART SIX – Dementia is a doorway

Chapter	Page

PART SEVEN – Education is more powerful than medication

Chapter	Page

Glossary can be downloaded from:
outwittingalzheimers.com/resources

Resources mentioned in the book can be downloaded from:
outwittingalzheimers.com/resources

References can be downloaded from:
outwittingalzheimers.com/references

About the author

Dr Helena Popovic MBBS is a medical practitioner (GP), award-winning author and international speaker. When her father was diagnosed with Alzheimer's, she began a decade of extensive research into improving brain function and preventing dementia. She is now a leading authority on brain health and peak performance and teaches patients, health professionals and the public how to boost their brain, turn stress into success and come alive and thrive. She is also a TEDx Fast Ideas finalist and popular TV and radio commentator.

Dr Helena graduated from the University of Sydney and she believes in slow ageing despite fast living. Her driving philosophies are that **education is more powerful than medication** and **our decisions are more powerful than our DNA**.

Although this is the sequel to her first bestselling book *In Search of My Father — Dementia is no match for a daughter's determination*, the books can be read in either order with equal suspense and enjoyment.

Her second book was *NeuroSlimming — Let your brain change your body*. *NeuroSlimming* won bronze medal in the international Living Now Awards for its contribution to positive global change in the health and wellness category.

Author's note

Always look on the bright side. That way, if something goes wrong, you can say the sun was in your eyes.

AUTHOR UNKNOWN

All names in this book (apart from mine and Dad's) have been changed to protect people's privacy. In some cases, I have merged several care-partners into one character so as not to overload the reader with unnecessary detail. One notable character, Felix (also not his real name), deserves a few words of explanation.

Felix is a private, unassuming, generous man with a quick wit and a penchant for puns. We met about two years after my previous partner and I had gone our separate amicable ways. When Felix entered my life, I didn't have time for a romantic relationship but that's precisely when they strike.

As I started writing this book, Felix requested that I only mention him when essential to the story. Thus, although I don't include him in many chapters, he has been an indefatigable uplifting support for Dad as well as for me.

* * * * *

The terms carer, caregiver, care-companion and care-partner are used interchangeably to mean anyone (a family member, friend or paid professional) who assists in the care of someone with dementia.

* * * * *

With respect to website links provided throughout the book, all web addresses have been checked and were accurate at the time of printing. However, some web addresses may change over time.

Once upon a time

Once upon a time we knew little about our brain,
the idea that it could change was considered quite insane.

That wrinkled lump of grey matter in our head,
just shrivelled and shrank until we were dead.

Nothing could be further from the truth we now know,
because research has shown that new brain cells can grow.

We can get smarter and better with age,
it's our beliefs about ourselves that have put us in a cage.

It's never too late and you're never too old,
and it doesn't matter what you've previously been told.

You can boost your brain and sharpen your mind,
you have so many untapped resources to find.

Take heed of what this book has to say
to discover the secrets your brain has hidden away.

After reading our story, you'll know what to do
to be wiser and healthier — and happier too!

DR HELENA POPOVIC MBBS
21 SEPTEMBER 2022 WORLD ALZHEIMER'S DAY

PREFACE

There's a way to do it better. Find it.
THOMAS EDISON (1847–1931)

Why did my father develop Alzheimer's dementia?

Does it mean I'm also doomed to get the disease?

Despite hundreds of failed drug trials, is there a way of curing the condition that has so far been overlooked?

Can a person's day-to-day lifestyle choices protect their brain from decline, even if they've inherited genes that increase their risk of Alzheimer's?

What is happening to the brain of a person with Alzheimer's that decimates their memory, personality and ability to function?

What is going on in the world that leads to a diagnosis of dementia **every three seconds?** In Australia alone, 250 people are being diagnosed every day.

Even before my father's diagnosis 15 years ago, I'd been searching for answers. I'm in the fortunate position of being a medical doctor who has spent most of her career scrutinising and interpreting research, disentangling hype from help, and working with patients and their dedicated care-partners. The most crucial things I've learned about dementia are recounted in this book — a chronicle of our adventure with dementia. Most importantly, our experience provides a step-by-step guide to outwitting Alzheimer's — a disease in which *education* **is more powerful than** *medication*.

PART ONE

Our decisions are more powerful than our DNA

*Circumstances don't make the man,
they only reveal him to himself.*

Epictetus (50–130 CE)

CHAPTER 1

In search of the car

Have you ever noticed that anyone driving ahead of you is an idiot and anyone driving behind you is a maniac?

AUTHOR UNKNOWN

'Wake up! Wake up! The car's been stolen!' My father's panic-stricken voice broke my slumber.

I reached across to the bedside cabinet and fumbled around for my watch. It was 3.55 am. Exactly the same time as last night. How does the human brain do that?

'Dad, it's okay. The car hasn't been stolen. It got written off in a car accident a week ago.'

'How? What happened?' The light from the hallway exposed his bewilderment.

I repeated my answer for the fourth consecutive night. 'On your way to church last Sunday you drove through an intersection at the same time as two other cars and ended up in a three-car pile-up.'

'What? No! How come I don't remember?'

'People often forget things when they experience a shock.'

'Was anyone hurt?' Another wave of panic swept over him.

'Thankfully not,' I tried to soothe him. 'Let me take you back to bed and we'll talk about it in the morning.'

I waited until he'd fallen asleep and tiptoed back to my room.

Interrupted or fragmented sleep, dream enactment and restless leg syndrome (RLS) are common features of Alzheimer's and other dementias. This is partly due to erosion of cells in an area of the brain called the suprachiasmatic nucleus (SCN) or master body clock. The SCN receives input from our eyes about whether it is light or dark and adjusts our state of wakefulness through production of a hormone called melatonin. Darkness causes melatonin levels to rise, which leads to feeling sleepy. Hence the importance of having bright natural light during the day and dimming the lights at night. Maintaining a consistent sleep–wake routine also helps to improve the quality of our sleep. Unfortunately, sleep disturbances worsen symptoms of Alzheimer's and can hasten progression of the disease. The more severe the disease, the worse the quality of sleep and a vicious self-perpetuating cycle can ensue. More about sleep and the SCN in later chapters.

The car accident was a blessing in disguise. Dad's dementia precluded him from driving, despite his insistence that he was perfectly capable. He struggled to find his way around familiar streets and was oblivious to road signs and kerb sides. He misjudged distances and braked perilously close to the vehicle in front of him. The handbrake was an afterthought and indicators were optional. Driving is a deceptively complex undertaking that involves many interrelated cognitive processes. These include acute powers of observation, appropriate planning and judgement, and rapid switching of attention from one thing to another. Erosion of all these skills is a common feature of many dementias. In Dad's case, he struggled to focus on his surroundings while he was preoccupied with the mechanics of driving. The deterioration in his driving skills also reflected a loss of ability to process multiple pieces of information coming at him simultaneously. But he had no insight into his condition, so it was understandable he resented his personal freedoms being taken away from him. His GP had sensitively recommended that he have an on-road driving assessment, but Dad had no recollection of the conversation.

Clearly his safety — and that of other motorists and pedestrians — was paramount. At the same time, I didn't want to diminish his self-confidence by insisting that he give up his driver's licence. It was a delicate balance that I dealt with by driving him everywhere myself. He didn't object because he didn't remember that I was always the one driving. On Sunday mornings I would leave him in the enthusiastic care of the candle-shop custodian at the local Serbian Orthodox church. He'd been an active member of the spirited congregation (pun intended) since the early days of our emigration to Australia more than 40 years ago. **Being surrounded by welcoming familiar faces was vital in preserving his social confidence and sense of belonging.** I used the time to catch up with my own friends and pick up a few groceries before collecting him when the service was over. One afternoon while I was driving us home, he became irritated by the sound of the indicator.

'What's that clicking noise?' he snapped.

'It's the blinker — the turn signal.'

'What's that?'

'It's a light that comes on at the front and back of the car to notify drivers around me that I'm about to make a left or right turn.'

'Stop it! It's none of anyone's business where you're going!' he exclaimed waggishly.

The previous Sunday I'd inadvertently slept in. Not wanting to disturb me, Dad drove himself to church. I was jolted awake by a phone call from ambulance officer James. 'Your father has been involved in a car accident — a three-car pile-up. He has no obvious injuries but we need to take him to hospital for a proper examination. He's refusing to come with us. Can you speak to him, please?'

After considerable negotiation, I managed to convince Dad to accompany James and assured him I'd be at the hospital to meet them. I walked in to hear Dad telling police that 'giving way (whey)' was something they should discuss with cheesemakers. Whey was not his area of expertise. He was an electrical engineer.

The upshot of it all was that Dad lost both his car and his licence. His car was a write-off. So was his licence after he admitted that he was speeding.

'Why were you speeding?' asked one of the officers.

'So that I'd get to where I was going before I forgot where I was going,' he winked.

* * * * *

Subtle changes in the way a person drives may indicate they are at risk of developing Alzheimer's up to 20 years before they start having memory problems. Canadian and US researchers from the Universities of Toronto and Washington used GPS devices to assess the navigational and driving abilities of 139 men and women over the age of 65 for 12 months from January to December 2019. None of the study participants had any symptoms of Alzheimer's and they all scored in the normal range on tests of brain function. The scientists also took samples of each person's cerebrospinal fluid (CSF) because abnormal ratios of two protein fragments called amyloid beta 42 (Aβ42) and amyloid beta 40 (Aβ40) in CSF are consistent with impending Alzheimer's (referred to as pre-clinical disease).

The results were staggering. Those with abnormal protein ratios, i.e. pre-clinical Alzheimer's, tended to:
• drive more slowly
• jerk the car
• brake harder and more suddenly
• accelerate more abruptly
• drive less at night
• drive shorter distances
• drive less overall
• stick to familiar routes
• avoid driving to new places.

Yet, in every other respect, their cognitive function seemed normal.

Destructive processes in the brain begin decades before any symptoms of Alzheimer's are evident. However, this study reveals that early brain changes can negatively impact complex tasks such as spatial navigation and driving, in minute ways that are undetectable unless they're closely monitored. Thus, tracking people's driving habits could become a useful method of identifying pre-clinical Alzheimer's — if a person wanted to know. This is not to suggest that everyone becomes hypervigilant about how we, our parents or grandparents drive. Anyone can occasionally have a bad day behind the wheel, hence the study examined people's driving over the course of a year using very fine measurements and complicated statistical analyses. The technology is still being refined and many more people need to be tested before definitive conclusions are reached. In other words, don't try this at home (or on the road).

My personal philosophy is that the earlier we detect declining brain function, the sooner we can take steps to improve our brain health and turn the situation around. Better still, don't wait for signs of decline. **We can be proactive about looking after our brain at every age and stage of life.** That's what this book is about.

CHAPTER 2

To tell or not to tell?

We suffer more often in imagination than in reality.

SENECA (4 BCE – 65 CE)

'If I ever get Alzheimer's like my mother, I'll swallow every pill in the medicine cabinet in one go. That should do the job, shouldn't it?' Dad looked self-satisfied with his proposition.

'Yes Dad, that would definitely finish you off.' Note to self: put a lock on the medicine cabinet and swallow the key.

'I don't want to be a burden on you. I don't want to live if I can't look after myself,' he brooded.

'Maybe that's how life unfolds,' I suggested. 'First you look after your children, then your children look after you.'

'No! And don't you ever put me into one of those homes for old people. I'll swallow every pill in their medicine cabinet as well.' His pronouncement seemed to mollify him.

'That would be very unfair to the other residents, Dad. If they don't have their medications, they'll get sick and die. Then you'd be charged with manslaughter.'

He looked puzzled for a moment before smugly announcing, 'But I'd be dead so it wouldn't matter.'

'It would matter to *me*. I'm in the business of keeping people alive and well. I can't have you undermining my good work!'

I don't know whether Dad had ever been cognisant of his diagnosis of dementia. Mum had never mentioned it. I only started piecing it together after she'd passed away and I found a box of Alzheimer's medications in the butter compartment of the fridge. Dad had been in denial about the terminal nature of Mum's lung cancer. Was he also in denial about his own condition? Or had he forgotten about his diagnosis because the condition erased his memory of it?

Alzheimer's dementia is notoriously difficult to diagnose. For a long time it was regarded as a 'diagnosis of exclusion'. In other words, a doctor made a diagnosis of Alzheimer's only after all other possible causes of the person's symptoms had been ruled out.

There are many and varied treatable conditions that can erode a person's memory and cognition. These include: strokes, brain tumours, hydrocephalus (accumulation of cerebrospinal fluid within the brain), sleep apnoea, urinary tract infections, pneumonia, dehydration, alcohol dependence, depression, hypothyroidism (underactive thyroid), vitamin deficiencies, autoimmune diseases, hypo- or hyperglycaemia and side effects of medications. All these potential causes of impaired mental functioning need to be tested for and remedied if possible.

Brain scans employing Computerised Axial Tomography (CT or CAT), Magnetic Resonance Imaging (MRI) and Positron Emission Tomography (PET) offer valuable clues about what is going on. Specific patterns of brain shrinkage can suggest — but not confirm — a diagnosis of Alzheimer's. Functional MRI (fMRI) and PET scans can demonstrate that certain areas of the brain are receiving less blood or using less glucose and are therefore less active than expected — another indication that a person might be developing Alzheimer's. Brain scans can also offer alternative explanations for a person's memory problems by revealing signs of stroke or tumours.

In research settings (and increasingly in dedicated memory clinics) doctors use PET scans with radioactive tracers to look for two proteins that are hallmarks of Alzheimer's dementia:
- amyloid beta ($A\beta$) plaques and
- neurofibrillary tau tangles.

However, even this type of PET scanning may not be definitive because not everyone with amyloid plaques and tau tangles gets symptoms of Alzheimer's. Sigh. It's complicated.

Therefore, diagnosis involves:
- taking a detailed medical and psychological history from the patient
- family members or friends reporting changes in the person's behaviour or mental abilities (if the patient consents to the involvement of support people)
- extensive neuropsychological assessment
- full physical examination
- blood tests
- brain scans
- other tests as required such as cerebrospinal fluid (CSF) sampling.

Even when a diagnosis of Alzheimer's is made, **each person's trajectory is unique.** To date, we are unable to predict how quickly the disease will progress — if at all. We can't predict the exact constellation of symptoms that a patient will experience. And we don't know if medication will be helpful until a person has been taking it for several months.

Our beliefs and expectations also modify the course of a disease. To the extent that Dad resisted Mum's prognosis, Mum resigned herself to it. As soon as Mum had been told she had lung cancer, she gave up hope of surviving longer than 18 months. She was a textbook case. Her disease progressed exactly as the statistics predicted because she knew the statistics and she subscribed to them. Too often we assume the identity of the labels we're given. Tragically, if our self-image conforms to a diagnosis, it becomes our destiny. **A diagnosis is a starting point, not an end point. A diagnosis can be a doorway to a healthier life** — if we choose to approach it that way. I'd lost one parent to a label; I didn't want to lose another parent in the same way.

Dad and I spoke about his memory lapses but not about his diagnosis. It was a subtle but significant distinction. Dad viewed declining memory as 'just getting old'. As such, he humoured my attempts at 'turning back the clock'. In contrast, he viewed dementia as a death sentence. Despite regaling him with evidence that lifestyle changes can ameliorate the disease, he insisted that he would 'will himself to death' if he ever showed signs of Alzheimer's. I was not prepared to call his bluff.

When I asked his permission to write my first book, *In Search of My Father — Dementia is no match for a daughter's determination*, I explained that I wanted to tell people our story to help them take care of their brain. Was he okay with that?

'I don't mind you sharing our story but you'll lose all your patients.'

'Why do you say that?' I was bemused by his response.

'No one's going to want to do everything you put me through,' he announced triumphantly.

As soon as the book was published, Dad asked for a copy to give to his friend Marko. The colour drained from my face. It had not crossed my mind that Marko would read it. For those who haven't read *In Search of My Father* (see the chapter 'O Brother'), Marko had been taking advantage of Dad's forgetfulness by siphoning money off him whenever they met. Fifty dollars to pay for dry-cleaning. Sixty dollars to pay for petrol. One hundred dollars to pay an insurance bill. And so it went on. My write-up of the situation was less than favourable and I was still trying to figure out how to put an end to the pilfering without putting an end to the friendship. Even though 'Marko' was not his real name, my account of events would make it obvious to the person who was 'Marko' that I was writing about him.

Every time Dad mentioned the book for Marko I tried to change the subject. I vainly hoped that he'd soon forget about it. It was the one thing he never forgot. Pester power nearly drove *me* to the pills in our medicine cabinet. Until one day I hit upon a solution: I'd write an edited version of the book just for Marko. I'd remove all mention of Dad's crafty comrade and print a one-off edition.

It took me a few days to make the necessary amendments. I forwarded the manuscript to my publisher.

'Why just one copy?' he asked.

'Marko is the only one who needs the modified version.'

'What about other members of the Serbian community who know Marko?'

'Not necessary. One copy will do.'

A week later, Marko dropped in to see us. 'Your father tells me you've written a book about him. I can't wait to read it.'

I proudly handed Marko his edited version.

Five days later I received a call from Marko's wife, Branka. 'Thank you so much for your heartwarming book. I couldn't put it down. I loved it and I'm going to buy a copy for everyone in our family. You've been so good to us, it's the least I can do to thank you and support your work.'

'Oh noooo! I couldn't possibly let you buy the book!' I protested. 'You're like family. It would give me great joy to bring you as many copies as you want.' Beads of perspiration were trickling down my forehead.

She stood firm. 'Oh no. You're too generous. I'm happy to buy the books.'

'I insist!' I was equally resolute. 'Besides, Dad would be mortified if I let you buy them. Don't deny him the pleasure of giving.'

'Well … all right then. How about I make your dad's favourite dish — *sarma* (stuffed cabbage rolls) and you join us for dinner at your earliest convenience?'

'That would be wonderful!' I hoped my stomach would stop churning by then. 'How many copies would you like?'

'Is six too many?'

'Of course not.'

I immediately rang my publisher again. 'How quickly can you produce another 10 copies of the edited version?'

'I took the liberty of printing 20 copies in the first place. I suspected this might happen.'

'You're a genius!'

Sometimes I wonder if I was being selfish by trying to hold on to Dad if he no longer wanted to live. Should I have sat him down and had an explicit conversation about his diagnosis? Would he have remembered the conversation the following day? In spite of the dementia, he lived a meaningful life. By all appearances, he was happy and contributed to the happiness of others. If he knew of his illness, he would have given up on life. He equated Alzheimer's with stigma, shame and helplessness. If I had told him that he had Alzheimer's and he had willed himself to death, I'd never have forgiven myself and I'd have spent the rest of my life in therapy. I was also convinced by solid scientific evidence that lifestyle interventions could slow down — and possibly reverse — the progression of his disease. I believed we had to give it a shot.

In 2022, more than 55 million people worldwide were living with dementia and 38 million cases (around 70%) were due to Alzheimer's. Currently, six million Americans and almost half a million Australians have a diagnosis of Alzheimer's and more than three times as many people are involved in their care (unpaid). In Western countries, Alzheimer's is the third leading cause of death — both directly and indirectly. Alzheimer's is as much a pandemic as COVID-19 — with no vaccine but with an uplifting list of preventative measures in sight.

Roughly 1% of people aged 60 to 64 years have Alzheimer's, and every five years until the age of 85 the number doubles. That means:
- 2% of 65- to 69-year-olds
- 4% of 70- to 74-year-olds
- 8% of 75- to 79-year-olds
- 16% of 80- to 84-year-olds
- 32% of 85-plus-year-olds.

Alzheimer's and other dementias can also occur at younger ages but much less frequently.

Did I make the right call not to discuss with Dad his diagnosis of Alzheimer's? It's a debate I continue to have with myself.

CHAPTER 3

In search of puzzle pieces

We are what we repeatedly do.
Excellence then is not an act but a habit.

ARISTOTLE (384–322 BCE)

Aristotle's dictum is a perfect summation of how our brain operates and develops. Our brain is the result of what we repeatedly do. Therefore, keeping our brain in excellent health is not an act but a lifelong habit.

This assertion frequently produces furrowed brows and worried questions:

'Does that mean I'm to blame for my dementia?'

'Did I cause my brain to develop Alzheimer's?'

No.

Recognising that our daily choices play a significant role in our health is about empowerment, not censure. It's about encouraging you to take whatever steps you can, to boost your brain and stop brain cells from dying. It's about not feeling helpless in the face of the world's most dreaded disease: dementia.

What is dementia? And how does it differ from Alzheimer's?

Dementia is an umbrella term for more than 100 different diseases, all of which lead to progressive decline in brain function that interferes with daily life. The symptoms can include memory loss, confusion, difficulty concentrating, repeating oneself in conversation, sensory deficits, communication problems, personality changes, errors of judgement and inability to plan or follow instructions. The word 'dementia' is analogous to the word 'cancer'. There are many subtypes with different symptoms. Appendix 1 lists the dementias you're most likely to encounter. To date there is no simple way to diagnose any of the dementias. It takes a battery of blood tests, brain scans, physical examinations and neurological assessments.

Alzheimer's is the most common type of dementia and accounts for 60% to 70% of cases worldwide. India has one of the lowest rates of Alzheimer's of any country. Why? Scientists speculate that extensive use of curcumin (the active ingredient in turmeric) may reduce brain inflammation and remove destructive amyloid plaques. Another theory is that over-use of hygiene products in developed countries kills key bacterial species in our gut that are required for optimal brain function. A third group of scientists believe that India's tightly knit family structures and high regard for their elderly protect their brains from decay. All three mechanisms are plausible and probably interact.

The second most common type of dementia is vascular dementia. As the name suggests, vascular dementia is due to inadequate supply of blood to the brain. This can result from major or minor strokes (even silent strokes), smoking, high blood pressure, generalised blood vessel disease (atherosclerosis) or heart failure.

When I tracked down Dad's GP, I learned that Dad had been diagnosed with vascular dementia at the age of 75 based on his history of smoking and heart disease. A few years later, the diagnosis was amended to Alzheimer's because MRI scanning showed extensive shrinkage in a region of his brain called the hippocampus. The two types of dementia often co-exist. The condition is then called mixed dementia. It's estimated that 45% of people with a diagnosis of one dementia actually have mixed dementia. This was most likely the case with Dad.

However, the most critical factor is not the diagnosis. **The most critical factor is the lifestyle choices we make every day for 30 years before a diagnosis is made.** If we live in a way that stimulates brain cell growth and repair, we may be able to avoid a diagnosis of dementia altogether. There are no guarantees, but we can certainly increase our odds of staying as sharp at age 90 as we were at age 30.

'Thirty years!' I hear you gasp. Does that mean if you're 70 it's too late to make a difference? Definitely not. We are able to continue creating new brain circuits for the entire duration of our lives. It's never too late to make positive changes and see them reflected in better health and improved cognition. There is always *something* we can do to improve a situation. Even the smallest things can have a big impact. Just try going to sleep with a mosquito in the room. It's also never too *early* to start making choices that improve brain performance and build what is known as cognitive reserve (the ability of our brain to resist functional decline). Brain deterioration starts decades before any symptoms appear. The earlier we implement brain-boosting habits, the sooner we nip any damage in the bud.

So where to begin?

Keeping our brain in good working order is like assembling a jigsaw puzzle with many pieces. There isn't just one factor responsible for optimal brain health. Nor is there one factor responsible for brain demise — short of falling off a roof and landing on your head or inheriting a very rare gene. There are multiple factors that improve or erode brain function. Many of these factors interact with each other and different factors can affect each of us differently.

Every aspect of our lives that influences brain health corresponds to one piece of the puzzle. For instance, getting regular physical exercise is a critical piece of the puzzle. So are social stimulation, good nutrition and having adequate levels of vitamin B12. Other puzzle pieces can include learning a foreign language and playing a musical instrument. Our genes also contribute several puzzle pieces because over 70 genes (discovered so far) may be linked to developing Alzheimer's.

If one puzzle piece is missing, it doesn't immediately lead to a drop in brain performance. It's like missing the last piece in a jigsaw. We can still make out what the picture represents. Even if several pieces are missing, it might not make a big difference to our quality of life. But if enough pieces — or if certain crucial pieces — are missing, the resulting damage to our brain starts to interfere with our ability to function.

For instance, smoking cigarettes increases a person's risk of dementia by 70%. But not all smokers get dementia. Type 2 diabetes doubles the risk of Alzheimer's. But not everyone with type 2 diabetes develops Alzheimer's. However, if you smoke AND have type 2 diabetes AND suffer from sleep apnoea, the combination of these three pieces might be enough to tip a brain into Alzheimer's. However, if that person also engages in brain-boosting activities such as daily physical exercise, a diet rich in real whole foods, meditation and a mentally stimulating social life, they MIGHT offset the smoking, diabetes and sleep deprivation. We simply don't have all the answers yet.

The other characteristic of jigsaw puzzles is that the pieces interlock and each individual piece shows only a tiny fragment of the whole. When all the pieces are correctly assembled, we see the complete picture. Most people start a jigsaw by trying to find the four corner pieces. Then they assemble the straight edges and finally all the sections in the middle. But there are no definitive rules for solving a puzzle. The main thing is to have fun. The point of a puzzle is the challenge and enjoyment of doing it, not simply the completion. The objective is engaging in the process.

The same goes for building up our brain. This book gives you the brain-boosting puzzle pieces we currently know about. I've collected the pieces through poring over research, caring for patients and, most of all, looking after Dad. The order in which you assemble the pieces is up to you. This isn't a book for you to merely read and reflect on. It's a book for you to act on.

I believe the four all-important foundations for a healthy brain (akin to the corner pieces of a puzzle) are (drum roll):
1. **having a sense of purpose, i.e. giving your brain a reason to stay sharp**
2. **consistent good quality sleep**
3. **meaningful relationships**
4. **regular physical exercise.**

These four puzzle pieces have a domino effect on every other aspect of our lives. I recommend you make sleep your first priority because it makes everything else easier. Motivation, energy, immune function, decision-making and even our capacity to empathise and forgive others are all enhanced by sleep. Just one night of sleep deprivation increases the number of amyloid beta (Aβ) plaques and tau tangles in our brain. If you're a mother with a newborn who won't let you sleep, don't panic. One night — even one year — of disrupted sleep won't give you Alzheimer's. However, the longer you leave it, the greater the risk. The message is to rectify the issue as soon as you can. I've dedicated several chapters to helping you get a good night's sleep.

When you've established the corner pieces of the puzzle, I recommend you work on the pieces that form the edges. These pieces relate to:
- lifelong mental stimulation
- what we eat
- whether we smoke
- how we manage stress
- type 2 diabetes
- midlife high blood pressure
- midlife abdominal obesity
- midlife hearing loss
- chronic depression.

Finally, there are all the pieces in the middle. These involve:
- head injuries
- alcohol consumption
- vitamins and minerals
- environmental toxins
- air pollution
- infections
- a host of other factors.

At first glance, the sheer number of puzzle pieces may feel overwhelming. Keep reminding yourself it's like opening a 500-piece jigsaw. (And there are far fewer than 500 things we need to do to keep Alzheimer's at bay!) **The very act of doing the puzzle — working on improving our brain — delivers benefits.** Every single piece you add makes a difference. Don't make it a chore. Make it a game. Striving to achieve something — whether or not you reach your end goal — increases connections between brain cells and sharpens our thinking. And the more you enjoy the process, the greater the benefits to your brain and body.

CHAPTER 4

Why this book?

Beliefs are choices. First you choose your beliefs.
Then your beliefs affect your choices.

ROY T BENNETT (born 1957)

Twelve years ago, when I wrote my first book *In Search of My Father — Dementia is no match for a daughter's determination*, I was a lone voice positing that Alzheimer's might be preventable. If we could make lifestyle choices to reduce our risk of heart disease, why not also brain disease? As it turns out, **what's good for the heart is also good for the brain.** I even went a step further and suggested that if someone already had dementia they could slow the rate of disease progression. I was met with accusations of giving people false hope. I responded by saying there was no such thing as 'false' hope. Hope is hope. It's not a guarantee; it's a window of possibility and it motivates us to try. As it turns out, **the mere act of trying leads to cognitive improvements.**

When I was in medical school we joked that neurologists didn't cure neurological diseases — they simply admired neurological diseases because there was nothing they could do about them. Alzheimer's was a disease of 'diagnose and adios' — you were told you had an incurable condition and needed to get your affairs in order. Today there are dozens of government, university and hospital websites offering courses on how to lower your risk of Alzheimer's. Most exciting of all is that the first ever Alzheimer's Prevention Clinic was founded at New York-Presbyterian and Weill Cornell Medical Center in the USA in 2013 by Dr Richard S Isaacson MD. This was unimaginable when I published *In Search of My Father*. The overriding opinion at the time was that dementia was a case of bad luck or bad genes and nothing could be done to sway the course. Over the next eight years, other Alzheimer's prevention clinics opened in Birmingham, Los Angeles, Puerto Rico and Florida. By the time you read this book, there will no doubt be more. This is incredible progress. In just one decade, Alzheimer's has gone from being an incurable curse to a modifiable malady.

What is the success rate of prevention programs? Based on numerous trials and statistical analyses involving people from all corners of the globe, **almost half of all Alzheimer's cases could be prevented.** That's phenomenal! One report calculated there would be three million fewer people in the world with Alzheimer's if seven risk factors were reduced by as little as 10% to 25%. These risk factors are smoking, type 2 diabetes, midlife high blood pressure, midlife abdominal obesity, depression and lack of mental stimulation. In other words, if 10% fewer people in the world had these conditions, there would be three million fewer people with Alzheimer's.

In July 2019 a landmark study presented at the Alzheimer's Association International Conference (AAIC) and published in the *Journal of the American Medical Association (JAMA)* demonstrated that a healthy lifestyle dramatically reduced the risk of developing Alzheimer's, even in people who had a higher genetic predisposition. This is especially good news if you have a close relative with Alzheimer's. It means that you are not doomed to follow the same path. **Our decisions — not our DNA — determine our destiny.**

Almost 200 000 people over the age of 60 were tracked for eight years. The factors that led to a reduction in Alzheimer's were:
- not smoking
- not drinking soft drinks
- drinking less than one standard alcoholic drink (10 grams or 100 mL of wine) per day
- eating a diet rich in unprocessed food, especially green and purple vegetables, fish, fruit, nuts, seeds and olive oil
- engaging in at least 150 minutes of moderate exercise or 75 minutes of vigorous exercise per week.

In May the same year, a randomised controlled trial (RCT) known as the Brain Health Champion Study tested whether people who already had Alzheimer's could improve their memory though physical exercise, diet, mentally stimulating activities and increased social interaction. Once again, the answer was YES!

A major review published in *The Lancet* in July 2020 confirmed 12 factors (puzzle pieces) that unequivocally increased the risk of dementia if not addressed:
1. cigarette smoking
2. low education
3. head injury
4. type 2 diabetes
5. midlife (age 40 to 65) hearing loss
6. midlife high blood pressure (hypertension)
7. chronic major depression
8. social isolation and loneliness
9. physical inactivity
10. waist circumference greater than 94 cm in men and 80 cm in women
11. alcohol consumption in excess of 10 standard drinks (100 g) per week
12. air pollution and second-hand tobacco smoke.

I created an acronym so I'd easily remember them:

HEADS TO HEADS

Hearing loss
Education deprivation (rhyme also enhances memory)
Alcohol excess
Diabetes type 2
Smoking

Traumatic brain injury
Obesity

High blood pressure (**h**ypertension)
Exercise deficit
Air pollution
Depression
Social isolation

I'll address all these factors in subsequent chapters and add several more of equal importance — chief among them being chronic sleep deprivation.

Unfortunately, these messages haven't reached the general public. Most people don't realise the extent to which the choices they make throughout the course of their lives influence the health of their brain. Hence my writing this sequel.

My first book established the basics of building a better brain as I blundered my way through looking after Dad. In this sequel I distil the staggering number of neuroscientific advances of the last 12 years to give you a deeper, more robust and eminently practical guide to staving off dementia, especially Alzheimer's. We have many more pieces of the brain puzzle now than we did a decade ago. Have we discovered all the pieces? Not yet. But we've discovered enough to become proactive about protecting our brain and dramatically reducing the number of people who develop dementia. Most of the research I discuss has been done in relation to Alzheimer's and vascular dementia, the two most common forms of dementia. Will the advice in this book also reduce your risk of other dementias such as frontotemporal and Lewy body? I can't say for certain but I suspect the answer is yes. Anything we do to improve our brain will help buffer us against all cerebral diseases.

Each chapter gives you one puzzle piece. Some pieces are immediately evident. Other pieces are embedded in an escapade with Dad. Some pieces are buried beneath tears and anguish. Some pieces are revealed through research. As with my first book, I've interwoven personal stories and scientific evidence to encourage you to embark on your own adventure to prevent dementia.

As you read, I invite you to go beyond passively absorbing the information. The more deeply we ponder, analyse and apply what we read, the more we build up connections in our frontal lobes and protect ourselves from Alzheimer's.

- What overarching themes can you extract from this book?
- What are various ways you can implement the ideas into your own life?

- Can you extrapolate the key messages to other health issues?
- If you were discussing the text in a book club, what questions would you pose to the group?

When you reflect on each chapter, if your knee-jerk response is something along the lines of 'I don't have time for that' or 'That sounds too hard' or 'The person I look after would never do that', brainstorm ways to overcome your perceived obstacles. You'll be surprised at the creative solutions you come up with when you challenge yourself to do so. And you'll be giving your brain another boost in the process.

Dire media predictions about an impending avalanche of worldwide Alzheimer's cases are outdated and contradict the science. We might not yet have a cure but we certainly know how to slow the train and even stop it from leaving the station. **Deteriorating brain health is NOT inevitable.** Each and every one of us has a role to play in arresting Alzheimer's — not only for ourselves but for our family and wider community. We all have unique strengths and passions. At the end of each chapter, ask yourself: how can I use my talents and interests to free the world of Alzheimer's?

It could be through:
- sharing your own story
- starting a conversation about brain health
- being a vibrant role model for your grandchildren
- taking someone with Alzheimer's for a picnic
- lobbying your local government for more green spaces
- creating a more brain-boosting work environment
- enrolling in an Alzheimer's prevention trial.

You'll come up with many more ideas as you assemble each puzzle piece. There are infinite ways we can be proactive about outwitting Alzheimer's. We don't need to wait for the next blockbuster drug. We already have solutions. **It's time to take action.** In fact, the very act of taking action will strengthen our neural networks and lead to better overall brain function. This is a win-win situation. Thinking about how to put all the puzzle pieces in place in your own life and that of the people you care about is giving your brain a boost. Strategic planning is one way to boost our brain; taking action is another. Things can only get better once you get started. Contrary to the doom and gloom that makes for news headlines, this is an incredibly hopeful situation.

As you embark on your adventure with dementia, I encourage you to think outside the page and ask probing questions. If you're not able to come up with satisfactory answers, submit your questions to outwittingalzheimers.com/contact. I'll notify you when I've responded in a blog, podcast or YouTube video. Reading this book can be the start of a dialogue between you, me, your doctor, family and wider community. Dementia affects all of us one way or another, be it by shaping our perceptions of ageing or engulfing us in the day-to-day challenges of being a care-partner.

When you've finished reading this book you can download a list of all the puzzle pieces at: outwittingalzheimers.com/resources. Before you do so, I recommend you give yourself a mental workout by figuring them out for yourself.

Another burgeoning field of research is how **beliefs influence biology.** Be careful what you think — our assumptions about ageing actually influence how we age. Harvard University psychologist Ellen Langer tested whether cultural stereotypes contributed to memory loss. Young and old residents of the United States, mainland China and an American deaf community were asked to list characteristics they associated with growing old. Chinese people and those who were born deaf were less likely to perceive memory loss as a feature of ageing. When they were subsequently given memory tests, young people in all three groups scored much the same. However, older Chinese and deaf people performed significantly better in memory tests than their hearing American counterparts. Their memory decline was not due to their biology; it was due to their beliefs.

If we forget something in our 20s, we don't give it a second thought. We attribute it to a big night out or a moment of distraction. If we forget something in our 70s, we worry it's a sign of decline. The anxiety triggers cortisol release, which causes brain freeze and destroys cells in the hippocampus (the memory and learning centre in our brain) — thus increasing the likelihood of more memory lapses. We become hypervigilant for further signs of weakening memory and start avoiding situations where our memory is put to the test. **Use it or lose it.** Before we know it, we've created a self-fulfilling prophecy.

Another study uncovered that one of the biggest determinants of healthy ageing was having sprightly grandparents. This was not attributable to genetics but to having vibrant role models. Children exposed to elderly people who are active and independent learn that **old age is associated with freedom, not frailty.** In many ways we are 'taught' how to age by those around us. The Japanese island of Okinawa is home to some of the longest living people in the world. Their culture equates ageing with wisdom and authority, not illness and irrelevance. This attitude guides their day-to-day lives and provides older people with meaning, purpose and vitality until the day they die.

Whenever Dad began protesting that his life didn't matter, I reminded him that his health and vitality were an example to others. 'Your engagement with life is not just about *your* quality of life but also that of people around you. You show them what's possible for a person of your age. You give them a vibrancy to aspire to. You're playing an important role in our community.'

Our beliefs are so ingrained and deeply rooted that we don't even perceive them as beliefs. We treat them as facts. Our beliefs are the lens through which we see the world and, if we never question our beliefs, we blind ourselves to the limitless possibilities within our reach.

CHAPTER 5

In search of acetylcholine

The true art of memory is the art of attention.

SAMUEL JOHNSON (1709–1784)

Dad and I always had a jigsaw puzzle on the go. He was initially dismissive of the idea. 'Puzzles are for children,' he retorted. I persisted nonetheless. We started with only a few hundred pieces because he was impatient to 'get the job over with'. In truth, his impatience was a symptom of his inability to focus. **Alzheimer's makes it increasingly difficult for a person to block out distractions and maintain a train of thought.** I could see him struggling to concentrate on the most basic of tasks. He would half set the table and then wander off to straighten a picture hanging on the wall. One minute we were raking the leaves from the front path and the next minute he was checking the mailbox. Back and forth between rake and mailbox he would go. Paying attention was akin to clutching at clouds. At least he was racking up his daily steps.

There was a biological explanation for his struggles: loss of acetylcholine.

Acetylcholine (abbreviated ACh) is a neurotransmitter — also referred to as a chemical messenger or signalling molecule. A neurotransmitter is released at the end of a nerve fibre and travels to other cells to instruct them to perform specific functions. Both brain cells and nerve cells (collectively referred to as neurons) produce neurotransmitters. The receiving cells include other neurons, muscle cells or gland cells. Acetylcholine has many different roles in the body. Specifically in relation to Alzheimer's, acetylcholine influences alertness, attention, motivation and memory.

In the late 1970s, postmortem examination of human brain tissue confirmed that people with Alzheimer's had less acetylcholine in their brains than healthy people. This explained many of the key symptoms of Alzheimer's: loss of motivation to do things they previously enjoyed, short-term memory problems and reduced ability to pay attention. This sparked a race among scientists to figure out how to increase acetylcholine levels in the brain.

Idea number one: give acetylcholine as a drug. No go. An enzyme called acetylcholinesterase (AChE) quickly breaks down acetylcholine and renders it ineffective. In addition, because of its molecular structure, acetylcholine can't enter the brain from the blood. Thus, even if the molecule remained intact, acetylcholine wouldn't get to where it was needed.

Idea number two: boost the brain's ability to produce its own acetylcholine. How? A key ingredient of acetylcholine is choline. Choline is made in the liver but not in large enough quantities to meet our daily requirements. Therefore, we need to obtain choline from food. By far the richest source of choline is beef liver followed by egg yolks and human breast milk. Other sources include red meat, salmon, pork and chicken. So far not looking good for vegans. But don't despair; you can also obtain choline from split peas, soy beans, shiitake mushrooms, almonds and broccoli, albeit in smaller concentrations. For a list of choline-rich foods visit: outwittingalzheimers.com/resources.

Research hasn't yet clarified exactly how much choline we need for optimal health. The functions of choline extend beyond acetylcholine production. Choline is also found in cell membranes and in a substance called myelin. Myelin insulates nerve fibres and ensures proper signalling between neurons. Our best guess is that men need at least 550 mg of dietary choline per day and women need 450 mg. Animal research suggests that women are able to use choline more efficiently than men because they have more oestrogen hormones. However, pregnant and breastfeeding women need about 900 mg of choline because it's essential for foetal brain development. Giving women choline supplements during pregnancy resulted in babies being able to process information more quickly and respond to stress more effectively. Choline was also able to mitigate some of the deleterious effects of prenatal alcohol exposure.

Adults who consume less than 50 mg of choline per day start to accumulate fat in their livers after only a few weeks. This can lead to a host of metabolic diseases including type 2 diabetes. Meanwhile, choline deficiency has been implicated in worsening brain function among institutionalised older people. This begs the question: could choline supplementation reverse some of the symptoms of Alzheimer's?

In trials across the USA and Europe, doctors gave Alzheimer's patients mega-doses of choline over many months and looked for improvements in memory and mental functioning. The outcome? Don't try this at home. It didn't work. Extra choline did not result in more acetylcholine production and no measurable brain-benefits were seen. We don't know why.

What can we conclude from this? Consume adequate amounts of choline throughout your life to maintain your brain health because mega-dosing after diagnosis won't reverse the damage. The reason I've made such a big deal about choline is because most people haven't heard of it and don't know if they're eating enough. Choline also supports the case for prevention over cure.

Idea number three: block the enzyme acetylcholinesterase from deactivating acetylcholine. Bingo! To a degree. In 1993 the first drug to treat Alzheimer's disease was approved. It works by reducing the breakdown of acetylcholine. Today there are three such drugs available. They are known as cholinesterase inhibitors or anti-cholinesterase drugs:
1. donepezil
2. galantamine
3. rivastigmine.

Unfortunately, these drugs are not a cure because the cells that make acetylcholine continue to die. Eventually there isn't enough acetylcholine being produced in the brain for the drugs to make a difference. But the drugs can delay or slow worsening of symptoms in the early stages of Alzheimer's. Benefits differ between individual patients and last for varying lengths of time — usually only six to 12 months. Dad had been prescribed rivastigmine shortly after Mum had been diagnosed with lung cancer. This was the medication that alerted me to his diagnosis. It was delivered via a thin plastic patch which I stuck to his back every night before bed. I kept my eye out for side effects: nausea, vomiting, diarrhoea and loss of appetite. No sign of problems. I heaved a sigh of relief.

If you or a loved one has recently been diagnosed with Alzheimer's, speak to your doctor about whether a cholinesterase inhibitor might be helpful. Even though they aren't a long-term solution, they could buy you some time.

Idea number four: put all your medications in a bag — including non-prescription remedies and supplements — and take them to your doctor. Tip them out onto his or her desk and ask the following question: 'Do any of these medicines have anticholinergic properties?'

If the answer is yes, ask for an alternative that does NOT have anticholinergic effects.

Many drugs — both prescription and seemingly harmless over-the-counter (OTC) preparations — can block acetylcholine in the brain and impair memory, attention and eye-hand co-ordination. They are known as anticholinergics. Taken long term they can increase the risk of Alzheimer's and other dementias. The higher the dose and the longer a person has been taking an anticholinergic, the greater their risk of cognitive decline, especially if over the age of 65. In the past, doctors believed that these side effects were short-lived and would resolve after stopping the medication. Worldwide research has now confirmed that anticholinergics are linked to a greater likelihood of developing dementia.

Anticholinergics include some (but not all) types of antihistamines, antidepressants and anti-incontinence drugs. They are used to treat a wide variety of conditions including:
- allergies
- coughs and colds
- insomnia
- anxiety and depression

- overactive bladder / urinary incontinence
- lung disease
- motion sickness
- diarrhoea and irritable bowel syndrome (IBS).

This is not to suggest that you immediately stop taking antidepressants. Chronic major depression also increases the risk of dementia and not all antidepressants have anticholinergic effects. A class of antidepressants known as tricyclics (e.g. amitriptyline) have the strongest anticholinergic effects and should not be prescribed to people over the age of 60. Another group of antidepressants are called selective serotonin re-uptake inhibitors (SSRIs) and an example of these is citalopram. Overall, they have a weaker anticholinergic effect, but some are nonetheless more anticholinergic than others. Newer antidepressants such as serotonin-norepinephrine re-uptake inhibitors (SNRIs) (e.g. venlafaxine) and atypical antidepressants (e.g. bupropion) have only minor anticholinergic effects.

NEVER stop taking a medication without first consulting your doctor. Many drugs need to be tapered off slowly before discontinuing them altogether. The point is to have a conversation about anticholinergics with your doctor. Any time you are prescribed a new medication, ask if it has anticholinergic side effects. Similarly, if you want something at a chemist that does not require a prescription, speak to the pharmacist and pose the same question: is this an anticholinergic? Make sure the person you are asking is not simply someone who serves behind the counter. Unless they are a pharmacist, they are unlikely to know the answer.

Idea number five: do jigsaw puzzles! Use it (acetylcholine) or lose it. **Train it and regain it.** Whenever we're absorbed in something that requires sustained attention, we stimulate our brain to produce acetylcholine. Memorising a poem, studying for exams, playing a musical instrument, doing origami, learning a new skill or focusing on finding a jigsaw puzzle piece — all trigger the release of acetylcholine. In addition, if the activity promotes a sense of achievement, we also release dopamine. Dopamine is another neurotransmitter that helps us focus. The more we're able to focus, the more we enjoy what we're doing and the greater our feeling of satisfaction. The positive cycle becomes self-reinforcing.

This is exactly what happened with Dad. The early days required a lot of coaxing. 'Dad, can you help me assemble this puzzle?'

'Why did you take it apart in the first place?'

'I didn't take it apart. That's how it came in the box.'

'Well, that was silly. Next time buy something that's already assembled. It will save you a lot of time.'

'Okay, thanks for the tip. But given the current situation, can you help me please?'

Soon he was engrossed in the task and I could leave him on his own while I went to cook dinner. He didn't always put the pieces in the right places. Alzheimer's had compromised his visual processing and his ability to distinguish colours and shapes. But it didn't matter. After he went to bed, I put the pieces in their correct positions and we continued with it the following day.

Sometimes I gave him an easy puzzle with large pieces so he'd finish it correctly without help. This gave him the opportunity to tell visitors, 'Look I finished that jigsaw puzzle all by myself in just a few hours.'

'That's excellent,' praised the visitor.

'Yes,' Dad would affirm. 'Especially as the side of the box says *four to five years*.'

It was his favourite joke. I don't know where he first heard it and I don't know how he remembered it. I'm not even sure he understood it. But he knew it would make people laugh. The positive emotional response seemed to have etched the joke into his brain. I wondered if the puzzles weren't more powerful than the medicine in enhancing his ability to focus?

CHAPTER 6

Are your medicines messing with your mind?

Nothing in life is to be feared; it is only to be understood.

MARIE CURIE (1867–1934)

About a month after Mum passed away, I was vacuuming Dad's bedroom and accidentally knocked over a family photo. When I went to pick it up, I saw a small box of tablets on the corner of his bedside cabinet. The label said Valium. I checked the expiry date. They were still potent. There were 10 tablets left from a total of 50. My heart started pounding. I went outside to find my father reading yesterday's paper.

'Dad, I just found these tablets in your room. Do you know anything about them?' I tried to sound blasé.

'Yes. I take them to help me sleep. Surely you know what they're for. You're a doctor.'

I gave him a sardonic smile. 'When was the last time you took one?'

'I take one every night.'

My heart was now violently pummelling the inside of my rib cage. 'How long have you been taking them?'

'I've always taken them.'

'You can't have always taken them. A doctor must have prescribed them and they're only meant for short-term use.'

He stared at me blankly.

'Do you remember who prescribed them?'

'A doctor — you just said so yourself.'

I shook my head. 'Since when have you had trouble sleeping?'

'I don't have trouble sleeping. I take a tablet at bedtime and I'm off before I know it.'

I sighed. 'Dad, these tablets are highly addictive and they cause problems with memory, concentration, co-ordination and balance. They might be the reason you've been feeling confused. It's a good thing you don't drink alcohol as that would have made the side effects even worse. You're also not allowed to drive if you take them.'

'Then I'll stop taking them,' he replied pragmatically.

'That creates another problem. You can't just suddenly stop taking them because you'll get withdrawal symptoms. Will you let me help you gradually reduce the dose?'

He nodded.

'Have you ever taken more than one tablet at a time?'

'No.'

'Okay, then I'll give you three-quarters of a tablet for a few nights and see how you go. Can I look after them for you?'

He smirked. 'Do I have a choice?'

'Of course you do,' I responded buoyantly. 'And I know you'll make the *wise* choice.'

'What if I can't sleep?'

'I'll read to you.'

'That should do the trick. Why didn't I think of that?'

* * * * *

Valium is one of many brand names for diazepam, which belongs to a class of drugs called benzodiazepines. It's used to treat a range of symptoms including anxiety, insomnia, muscle spasms, restless leg syndrome and seizures. The older we get, the more sensitive we become to the effects of benzodiazepines and the greater the risk of a fall or cognitive impairment. Diazepam should not be given to people over the age of 65 unless they are carefully monitored in hospital. If special circumstances warrant their use at home, the dose should be half that for younger people, and the duration of treatment should be no longer than two weeks.

Dad was 78 at the time and had been taking 5 mg a day for who knows how long. I was terrified he'd developed tolerance and would suffer withdrawal symptoms. If he'd had sleep apnoea, diazepam would have further compromised his breathing, which would have further compromised his brain function. And worst of all, even after stopping the drug, cognitive problems can persist for over six months. I was too devastated to cry.

Over the next fortnight we reduced his dose by a quarter of a tablet every five days and I watched him carefully for signs of withdrawal: anxiety, restlessness, headaches, abdominal cramps, vomiting, shaking, muscle pain, loss of appetite, the list went on. Fortunately, he exhibited none of these. In place of Valium I applied a drop of lavender oil on his temples and wrists and started the habit of reading to him when he went to bed. I began with a soothing book we'd both loved in the past: *Tuesdays with Morrie* by Mitch Albom. The transition to drug-free sleep was a success but the incident continued to plague me.

How long had Dad been taking Valium? How often had he taken benzodiazepines throughout his life? Could this have contributed to him developing Alzheimer's? The thought was crushing. Benzodiazepines were initially believed to be safe and free of side effects. Decades of research have now revealed that frequent use of these drugs throughout life — not just after a certain age — increases the risk of dementia. If you absolutely need to take them, use the lowest effective dose for the shortest amount of time. Always have a conversation with your doctor about the side effects of any medication you're prescribed. And be on the lookout for undesirable reactions — physical, mental or emotional. The same medicine can affect different people differently.

Benzodiazepines and anticholinergics are the commonest drugs linked to an increased risk of Alzheimer's. However, many other drugs such as anticonvulsants, antacids, heart medications, corticosteroids and non-steroidal anti-inflammatory agents (NSAIDs) can cause acute (and less commonly chronic) confusion. Most disturbing of all is that **almost any drug can disrupt brain function in an older person** and give rise to disorientation, agitation or hallucinations.

The medical term for drug-induced confusion (or other reversible causes) is delirium. If delirium is not diagnosed and the offending drug not stopped, it can be mistaken for dementia. As we age, our liver and kidneys get slower at removing drugs and toxins from our body, which means the effects tend to be stronger and last longer. Most people also lose muscle and gain fat, which changes how drugs are distributed and broken down in our tissues. In addition, there is a weakening of what is known as the blood–brain barrier (BBB) so drugs are able to enter the brain more easily than when we were younger. Paradoxically, because of increasing health problems, older people are often on multiple medications (prescription and over-the-counter), which can interact with each other and cause harm in unexpected ways. Mixing medicines can be akin to mixing drinks. All these factors add up to older people experiencing substantially more nasty effects from taking medicines than younger people.

My message is not to avoid medications altogether. My message is to be a careful and conversant consumer. Be aware that drugs can mimic or exacerbate dementia. **If an older person starts exhibiting symptoms of mental decline, the first thing to rule out is side effects of medication.** Even if they've been taking a drug for a long time, the dose they were on when they were younger might now be too high. Ask your doctor: 'Could the symptoms be due to **medication fog**?' Review all the medications and supplements that a person is taking and see if the solution might be stopping, rather than starting, something — always slowly and under medical supervision.

CHAPTER 7

In search of signs

The good physician treats the disease;
the great physician treats the patient who
has the disease.

SIR WILLIAM OSLER (1849–1919)

Jasmin was a perceptive medical student whose grandmother had recently been diagnosed with Alzheimer's. Jasmin had waist-long glossy brown hair that looked like she'd just walked off the set of a shampoo commercial. She was eager to learn everything she could about the disease that was stealing her nan away. She approached me at the end of a presentation I'd given on *How to boost your brain and defy dementia*.

'I'm sure you're asked this question all the time,' she opened our conversation, 'but what are some of the earliest warning signs of Alzheimer's? I know the obvious things to look for are forgetting recent events, repeating oneself in conversation and misplacing things, but what else should I be aware of? Sometimes I walk into a room and draw a blank about why I entered. Should I be worried?'

'No,' I reassured her. 'That's actually a survival mechanism. Doorways signify entering a new environment and our brain is wired to regard any change in our surroundings as potentially dangerous. We tend to forget what we've just been thinking about because we need to pay attention to what lies ahead. We file away our thoughts and memories from the previous room, in order to create a blank slate to take in new information from the new room. Rationally, we know there's nothing to be afraid of but we're not able to switch off our automatic evolutionary response. The process is referred to as "triggering an event boundary in our brain". In experiments conducted at the University of Notre Dame in Indiana, USA, people were asked to choose a number of items from a table and put them in a backpack. The backpack was then removed and the participants were distracted for a short while before being asked to write down from memory the items they'd chosen. If they'd been made to walk through a doorway before writing down the items, they remembered fewer items than when they sat the test in the same room.'

'That's a relief!' she laughed. 'What about when a word is on the tip of my tongue but I just can't recall it?'

'That's also nothing to worry about if it only happens from time to time. The tip of tongue phenomenon occurs once or twice a week in our 20s and up to four times a week in our 70s and beyond. My concern is how we respond to it. In our 20s we shrug it off. In our later years we label it "a senior moment" or wonder if it's the beginning of the end. Feeling stressed impairs memory and makes it more likely to happen again. This has the potential to set off a self-perpetuating spiral of worsening memory.'

'My grandmother is getting her words mixed up. She'll say things like "I poked some flowers in the garden today" when she means "I *planted* some flowers". That's typical of Alzheimer's, isn't it?'

'Yes, people with Alzheimer's often have difficulty finding the right word so they substitute a similar-sounding word. In the early stages, they often realise what they're doing but they still can't help it. Later they are unaware that their speech becomes incoherent to others.'

'What other kinds of memory lapses are harbingers of Alzheimer's?'

'Alzheimer's can present in many different ways depending on the part of the brain that is affected. The hippocampus — involved in memory, learning and navigation — is often one of the first regions of the brain to suffer damage, hence the association of Alzheimer's with short-term memory loss, disorientation and difficulty learning new things. But there are many other signs that brain function may be deteriorating; for example:

- getting easily confused, especially about dates, days and times
- getting facts mixed up
- inability to follow simple instructions
- loss of interest in doing things the person previously enjoyed
- difficulty making decisions or plans
- diminishing attention span
- poor judgement
- personality changes
- inappropriate remarks
- mood swings or snappiness that are unusual for the person
- becoming withdrawn and not wanting to socialise.'

'Some of those traits describe *me* on a bad day!' Jasmin exclaimed.

'The key is noticing a *change* from previous behaviour,' I clarified. 'If someone has always been indecisive or inappropriate, it isn't suggestive of dementia. However, if a person who was previously tidy and well-mannered becomes disorganised and starts swearing, I would sit up and take notice. Listen carefully to what friends and relatives tell you. Comments such as "He used to be so easy-going. I don't know what's come over him" or "She's acting out of character" are red flags for some sort of brain pathology and require scans and blood tests.'

'Many of the things you listed are also features of depression,' she observed.

'Yes, that's right. Over the age of 60, depression can cause similar cognitive impairment to dementia. This makes it very tricky to differentiate between depression and dementia. In fact, depression that mimics dementia is called **pseudo-dementia**.'

'Sorry, I don't understand,' Jasmin furrowed her brow.

'Depression and dementia can present with the same symptoms. When an older person has depression but it looks like dementia, their depression is given the name pseudo-dementia — in other words, depression masquerading as dementia. When the person receives appropriate therapy for their depression, their cognition can return to normal. If their depression is mistakenly assumed to be dementia and is not treated, the depression becomes a risk factor for developing dementia! Therefore distinguishing between the two conditions is critical.'

'How does one distinguish between the two?'

'The person needs a comprehensive assessment by a psychiatrist, psychogeriatrician or neuropsychologist. Sometimes the only way to know what's going on is to give someone a trial of antidepressants and see if their symptoms improve.'

'It all sounds so complex,' she sighed.

'The important thing is not to fall into the trap of automatically assuming that cognitive decline in an older person is dementia. It could be depression, a brain tumour, side effect of medication, infection or any number of other conditions.'

'Noted,' she promised.

'The opposite is also true. Never assign memory decline to "just getting old". Listen to a person's concerns and ask them to give you examples of their memory lapses. If someone says "A week ago when I came home from a sip-wine-and-paint-party I couldn't remember if I'd watered the garden that morning" they are unlikely to have memory problems. It's probably the result of a busy day finished off with a glass of wine. But if someone doesn't have any recollection of going to the party in the first place, that's something that warrants further investigation.'

'It would also depend on how often a person forgets or misplaces things. Once in a while is okay but every day is not.'

'That's right. You also need to be aware of what's known as **mild cognitive impairment** or **MCI**,' I continued.

'What's that?'

'MCI is a condition in which a person's thinking skills have declined but not to the extent that it interferes with their daily life. In some cases, MCI can be the start of Alzheimer's or other dementias. In other people, the condition stays stable or they revert back to normal functioning after an unspecified period of time.'

'Is there a way of knowing if a person with MCI will progress to Alzheimer's?' Jasmin pondered.

'That's the subject of ongoing research. There are two types of MCI:
1. amnestic (aMCI) — the main symptom is memory loss
2. non-amnestic (naMCI) — this includes problems with reasoning, communication, decision-making, distance perception and navigation.

'People with amnestic MCI tend to progress to Alzheimer's, while people with naMCI are more likely to develop other forms of dementia such as dementia with Lewy bodies (DLB).

'One group of scientists found that the longer it takes a person with MCI to process written words — referred to as language processing speed — the more likely they are to progress to Alzheimer's.'

'How do you measure language processing speed?' Jasmin was intrigued.

'By attaching electrodes to a person's scalp and measuring the electrical activity in their brain while they look at a series of words on a computer screen.'

'Are you referring to an electroencephalogram (EEG)?'

'Yes. An EEG shows a particular pattern of brain activity when we read. The average person takes 250 milliseconds to process a written word. In people with MCI who go on to develop Alzheimer's, the pattern of electrical activity in their brain is distorted and it takes them longer to comprehend what they're reading. A person with MCI whose EEG shows normal language processing despite other memory glitches tends not to progress to Alzheimer's.'

'Now I understand why it took Granny so long to read her birthday card. I thought she simply wasn't interested in what I'd written. It's more likely that her brain was slow in processing the words.'

'And because she was exerting so much mental energy in trying to comprehend what she was reading, she had no energy left to remember the words. So she probably kept going back and re-reading the previous sentence.'

'How exhausting!' Jasmin looked dejected. 'Does that mean that everyone with MCI has an EEG to diagnose whether or not they are likely to progress to Alzheimer's?'

'No. Unfortunately EEG measurements of language processing are not routinely done. It takes a long time for discoveries in a laboratory to make their way into medical practice. Sadly, doctors are currently not able to predict the course of MCI. If MCI progresses to Alzheimer's, it was the start of Alzheimer's. If MCI never gets any worse or if the person improves, then the diagnosis remains MCI. The point is that not everyone with MCI will get Alzheimer's. **MCI is a window of opportunity** to stop the onslaught of Alzheimer's. It's a cue to re-evaluate our life and do everything we can to boost our brain such as:
- ensure regular good quality sleep
- quit smoking
- stay socially active
- engage in daily physical exercise
- audit our diet and alcohol consumption
- take up a new hobby
- start doing volunteer work.

'Of course, you also need to see a doctor and get tested for vitamin deficiencies, liver, kidney or thyroid dysfunction, high blood pressure, infections and tumours. Make brain health the number one priority in your life — otherwise you might find your life slipping away from you.'

'That's your key message, isn't it?' she reflected. 'Alzheimer's is not inevitable, even when the first indications of brain disease start to appear. **Education is more powerful than medication,** especially when it comes to dementia. And I gather **the sooner we intervene, the more likely we can arrest further decline.'**

'Yes,' I confirmed. 'That's why you need to be on the lookout for the subtlest signs that something is amiss. For instance, specific tests have revealed that **changes in a person's sense of humour** can appear nine years before any other symptoms of dementia.'

'Why?' Jasmin's eyes widened.

'Humour is a particularly sensitive way of detecting dementia because it puts demands on many different aspects of brain function. To understand humour, you need to be able to grasp double meanings, think laterally and recognise when something is out of place. People with Alzheimer's and frontotemporal dementia (FTD) are especially prone to losing their ability to comprehend satirical humour because they take things literally and don't recognise irony or exaggeration.'

'I've noticed that my grandmother takes everything at face value,' Jasmin agreed.

'That happens with many dementias. On the flip side, people with FTD tend to laugh at things that others would not normally find funny, such as a serious news story or creaky stairs.'

'I've heard that losing your sense of smell could also be a sign of impending Alzheimer's. Is that true?' Jasmin asked.

'Yes, the nose knows! The medical term for loss of smell is anosmia or olfactory loss. You can assess a person's sense of smell using a standard tool called the Sniffin' Sticks Odour Discrimination Memory Test (SSODMT) in which people have to correctly identify 16 distinct scents. Extended versions of the test use 32 scents. The less a person is able to identify smells, the more likely they are to have memory problems and develop Alzheimer's. Sniffin' Sticks could be another way of distinguishing MCI from Alzheimer's.'

'I find that certain smells can evoke specific memories. The scent of gardenias always takes me back to my childhood because we had a big bush in our backyard. And a particular perfume immediately brings to mind one of my school teachers,' Jasmin reflected.

'The part of the brain responsible for olfaction lies close to our memory warehouse — the hippocampus — and there are multiple interconnecting pathways between the two brain regions.'

'What are some of the smells that people are asked to identify?'

'Apple, banana, cinnamon, cloves, coffee, garlic, fish, leather, lemon, orange, peppermint, pineapple and turpentine,' I listed.

'Could I try this at home?' Jasmin asked earnestly.

'Pantry items can alert you to severe loss of smell but Sniffin' Sticks are much more reliable at picking up subtle changes because they measure three aspects of olfaction:
1. the threshold at which you detect a smell
2. your capacity to distinguish between different smells
3. your ability to accurately name what you're smelling.

'Of course, there are other causes of anosmia such as colds and flu, nasal polyps, side effects of medications, tumours, head trauma, Parkinson's disease, radiation, zinc deficiency and cocaine abuse. **Women tend to perform better in tests of smell than men** but that doesn't mean men are more likely to develop Alzheimer's. Don't assume the worst. Sometimes reduction in smell is simply part of ageing — like needing glasses to read. **One symptom does not make a disease.** You need to look at the overall picture of someone's functioning before making a diagnosis.'

'Are there any simple tests I could administer to help diagnose Alzheimer's?' Jasmin implored.

'Ask someone to **draw a clock face** showing the time of 10 minutes past 11. If they struggle to put numbers in the correct places or they draw only one clock hand, it definitely warrants more medical tests. Even simply refusing to do the test can be indicative of a problem.'

'Why would drawing a clock represent such a big challenge?'

'Time is an abstract concept. It requires a high level of intellectual functioning.'

'Are there other quick tests a doctor can do?'

'Have you heard of the Stroop test?'

'No,' she shook her head.

'To set up the test, write a list of 10 or more colours — red, yellow, orange, blue, green, black, purple etc. — and write each word on a separate sheet of paper. The catch is that you write the words in the wrong colour. For example, when you write the word *red*, use a blue-coloured pencil; when you write the word *orange*, use a green-coloured pencil. It doesn't matter which colour you use to write the word, just keep mixing it up. Then show each piece of paper in turn to the person whom you're testing and ask them to tell you the colour *not* the word. When they see the word *red* but it's written with a blue pencil, the correct answer is blue. People with no cognitive impairment will answer correctly. As we age, we get slower but we still get it right with maybe one or two errors. A person with Alzheimer's will not only be much slower, they will make a lot more mistakes because they find it harder to focus on one thing (the colour) when they're being distracted by something else (the word). You can also create this test on a computer using PowerPoint or Keynote slides.

'Don't use this test with someone who already has established Alzheimer's because it will only frustrate and exhaust them. The Stroop test is useful as a screening tool when you're not sure if a person's executive functioning (planning, reasoning, problem-solving) is on the decline. Always remember that **doctors treat people, not diseases**. First and foremost, put every patient at ease. Make them feel comfortable and don't let it become a pass-or-fail situation. Talk about the test as a game. Establishing a trusting and compassionate relationship is the most healing thing you can do for someone.

'And here are two acronyms to help you remember potential signs of dementia:

Are they having problems with **JUMPING**?
Judgement
Understanding instructions or directions
Memory, misplacing things and mood swings
Planning and problem-solving
Inappropriate words or remarks
New environments cause anxiety or confusion
Getting lost

'Be **WARNED** of the following changes:
Withdrawal from social activities or other things they used to do
Apathy
Reduced attention span
New behaviours
Evolving personality changes
Difficulty drawing a clock face.'

CHAPTER 8

In search of memory

Life isn't about finding yourself. Life is about creating yourself.

GEORGE BERNARD SHAW (1856–1950)

Dad and I were attending a six-monthly review with his neurologist, Dr Penny. Dad accepted that routine memory check-ups went hand in hand with turning 80.

'You've parked in the wrong spot,' Dad announced as soon as we got out of the car.

'What do you mean?' We were in the underground hospital carpark.

'It says *Patient Parking*. You need to find a spot marked *Impatient Parking.*'

Dad was always at his chivalrous best with perceptive Dr Penny. She began by measuring his waist circumference and then asking him to step on the scales.

'I thought you were examining my brain, not my belly,' he remarked.

'Your brain and belly are closely related,' she explained. **'The bigger your belly, the smaller your brain.** People who have excess fat around their internal organs — known as visceral fat — produce chemicals called cytokines that increase brain inflammation.'

'How can chemicals produced in my belly interfere with my brain?' Dad was skeptical.

'Pro-inflammatory cytokines are carried to your brain in your blood. Once they enter your brain they can promote brain insulin resistance, mitochondrial dysfunction and accumulation of amyloid beta ($A\beta$) plaques. All these factors reduce the functioning of your brain. The good news is that your waist circumference is less than 94 cm and your body weight has remained stable. That tells me you're maintaining your muscles and not gaining visceral fat. Keep up the good work — both of those parameters are critically important. Men with a waist circumference over 94 cm and women with a waist circumference above 80 cm start to increase their risk of all chronic diseases including Alzheimer's. Going to the gym doesn't just build muscle, it builds memory.'

'My daughter set you up to say that,' he accused playfully.

'No, she didn't. It's a medical fact,' Dr Penny upheld. 'Now can you tell me what day it is?'

Dr Penny swiftly transitioned to what's known as the Mini-Mental State Examination (MMSE) or Folstein test — so called because it was created by Marshal and Susan Folstein. It's a blunt test of cognitive impairment used to establish a baseline and track changes in mental functioning over time. It takes less than 10 minutes and involves answering 11 questions relating to time, place, memory, arithmetic and ability to follow instructions. Each task is allocated a specific number of points and the maximum score is 30. Anything less than a score of 24 warrants further tests. It does not automatically mean a diagnosis of dementia. See Appendix 2 for a copy of the MMSE.

Dad was looking uncertain.

'Do you know what day it is?' Dr Penny repeated kindly.

'It's a beautiful day! Any day I spend in the company of a beautiful woman is a beautiful day,' he beamed.

'I'm glad you're having a beautiful day,' she responded warmly. 'Do you know what day of the week it is?'

Dad turned to me for a hint. I shrugged.

'Why does it matter what day of the week it is?' he quipped.

'You're right. It doesn't matter,' affirmed Dr Penny. 'Maybe you can tell me the date?'

'At my age it's better not to know.'

'What about the month or the year?'

'All that matters is the present.'

'Right again,' she nodded. 'When is your birthday?'

'July 25th,' he remembered correctly.

'Excellent. And what year?' she coaxed.

'Every year,' he replied confidently.

'You're a very intelligent man,' Dr Penny was genuinely respectful. 'Do you know where you are?' she continued questioning him.

'I am wherever my daughter wants me to be.'

'And where's that right now?'

'A hospital.'

'Great. What country are we in?'

'Australia.'

'Which state of Australia?'

'New South Wales.'

'You're doing very well. And which city?'

'Sydney.'

'Fabulous! Did you notice which floor of this building we're on?'

'No. My daughter made me take the stairs. I lost count.'

'You must be very fit!' She was visibly impressed.

'Or very stupid,' he grinned.

As she continued with the test, it was evident that Dad's comprehension and arithmetic were intact but his short-term memory was AWOL.

'I think we should start you on a medicine to improve your memory,' she suggested. 'It's called memantine.'

'I have my daughter to remember things for me,' he declared sanguinely.

'I know you have your daughter,' she continued unperturbed, 'and you're also taking rivastigmine. But memantine is a different type of drug. It might offer some additional benefit.'

Memantine is the fourth and only other drug in Australia currently approved for treating Alzheimer's disease. The other three are the cholinesterase inhibitors discussed in Chapter 5 'In search of acetylcholine'. Memantine works by reducing the amount of a neurotransmitter in the brain called glutamate. Glutamate is necessary for normal brain functioning but Alzheimer's disease and stroke are associated with too much of it. When glutamate attaches to cell membranes via a receptor called NMDA (N-methyl-D-aspartate) it allows calcium to enter the cell. Too much calcium causes damage and eventual death of brain cells by a mechanism known as excitotoxicity — akin to over-stimulation or too much of a good thing. Memantine blocks the NMDA receptor and is therefore called an NMDA-receptor antagonist. Some people with moderate to severe Alzheimer's who take memantine show modest improvement in memory, attention, reasoning and language skills. Memantine can also reduce symptoms of agitation, irritability, delusions and hallucinations. In a subset of people, the drug makes no difference at all. In a third group of people, the combination of memantine plus a cholinesterase inhibitor offers greater improvement than taking one drug alone. The only way to find out is to try it.

My overriding philosophy is first do no harm. 'What are the potential side effects of taking memantine?' I wanted Dad to be aware of both sides of the equation. He was capable of making an informed decision even though he'd forget the conversation by the time we arrived home.

'Have you ever had a seizure?' Dr Penny was excluding contra-indications to taking the drug.

'What's that?' Dad asked.

'Epilepsy,' I simplified. 'No, he hasn't.'

'Good. You wouldn't be able to take memantine if you had a history of epilepsy. Like all medications, there are potential side effects but memantine is usually well tolerated. Only one in 100 people report an adverse experience such as confusion, dizziness, sleep disturbances or headaches.' She paused after each word to allow Dad to process the information.

'My headache is sitting in the chair behind me,' he mock-whispered.

She laughed before proceeding slowly and deliberately with her list, 'Even fewer people experience anxiety … vomiting … bladder irritation … or a strange feeling in their muscles. Of course, the response is very individual and it can take several months to see a benefit.'

Dad suddenly became serious and leaned towards her as he lowered his voice, 'If it means I'll be less of a burden on my daughter, I'll take the tablets. I'll put up with the side effects so she doesn't have to put up with my nonsense.'

I looked away from him as I blinked back tears.

'I'm sure your daughter doesn't see it that way,' Dr Penny reassured him.

'I'll take the tablets if you think they'll help my memory.'

Six months later, Dad was showing no evidence of side effects. Whether it was memantine, mulberries or mambo lessons, something was keeping his Alzheimer's at bay. At least for now.

CHAPTER 9

Are you in debt?

Both optimists and pessimists contribute to society.
The optimist invents the aeroplane, the pessimist
the parachute.

GEORGE BERNARD SHAW (1856–1950)

Mum's weekly bulletin should have alerted me to Dad's waning cognition. I lived 900 km away and we spoke on the phone every Sunday evening.

'Your father has always been absent-minded but he's getting worse. He must think there's an impending war. When I opened the bathroom cupboard yesterday, there was a stockpile of toiletries — at least a dozen bottles of shampoo and twice as many bars of soap.'

'They must have been on special,' I replied, unperturbed. I thought nothing of it. When Mum said 'dozen' she probably meant four. When it came to Dad, Mum was prone to hyperbole. I now realise that Dad must have kept forgetting what he'd bought on previous shopping trips so every time he went to the grocery store he bought more of the same.

'Your father is getting very gullible. I only just managed to stop him giving his credit card details to a scammer on the phone.' I could visualise Mum shaking her head in exasperation.

'How do you know it was a scammer?'

'The caller claimed we'd won a trip to Port Douglas and needed our credit card details to secure the hotel booking. When I grabbed the phone and started questioning the man, he promptly hung up on me.'

Many dementias affect the frontal lobes of the brain, which govern judgement and rational thinking. This can have several consequences. On the one hand, a person with dementia can be swayed into believing something that is ill-founded. This occurs because they lose trust in themselves and stop questioning things, even if they seem odd. On the other hand, if things no longer make sense to a person, they may become paranoid and lose trust in those around them who genuinely have their best interests at heart. Dad approached everyone with kindness and generosity. It was the only way he knew how to be. Unfortunately, dementia turned his benevolence into vulnerability — Marko being a case in point.

I had made the decision not to do anything about the money laundering, I mean lending. It was Dad's money and he could spend it as he chose. Even though I felt that Marko was taking advantage of Dad's charity and forgetfulness, I kept telling myself the net result was positive: Dad's mood, confidence and cognition were all bolstered by his friendship with Marko. Social activities are one of the biggest buffers against developing Alzheimer's and, if I confronted Marko, I might jeopardise their relationship. Besides, who was I to judge Marko? Maybe he was in genuine need and had every intention of repaying Dad at a later date. Of course, my father would never take the money back, even if he remembered giving it to him … and Marko knew it …

There I go again. I had to stop jumping to negative conclusions. Everyone is doing the best they can with the resources they have. I had no idea what pain or private struggles Marko might be going through. He was a proud man and might be too embarrassed to reveal the true nature of his hardship. Maybe he was helping a family member who had crippling medical bills? Maybe he was paying for a grandchild's speech therapy? These were situations that Marko would never admit to. At any rate, it wasn't doing my brain any good dwelling on it.

Researchers at University College London found that repetitive negative thinking (RNT) — the fancy name for which is perseverative cognition — can change the structure of our brain and predispose a person to Alzheimer's. A study of 350 men and women over the age of 55 revealed that those who habitually criticised themselves, focused on regrets, ruminated about past failures and worried about the future had greater decline in memory and thinking skills than people who were more positive and optimistic. The ruminators also had higher amounts of two aberrant proteins in their brain: amyloid beta (Aβ) plaques and tau tangles. These are the hallmarks of Alzheimer's disease. More about these two proteins in subsequent chapters.

The key word is 'repetitive'. Everyone sometimes feels despondent but if it becomes a person's default mode of thinking, **pessimism erodes brain function.** This is an astonishing finding: **our thoughts have a physical impact on our brain. Toxic thoughts produce toxic molecules.**

Scientists refer to this as the Cognitive Debt Hypothesis: persistent negative states of mind induce a chronic stress response that erodes brain function. The mechanisms through which stress promotes neuronal death involve reduced brain blood supply (known as cerebral hypoperfusion), increased inflammation and a hormone called Corticotropin Release Factor (CRF).[1] Negative thinking also depletes the brain of energy and leaves it with less fuel for other tasks. Hence memory, focus and cognition can all begin to suffer. Persistent negative states of mind can be due to depression, anxiety, insomnia or post-traumatic stress disorder (PTSD). All these conditions make a person more vulnerable to developing Alzheimer's and vascular dementia later in life.

Fortunately, all these conditions are amenable to counselling, cognitive behaviour therapy (CBT) or specific psychotherapies such

---

[1] CRF is a peptide (a short chain of amino acids) released during stress from an area of the brain called the hypothalamus. There are several ways in which CRF is implicated in Alzheimer's. One way is that CRF leads to the release of cortisol from our adrenal glands. Cortisol travels back into the brain via the bloodstream and attaches to cells in the hippocampus. This makes the cells more vulnerable to decay. CRF can also directly bind to cells in the hippocampus. This triggers phosphorylation of tau proteins and subsequent accumulation of neurofibrillary tangles — one of the hallmarks of Alzheimer's. Scientists are currently working on developing drugs to block CRF from attaching to cells in the hippocampus to prevent the build-up of tau tangles.

as EMDR.[2] They may take months or even years to heal, but with dedicated effort and a qualified therapist, we can literally change our mind. The first step is becoming aware of our dominant way of thinking. If you discover that you engage in repetitive negative thinking (RNT), I recommend two invaluable brain-boosting books:
1. *Learned Optimism* by Martin Seligman
2. *Positivity* by Barbara Fredrickson.

I have no affiliation with either of these brilliant authors. I read their books after hearing them speak at a conference and I think both titles should be on the reading list for secondary school students.

Chronic depression, anxiety and insomnia have a bidirectional relationship with many forms of dementia. As mentioned, longstanding untreated depression, anxiety and insomnia make it more likely that a person will develop dementia. Conversely, dementia makes a person more likely to develop depression, anxiety and sleep disturbances. To complicate things further, depression in an elderly person shares many of the symptoms of Alzheimer's: apathy, confusion, memory loss, diminished self-confidence, social withdrawal, irritability and reduced capacity to plan and problem-solve. This is known as pseudo-dementia: depression that is mistaken for dementia. The first rule of dementia is to elicit whether the person is suffering from depression. Sometimes when the depression lifts, the dementia disappears along with it.

Many studies have found that chronic midlife stress contributes to brain shrinkage and memory impairment, especially in women. Why stress should have a greater impact on women's brains is yet to be elucidated. Stress in this context is defined as emotional or psychological suffering, not the positive stress associated with rising to a challenge. Sources of chronic stress include family discord, hostile work environments, being bullied, severe financial hardship and serious illness in a loved one. Modern-day living is inherently stressful and most people can identify with at least one of the aforementioned. This does not mean that everyone's brain is precipitously shrinking. What it means is that learning to deal

---

[2] EMDR stands for Eye Movement Desensitisation and Reprocessing. It is currently one of the most powerful ways to heal PTSD.

with stressful situations is critical to long-term brain health. It's the perception of an experience as distressing that causes damage, not the experience itself. We can't always change what's going on around us but we always have a choice in how we respond. **As kryptonite is to Superman, stress is to humans.** In the same way that lead can protect Superman from kryptonite, stress-management strategies can protect us from stress. One of the most effective and well-researched approaches to reducing stress is Mindfulness-Based Stress Reduction (MBSR). This is an eight-week face-to-face or online program developed by Jon Kabat-Zinn in the 1970s, which has stood the test of time and science. I signed up for the program myself and found it immensely helpful in every area of my life.

Complementing the Cognitive Debt Hypothesis is the Cognitive Reserve Hypothesis: higher education, lifelong engagement in mentally stimulating activities, rich social experiences, overcoming obstacles, conscientiousness, optimism and learning new skills into old age create multiple new pathways between brain cells and protect against cognitive decline. PET scans have demonstrated that a person can remain mentally intact despite having Aβ plaques and tau tangles throughout their brain. How is this possible? They have forged brain circuits that bypass the areas of damage. Hence the description cognitive reserve. Cognitive reserve is like having money in a savings account to keep us afloat when our regular account is overdrawn.

Cognitive debt and cognitive reserve are two opposing pieces of the Alzheimer's puzzle that we can turn to our advantage. In fact, there are infinite ways to boost cognitive reserve. A few examples include:
- taking up a new hobby
- joining a book club or local community group
- learning to speak a foreign language or play a musical instrument
- enrolling in a creative writing class — or any class that sparks your interest
- doing anything that you find challenging and enjoyable.

A life of joy, appreciation and fulfilment simultaneously lowers cognitive debt and increases cognitive reserve.

In the interest of reducing my cognitive debt, my cynical rumination about Marko had to stop. The best way I knew to do this was to practise **gratitude**. I took a deep breath. I'm grateful that Dad wants to spend time with Marko. I'm grateful that Marko wants to spend time with Dad. I'm grateful that Marko makes Dad laugh. I'm grateful that Dad is always cheerful after spending time with Marko. I'm grateful that Marko's wife Branka cooks traditional Serbian dishes that Dad loves to eat. I'm grateful that Branka often sends Dad home with leftovers. I'm grateful that Dad insists on sharing the leftovers with me … Yep, I was feeling better already.

CHAPTER 10

Let reading be your medicine

Books are the quietest and most constant of friends;
they are the most accessible and wisest of counsellors,
and the most patient of teachers.

CHARLES W ELIOT (1834–1926)

'Your father is losing interest in the garden,' Mum lamented during one of our Sunday phone calls. 'He used to be so proud of his roses. Now he just wants to sit inside and read the paper all day.'

Apathy is a red flag for dementia. Too often it's mistaken for 'just getting old'. Apathy is NOT a normal feature of ageing. Apathy is NOT laziness, tiredness or depression (though it can be a feature of depression). Apathy is defined as a lack of motivation and loss of interest in pursuing meaningful or pleasurable activities. MRI scans reveal that apathy is associated with damage to small blood vessels in the white matter of brain regions associated with motivation and planning. Furthermore, neuroscientists from the University of Cambridge, UK, found that people with higher levels of apathy or increasing apathy over time were at greater risk of developing both Alzheimer's and vascular dementia. Does apathy cause dementia or does dementia cause apathy? It's likely a bidirectional relationship in which one condition exacerbates the other. In addition, neurologists at the Academic Medical Center in Amsterdam found that high levels of **apathy more than doubled the risk of early death**.

Structural changes in the brain are not the only cause of apathy. Loss of confidence is another contributing factor. If a person starts forgetting how to do things they could previously accomplish with ease, they become frustrated and give up. Confusion and clumsiness — also features of Alzheimer's — are a further assault on a person's sense of competence. When we're afraid of making mistakes, we shy away from activities that might expose our shortcomings.

This makes apathy a dangerous downward spiral. It accelerates cognitive decline because withdrawal from meaningful pursuits means less stimulation means further decline. It also increases the physical and emotional burden on care-partners. As their loved one does less and less, care-partners find themselves having to do more and more.

Is it possible to reverse apathy and restore a person's enthusiasm for life? Several medications such as methylphenidate (commonly known as Ritalin) are being tested in people who have mild Alzheimer's along with apathy. The results show promise but, like all drugs, there are side effects.

Personally, I believe that **humanity trumps pharmacology**. This was borne out in a two-year trial involving 1000 people with dementia in 70 care homes across the United Kingdom. When staff were taught to introduce personalised activities tailored to the individual's interests, it dramatically improved motivation, cognition and longevity. Known as the WHELD study (Wellbeing and Health for People with Dementia), it demonstrated that apathy can be reversed by taking the time to discover a person's former passions, hobbies and favourite topics of conversation. Empathic encouragement and positive reinforcement slowly led to re-engagement with life. The result was a reduction in the use of anti-psychotic medications and a 30% drop in mortality.

In retrospect, another reason Dad spent all day reading the paper was because he couldn't retain what he'd read. All his life he'd been an avid reader of fiction and non-fiction, art and archeology, history and mythology, classics and comedy. He was the parent who introduced me to C S Lewis, Charles Dickens, George Orwell, H G Wells, Jane Austen, the Bronte sisters, Alexandre Dumas, Thomas Hardy, F Scott Fitzgerald and countless more authors who filled my nights with intrigue and adventure. Whenever Mum spotted the incriminating shaft of light under my bedroom door, she'd threaten to confiscate my precious book. Dad couldn't allow this to happen so he secretly bought me a tiny book light that enabled me to read without fear of detection. He understood the allure of worlds woven from words.

From my earliest memories, Dad and I had been confederates. He instilled in me his love of reading. He found any excuse to buy me a book: birthdays, Christmas, Easter ('Books are better than chocolate'), Mother's Day ('This book will help you understand your mother'), Father's Day ('This book can teach you things your father can't'), and any day I was sick from school ('This book will help you heal. A healthy mind means a healthy body.')

'What am I going to do with the two of you?' Mum shook her curlers in mock reproach. 'Buying her books when she's sick will only encourage her to feign illness so she can stay home and read!'

Dad replied with corresponding faux gravity: 'Don't put off until tomorrow what you can read today!'

Dad seized on every pretext to take me to the library: to find information for a school project, to learn about a bird that was nesting in our bottlebrush or to settle a debate we'd started that morning. We'd spend hours exploring aisle after aisle, one theme leading to another, until we'd forgotten why we came in the first place. Every visit to the library was an enthralling treasure hunt.

Decades later, when I was invited to be ambassador for an annual event called *Australian Reading Hour*, I jumped at the chance to expound the extensive brain-benefits and joys of reading. *Australian Reading Hour* invites everyone in the country to stop for one hour, on a designated day in the year, to pick up a book and simply read for pleasure. It's also an opportunity to read aloud to a young child, an elderly person or someone who has not been afforded the privilege of literacy. When asked for the top 12 ways that reading boosts brain function and staves off dementia, here is what I said:

Top 12 brain-benefits of reading backed by neuroscience

1. The more books in a home as a child is growing up, the less they experience cognitive decline as they age, even when factors such

as socio-economic status and physical health have been taken into account (both of which are associated with better brain health). It seems that extensive reading in early life creates a lasting butter against mental decline.

2. Fortunately, it's never too late to pick up a book and reap the benefits. Voracious reading in old age not only reduces the risk of Alzheimer's, it has been found to prolong life — just 30 minutes of reading a day starts to provide a survival advantage. Books are better brain-boosters than newspapers or magazines. Books engage broader memory and thinking skills because they are more immersive and require the reader to juggle intertwined themes, ideas and characters for an extended period of time.

3. Reading a wide range of genres improves problem-solving skills. Absorbing ourselves in something completely different from our work activates regions of the brain we are not in the habit of using. The more diverse the books we read, the more we are able to think in diverse ways.

4. Research from the University of California found that when we experience awe by watching or reading something that transports us out of our day-to-day lives, it quiets the critical voice in our head and reduces the production of inflammatory cytokines.[3] This improves physical, as well as mental, wellbeing.

5. Stanford University researchers found that when we read an inspiring story, we are subsequently more ethical and generous, more likely to help a stranger, and feel more connected to other people.

6. Functional MRI scans demonstrate that when we read about a character's experiences, the same regions of our brain are activated as if we were in the situation ourselves. This enhances our capacity to empathise with others in real life. Reading also makes us more empathic by broadening our outlook and challenging our assumptions.

7. Brain scanning also shows that reading different styles of literature for different purposes (for example, relaxation versus critical

---

[3] Cytokines are small proteins secreted by specific cells of the immune system that exert an effect on other cells. Cytokines facilitate communication between cells and stimulate migration of cells to sites of trauma, infection and inflammation. The term originates from two Greek words: *cyto* meaning 'cell' and *kinos* meaning 'movement'.

analysis) activates different regions of the brain. Both types of reading are advantageous.

8. Challenge yourself with complex literature. When we put demands on our brain to figure something out, it stimulates the growth of new brain cells and sharpens our thinking.

9. Read to educate yourself. Nobel prize-winning scientist Eric Kandel demonstrated that when we learn something new, the connections between brain cells are increased. This helps to build what is known as cognitive reserve — back-up pathways within the brain that help to protect against dementia.

10. Reading can help us unwind, reduce stress and deal with uncertainty. In addition to switching off unproductive rumination, reading fiction improves information processing and creativity.

11. Reading can be a way of accessing feelings we try to hide from ourselves. Throughout life there are times when we suppress negative emotions because we feel pressured to put on a brave front or stay upbeat for the people around us. Reading a moving story gives us permission to get in touch with buried emotions and cry if we need to.

12. Finishing a great book provides a sense of satisfaction and accomplishment, along with a healthy hit of dopamine.

How can reading help someone who already has dementia?

The science is conclusive: don't stop reading! Psychologist Marina Guitartand — co-ordinator of the Day Care Unit at Fundació ACE (Alzheimer Centre Educacional) in Barcelona — reports that reading every day helps to preserve language and memory. People with Alzheimer's find it difficult to focus and are unable to remember the thread of a story. Despite this, they often maintain their ability to read, at least in the early stages. Sadly, they often give up reading because it becomes an exhausting mental effort. In order to inspire and support their dementia clients to keep reading, the Day Care Unit developed the following guidelines with great success:

- Therapists, caregivers and family members are encouraged to read alongside people with dementia.
- The books that work best for dementia have photos, large clear text and humour.

- Books, magazines and newspapers are placed throughout the residence so they are always readily available.
- The caregiver makes notes about the plot and always reviews what was read the previous day.

Choose different books for different stages of dementia. This is similar to selecting age-appropriate books for children.

- For people with mild dementia: uplifting news articles, books of short stories or pithy novels are the most engaging option.
- For moderate dementia: fun, amusing rhymes and poetry work best.
- For advanced dementia: read familiar proverbs that spark conversation. For example: 'Actions speak louder than words' and 'Every cloud has a silver lining'.
- Even if someone is no longer able to respond, reading to them can still prompt recognition and evoke positive emotions.

A study from Essex Meadows Health Center in Connecticut, published in the 2017 issue of *Advance Senior Care (IASC)*, showed that the best way for a person with mild to moderate dementia to maintain focus while reading was to use hard-cover books with the following features:

- captivating pictures that support the text
- large margins
- headings printed in bold
- 10 to 15 lines of text at a time.

When reading books with this format, study participants experienced less brain-strain, lower levels of fatigue and longer reading times. This is because images, titles and text stimulate different regions of the brain and work synergistically to increase engagement and understanding.

On a personal note, reading to Dad was a way of staying connected, even when his cognition was at its lowest ebb. It brought us both into the present moment — our attention anchored to the words on the page. For him, each word might only last an instant, but another soon filled the void. We both found our nightly ritual soothing and comforting — we could relax while eavesdropping on someone else's thoughts.

Why reading is a wonderful habit for anyone

Reading has invigorated the greatest minds throughout history. Here are some of my favourite reflections on reading.

Socrates (470–399 BCE): *Employ your time in improving yourself by other men's writings so that you shall come easily by what others have laboured hard for.*

Seneca (4 BCE – 65 CE): *Reading nourishes and refreshes the mind. It should be an indispensable part of one's daily routine.* Seneca encouraged his students to read deeply, repeatedly and forcefully.

Descartes (1596–1650): *The reading of all good books is like conversation with the finest people of the past centuries.*

Napoléon Bonaparte (1769–1821): *Show me a family of readers, and I will show you the people who move the world.*

Stendhal (1783–1842): *A good book is an event in my life.*

Margaret Fuller (1810–1850): *Today a reader, tomorrow a leader.*

What do I love about reading?

I'm very fortunate that reading brings me unadulterated joy — and anything that sparks joy boosts brain function through a multitude of chemical and neurological pathways. Reading a few paragraphs of inspiring literature is an uplifting way to start each day. It is likewise a lovely way to end the day. If my mind is churning, a good book can switch off the worry cycle and help me get to sleep.

Books are like friends. There is always a protagonist who has gone through the same trials and tribulations that I'm going through, so I never feel alone. It's like a reassuring voice saying 'Me too'. Whatever is happening in my life, there's always a good book to help me get through it.

CHAPTER 11

In search of keys

Since you alone are responsible for your thoughts,
only you can change them.

PARAMAHANSA YOGANANDA (1893–1952)

Dad's neurologist had ordered an MRI (magnetic resonance imaging) scan of Dad's brain. Shrinkage of two specific areas that are critical for memory function — the hippocampus and entorhinal cortex — are strongly linked to Alzheimer's.

We arrived at the radiology centre on a sweltering Sydney afternoon.

'Where's your jacket?' Dad asked as soon as I'd parked the car.

'I don't need a jacket today, it's too hot,' I replied.

'You're showing too much flesh. You should cover your shoulders.'

'It's fine,' I reassured him. 'There's no dress code and this dress is far from revealing.' I was wearing a knee-length, sleeveless floral cotton frock with a conservative neckline.

'It doesn't matter if other people don't have a dress code. YOU should have a dress code. You're a professional. A *medical* professional. No one will take you seriously in that dress.'

'I'm not here in the capacity of a medical professional. I'm here as your daughter. Another doctor ordered the scan.'

'But you're still a doctor and you need to dress appropriately.'

Dress codes had recently become one of Dad's preoccupations. I knew better than to argue with him so I rummaged around the boot of the car (boot = trunk for my North American readers) where I always kept a light jacket. 'Here it is,' I smiled as I draped it over my shoulders.

'Put it on properly.'

I prayed the air conditioning would be on maximum cooling.

After completing the lengthy paperwork and reminding Dad over and over that he would need to remain perfectly still while enclosed in a tunnel listening to soft music through padded headphones, he was taken into the scanning room. I heaved a sigh of relief as I peeled off my jacket. I was about to settle down to a peaceful half-hour of reading when I realised I'd left my book in the car. I informed the receptionist I'd return in a few minutes.

Back at the car, I reached into the side pocket of my handbag where I always kept my keys and … my keys were not there. I must have been distracted by the jacket kerfuffle and dropped the keys into the middle of my bag instead of the side pocket. I sifted through the entire contents to no avail. Three times. I checked the car doors and confirmed they were locked. It's impossible to lock the car without using the key … unless I'd clicked the boot open *after* locking the car and absentmindedly placed the keys in the boot while putting on the jacket. I then could have slammed the boot shut and the keys would be locked inside.

But didn't I remember clicking the car remote as we were walking towards the radiology clinic? Did I or didn't I? I began to worry that Alzheimer's might be contagious. The more I worried, the less I remembered. I retraced my steps and scanned the ground in case I'd dropped them. This was unlikely because the car remote was on the same keychain as the garage remote and two house keys (front and side doors) and I would have heard a loud clang if they'd landed on concrete. I returned to the radiology clinic and checked where I'd been sitting. I scoured the floor and reception area before asking everyone in the waiting room if they'd seen a bunch of keys. Everyone shook their head apologetically.

There was only one thing left to do. I rang Roadside Assistance and explained that I'd locked the keys in my car. Could they help? Of course they could. However, as they were currently receiving an unprecedented number of calls, I would probably have to wait 90 minutes before anyone was available. Dad would never let me live this down. To my jubilant surprise, within 10 minutes I received a call from John who was about to arrive at the car park to break into my car. I skipped to the car in anticipation of meeting my hero.

I couldn't believe how easily he popped open the passenger door. Yes, it literally popped. 'I'm glad you use your powers for good and not evil,' I effused. 'I can't thank you enough.'

I waved him off and immediately dived into the boot. I took out shopping bags, umbrella, gym mat, skipping rope and newspaper … but no keys. I shook out every item. Still no keys. Where on earth could they be? I looked under the car. I looked under all the cars that were parked between my car and the clinic. Nothing. Someone must have found them and taken them to the police. Or was someone sinister hiding and watching me this very minute … waiting for me to leave the car unattended so they could use it as a getaway vehicle after robbing a bank? What should I do next? I left the car unlocked and entered the clinic just as my father was escorted back into the waiting room.

'That was very relaxing,' he beamed. 'Can I have another go? I love the peace and quiet,' he winked at the radiographer.

The radiographer returned his grin. 'You're welcome any time, mate. Oh and don't forget your keys. You left them in the locker.' He handed Dad *my* keys.

'What?' I gasped.

'Nothing metallic can be worn in the scanner. These were in your father's pocket.'

To stop myself from hyperventilating, yelling or doing something else I'd later regret, I resorted to **box breathing**. Also known as square breathing, it's a technique for relieving stress and anxiety or improving concentration and performance. Start by inhaling slowly and deeply to the count of four. Hold your breath for another slow count of four. Exhale through the mouth for four. Hold for another four. Repeat the four-step cycle until the urge to commit dastardly deeds subsides.

Slow breathing and breath-holding elevate blood levels of carbon dioxide and stimulate the vagus nerve to lower blood pressure and induce a sense of calm. Within a few minutes, box breathing had worked its magic. The technique can also improve mood, reduce pain and help with insomnia. Moreover, it was a trigger for me to recall the words of Ralph Waldo Emerson: 'For every minute you are angry, you lose 60 seconds of happiness.' I needed to employ it more often, rather than reserve it for special occasions.

Much as I was intensely curious about how my keys had ended up in Dad's pocket, I made no mention of them. Besides, he probably had no recollection of picking them up. We drove home playing 'I spy with my little eye, something beginning with … A/B/C.'

CHAPTER 12

To test or not to test?

The best way to predict the future is to create it.

This quote is often credited to ABRAHAM LINCOLN (1809–1865) but I am not able to verify the attribution. Whoever said it was spot on.

'Why do you want to know?' Dr Mills asked kindly as she picked up her delicate rose-gold glasses.

'My father has Alzheimer's; his mother and uncle also had Alzheimer's. It makes me suspicious of an underlying genetic predisposition.' My voice unexpectedly faltered. I hadn't anticipated feeling emotional about requesting a gene test.

'How old was your father when you first started noticing changes in his cognition?' Dr Mills rested the edge of her glasses against her matching-colour blouse.

'I wasn't living with my parents at the time so I can only guess from my mother's description. I'd say in his mid-70s.'

'What about your paternal grandmother?' she continued in the same even tone.

'Also in her 70s.'

'Has your father had any gene tests for Alzheimer's?'

'No. He doesn't want to know because he believes it would seal his fate.'

'Finding out your gene status would also shed light on your father's genes. How do you feel about knowing something he doesn't want you to reveal?'

'I would respect his wishes not to know. I haven't told him I'm having the test and I won't tell him the results.'

'Do you have siblings or children? Your results will also impact other family members who may or may not want to know their gene status.'

'I don't have any children or siblings.'

'Are you aware that if you apply for a new life insurance policy — including disability and income protection — you would need to disclose the results of an Alzheimer's gene test?'

'Yes.'

'If you discovered that you had a gene that increased your risk of Alzheimer's, would you become hypervigilant and paranoid about every memory glitch being a harbinger of dementia?'

'Maybe … I'm not sure,' I gave her a wan smile.

'Is there a danger you would turn your result into a self-fulfilling prophecy?' she persisted. 'If you thought you were on the path to Alzheimer's, are you likely to become depressed and withdrawn? In which case, you'd increase your probability of developing Alzheimer's even in the absence of a predisposing gene.'

'No,' I was sure of my answer. 'It would have the opposite effect. I would become all the more proactive about doing everything I possibly could to ward off the disease.'

'Aren't you doing that already?' she challenged.

'Yes, I feel that I am,' I paused. 'So in theory it shouldn't make any difference. But what I would do differently is learn everything I can about the specific measures that someone with an APOE4 gene needs to take.'

She folded her glasses and placed them back on her uncluttered desk. 'I understand you're a doctor and you've no doubt done your research. But I still have to go through all aspects of genetic counselling with you.'

'Of course,' I felt relieved to simply listen for a while.

'There are two categories of genes related to Alzheimer's. One category of genes is referred to as deterministic. This means if you inherit the gene, you are guaranteed to get Alzheimer's. We know of three genes in this category. They are called:

- Presenilin 1 (PSEN1) on chromosome 14
- Presenilin 2 (PSEN2) on chromosome 1
- Amyloid precursor protein (APP) on chromosome 21.

'If either of your parents carries one of these genes, there's a 50% chance the affected parent will pass the gene on to you. If you inherit one of these genes, you will almost certainly be diagnosed with Alzheimer's before the age of 60. Fortunately, these genes are very rare and account for less than 1% of Alzheimer's cases worldwide. You've told me that your family members all developed Alzheimer's after the age of 70. Therefore, we can rule out these three deterministic genes.'

I nodded.

'The second category of genes is referred to as risk factor genes. If you inherit a risk factor gene, you are more prone to getting Alzheimer's than someone without the gene — but you are by no means destined for the disease. Furthermore, these risk factor genes interact with other genes that modify their impact. Hence Alzheimer's is described as a polygenic disease — multiple genes work together to pull you in one or another direction. And of course, environmental factors also play a major role in how genes behave — referred to as epigenetics. It's a very complex picture and I suspect that no two people follow the exact same path to Alzheimer's.

'The best-known gene related to Alzheimer's is Apolipoprotein E (APOE) on chromosome 19. This gene exists in three different forms — technically referred to as alleles or variants. The three forms are called APOE2, APOE3 and APOE4. Everyone inherits one form from each parent. That means each person ends up with one of six possible combinations of APOE. All other things being equal, people who have one or two copies of the E4 variant are more likely to get Alzheimer's or vascular dementia than people without the E4 variant. They are also more likely to get dementia at an earlier age than if they didn't have the gene, and the disease tends to progress more quickly. But of course, "all other things" are never equal. Ethnicity also plays a role in how the APOE4 gene affects brain health. For instance, people with the E4 gene who are Nigerian, Hispanic or Latino are much less likely to develop Alzheimer's than E4 carriers of Caucasian or Japanese descent.'

'Why is that?' I asked.

'The prevailing theory is that the APOE4 gene is linked to a set of genes that are usually inherited along with it. Different ethnicities have different combinations of genes linked to APOE4. Variations in adjoining genes have a differential influence on how APOE4 behaves. Thus APOE4 by itself isn't enough to give you Alzheimer's. It might need to be inherited together with a set of other predisposing genes that we're not yet aware of. Or maybe certain environmental factors have to interact with APOE4 in order for it to start causing problems. We know that **if an APOE4 carrier develops type 2 diabetes, their risk of Alzheimer's skyrockets.**

'The best I can offer you at this stage of our understanding is the following table. It lists the APOE gene combinations in order of lowest to highest risk of Alzheimer's for someone of Caucasian origin such as yourself.'

Gene combination	Risk of getting Alzheimer's	Percentage of population carrying this gene combination	Other features of this combination
E2 + E2	These people have the lowest risk of getting Alzheimer's — estimated to be 40% less likely than people carrying E3 + E3.	1%	These people tend to have higher blood triglyceride levels and an elevated risk of stomach ulcers, blood clots, aneurysms, recurrent miscarriages and hammer toe (hallux valgus).
E2 + E3	These people also have a lower risk of Alzheimer's than those with E3 + E3 — also close to 40% lower risk.	10–15%	Nil of note.
E3 + E3	Neutral risk	60%	Nil of note.
E2 + E4	These people have one anti-Alzheimer's gene and one pro-Alzheimer's gene. This tends to put them at a slightly higher risk of Alzheimer's than those with E3 + E3.	2%	Carrying one E4 gene appears to be associated with a higher risk of stroke.
E3 + E4	Two-to four-fold higher risk than someone with E3 + E3 BUT these people can neutralise the effect of having an E4 gene through physical exercise and other lifestyle measures.	20–25%	Some studies indicate that having one copy of E4 may pose a greater risk of Alzheimer's to women than to men. Having two copies of E4 seems to affect men and women to the same degree.
E4 + E4	>10-fold higher risk than someone with E3 + E3 BUT these people can also neutralise the effect of having E4 genes through physical exercise and other lifestyle measures.	2–3%	These people tend to have higher LDL-cholesterol levels but a lower risk of obesity, liver disease and chronic airway obstruction.

'However,' she leaned forward for emphasis, 'as I said earlier, **a single gene NEVER tells the whole story.** Your risk is very much influenced by other genes you've inherited along with your APOE. In other words, the APOE4 variant behaves differently depending on its neighbouring genes. Many people with one or two copies of the E4 gene never develop Alzheimer's because somewhere in their DNA they also carry protective genes or they lead a healthy lifestyle. On the flip side, people without an E4 variant can still get Alzheimer's if they carry other Alzheimer's risk genes that we don't yet know about or they're exposed to environmental or lifestyle factors that compromise their brain function. This is why most doctors will not recommend having an APOE test. It is not a reliable predictor of Alzheimer's because there are too many other variables at play. I also need to warn you not to become complacent if you discover you've inherited E2 + E2. It doesn't mean you can throw all caution to the wind and get away with eating junk food. I've seen people with E2 + E2 develop Alzheimer's despite having these so-called protective genes.' Dr Mills paused to allow me to review the table.

'I'm aware that inheriting E4 + E4 is not all bad news,' I confirmed.

'Good,' she seemed satisfied with my assurance. 'So let's take a closer look at what APOE actually does. APOE genes instruct your brain and liver to produce a protein called — surprise, surprise — Apolipoprotein E or ApoE for short. When scientists are referring to the gene, they use capitals: APOE. When they're writing about the protein, they use lower-case letters: ApoE. The ApoE protein has many different functions. This protein plays a role in:
- transporting cholesterol in the blood and the brain
- clearing amyloid beta (Aβ) plaques from the brain
- regulating brain inflammation
- maintaining the health of blood vessels throughout the brain
- keeping the blood–brain barrier (BBB) intact
- glucose utilisation by the brain
- mitochondrial function.

'The E2, E3 and E4 versions of this protein are very similar. However, minor differences in structure produce major differences in function.

For instance, the ApoE4 protein is not as good as the E3 and E2 proteins in preventing the build-up of Aβ plaques. ApoE4 also activates a stronger immune response in the presence of head trauma and infection. In addition, ApoE4 binds to genes that drive insulin resistance, oxidative damage and accumulation of tau tangles. The picture is very complicated but what I'm trying to convey is that many of the toxic processes generated by ApoE4 can be mitigated by diet, exercise, sleep and stress management.'

'That's exactly why I want to have the test,' I affirmed. 'I don't want to know whether I have an APOE4 gene in order to predict my risk of Alzheimer's. I want to use the information to guide my lifestyle choices and to participate in clinical trials that call for my genotype.'

'That's highly commendable,' she approved. 'One of the most positive and empowering things a person can do is to participate in Alzheimer's research. When you volunteer for a study, you're not only playing an active role in improving your own health, you're paving the way for a potential cure for others. Are you aware of a service called Step Up for Dementia Research?'

'No.'

'As the name suggests, Step Up for Dementia Research (visit: stepupfordementiaresearch.org.au) enables you to register for upcoming studies and trials to advance our understanding of dementia. Their tagline says it very succinctly: "A dementia breakthrough, powered by you". When a suitable trial comes up, you'll be contacted and asked if you're interested in taking part. I think it's exactly what you're looking for.'

'Yes, definitely. I'll sign up as soon as I get home.'

'The Alzheimer's Association in the US has a similar service called TrialMatch that allows people to see which trials would be a good fit for them or a family member.'

'I've tried to find studies that would be suitable for Dad but for one reason or another, he hasn't been eligible,' I sighed.

'Don't give up,' she encouraged. 'In the meantime, do you have any questions?'

'Apart from APOE, can you test for any other genes believed to increase — or decrease — the risk of late-onset Alzheimer's?' I pulled out my list of cryptic gene names. 'ABCA7, CLU, CR1, CD1E, CETPI405V, GLIS3, LDLR, MTHFR, PICALM, PLD3, PTPRC, SORL1, TNFα, TOMM40, TREM2, TREML2 ...'

'No, no and no,' she interrupted. 'The role of the other 30 or so genes that are implicated in Alzheimer's is so nuanced and complex that testing is usually reserved for research purposes only. We don't yet know enough about these genes to be able to provide meaningful advice. Scientists need to do more probing to understand why these genes increase the risk of Alzheimer's. For instance, a particular variant of the ABCA7 gene appears to be a major risk factor for Alzheimer's in African-Americans but not in Caucasians. Like APOE, the gene is involved in cholesterol metabolism and amyloid precursor protein (APP) transport but its precise mechanism of action is not known. Can you see why making predictions based on APOE alone is fraught with difficulty?'

'Yes.'

'I urge you to think through all the implications we've discussed before making a decision,' she cautioned. 'The test is not covered by Medicare and will cost $154. I should receive the result in five business days. Please make two more appointments to see me. In our next appointment I'd like to discuss what you would do differently if the test revealed you had one or two copies of the APOE4 gene. This is a conversation we need to have before you have the test. Then, if you decide to go ahead, you will need to see me in person to receive the result.' She studied my countenance before reiterating, 'No matter what the result, I will need to see you face to face for post-test counselling. If you change your mind after having the test and decide that you don't want to know your result after all, the information will remain confidential until such time as you wish to discuss it.'

'Your approach is in stark contrast to at-home genetic testing where people simply send off a specimen of saliva and receive their results by email,' I observed.

My calm genetic counsellor suddenly became animated. 'Don't get me started on direct to consumer (DTC) genetic testing!' she exclaimed. 'It's irresponsible, inaccurate and potentially damaging. Most of the time the consumer has no idea what is being tested or what the results really mean. They believe they'll discover the elixir to eternal life by "knowing" which types of food, exercise and skin products are best for their specific genetic make-up. What nonsense! You might as well be guided by your star sign. Hype and manipulative marketing — that's what it's all about. For a start, blood is more accurate than saliva because saliva can be contaminated by a recent meal or by bacterial genes. One company failed to identify that a prankster had sent in their dog's saliva. Other audits have shown that up to 40% of reports contain false positives. In other words, a person is told they have a particular trait or condition but they don't actually have it. The mistakes are not deliberate but they point to a lack of precision in testing procedures and data interpretation.

'Most DTC tests do not sequence your entire genome — your genome being the complete set of genes that you carry. Instead, these companies simply examine areas of your DNA that are known to carry interesting information and then compare what they find with their existing DNA database. Multiple different genes can influence your response to specific foods and they interact in intricate and as yet undetermined ways. To suggest that a gene test can guide your dietary choices is stretching the truth. It's something we're working towards but we're not there yet. What makes me laugh is that the advice these companies dish out is nothing more than standard healthy lifestyle recommendations: don't smoke, eat more vegetables, cut out sugar and engage in regular physical exercise. Wow! I never would have predicted that,' she declared sarcastically.

I was amused by her sudden outburst.

'If that were all,' she continued, 'DTC gene testing would be harmless. Unfortunately, people don't just learn useless information about their propensity to produce gooey earwax; they can also discover things they were unprepared for — such as their APOE status. Too often, the consumer reads that they've inherited E4 + E4 or even just one copy of E4 and they haven't been given any explanation or counselling. So they ask Dr Google and suddenly they think they're doomed to get Alzheimer's. I end up having to counsel these people after they turn up to their GP with anxiety and panic attacks. It makes me very angry when I see needless suffering. One woman had outright PTSD after learning that she was an E4 + E4 carrier. She had no idea what it meant until she received her result and started searching the internet for answers. Now tell me that isn't reckless and unethical on the part of the company administering the tests.'

I agreed that it was reckless and unethical. Did I dare otherwise?

'Knowledge is only power if it's delivered in an empowering way. People need to be given a choice about whether or not they want to know something that has wide-reaching consequences. Studies such as the NIH REVEAL Project show that if people are given in-depth pre- and post-test counselling, they do not suffer long-term psychological or emotional problems from learning their APOE gene status. In some cases, the initial shock can produce short-term distress but, with appropriate support, most people assert that knowing they are more susceptible to Alzheimer's has motivated them to make long-term healthy lifestyle changes. They also admit to seeking out more joy and not taking things for granted. Having said that, there is always a small percentage of people who will suffer prolonged negative impacts. My job is to make sure you're not one of them. I recommend you sleep on it.'

CHAPTER 13

Genes are like teens

Men are not prisoners of fate, but only prisoners of their own minds.

FRANKLIN D ROOSEVELT (1882–1945)

When I arrived for my second appointment with Dr Mills, I was asked to complete a questionnaire.

On a scale of 1 to 5, how much do you agree or disagree with the following statements in relation to yourself?
1 = strongly disagree
2 = somewhat disagree
3 = neither agree nor disagree
4 = somewhat agree
5 = strongly agree

(a)   *I can feel myself getting older.*
(b)   *Slowing down is an inevitable part of ageing.*
(c)   *Life gets harder as you get older.*
(d)   *Old age tends to bring increasing health problems.*
(e)   *As you get older you become less useful.*
(f)   *As you get older you become more forgetful.*
(g)   *Things go steadily downhill as you age.*
(h)   *It's harder to make friends as you age.*
(i)   *Old people tend to be lonelier than young people.*
(j)   *Old age is associated with loss of independence.*
(k)   *Old age is associated with loss of confidence.*
(l)   *Old age is associated with increasing aches and pains.*
(m)   *Old age is associated with physical and mental decline.*

(n)   *I worry about getting old.*
(o)   *Getting old is depressing.*
(p)   *How well a person ages is largely determined by their genes.*
(q)   *Old people can continue to enjoy as many opportunities and experiences as young people.*
(r)   *Old people manage stress better than young people.*
(s)   *Old age brings many freedoms.*
(t)   *Old age brings wisdom and insight.*
(u)   *Old people can be just as happy or happier than young people.*
(v)   *Old people are able to learn new skills and become highly proficient at them.*
(w)   *Life continues to be interesting and I continue to grow as a person.*
(x)   *Our daily habits and life choices play a big role in how we age.*
(y)   *I plan to age well.*

Dr Mills had my scores in front of her when I walked into her office. 'You have an extremely positive attitude towards ageing,' she remarked. 'Where do you think that comes from?'

'Being raised by my sprightly maternal grandmother who lived to the age of 92,' I remembered with great fondness. 'She was a wonderful role model.'

'Yes, having active and involved grandparents has a strong influence on our perceptions of ageing,' she concurred.

'Research on ageing also corroborates that we have the potential to remain sharp, active and healthy until our last breath. It takes a pro-active lifestyle but not a gargantuan effort.'

'Please elaborate,' she prompted as she peered over her glasses.

'Of course, our genes and life circumstances play a role but **old age per se does not cause our bodies to malfunction.** Accumulated damage to our brain and body from environmental or self-inflicted insults is the culprit. I see plenty of 80-year-old patients who are fitter and stronger than some of my 18-year-old patients because the 80-year-olds do regular exercise, have a rich social life, spend time in nature and eat home-cooked meals. In contrast, the 18-year-olds do little exercise, spend all their time indoors, live on fast food and don't really feel connected to any of their so-called friends on social media. I'm describing two extremes but you get the picture. One of my pet-hates is the term "anti-ageing". Why should we be anti-ageing? It sends the message that ageing is a bad thing. It's absurd to view ageing as bad when ageing is unavoidable. Ageing can lead to increasing fulfilment. I'm emphatically pro-ageing because the alternative is dying young. Smoking is avoidable. Junk food is avoidable. Excessive alcohol consumption is avoidable. Ageing is not avoidable unless you jump off a cliff at whatever age you believe that ageing starts. So instead of trying to escape the inescapable, I want to celebrate ageing. **We have to stop blaming our age for our limitations.'**

'Likewise, we have to stop blaming our genes for our limitations,' Dr Mills responded, 'which brings us to the point of the questionnaire. **How we think about ageing affects how we age.** Carriers of the APOE4 gene who have a positive view of ageing — that is to say, they largely disagree with the first 16 statements and agree with the last nine statements — do NOT develop Alzheimer's at a higher rate than non-carriers of the gene. In other words, **an optimistic view of ageing cancels out the negative effects of the APOE4 gene.'**

'That's remarkable!' I gasped.

'It gets better,' she continued, 'or worse, depending on your outlook. A study by Yale University and the US National Institute on Aging (NIA) found that people with longstanding beliefs that ageing was associated with physical and mental decline had three times the rate of shrinkage in their hippocampus — the brain's memory centre — compared with people who felt that ageing can bring fulfilment and joy. **Your brain shrinks three times faster if you feel pessimistic about getting old.** The same study also found that people who felt negatively about ageing had more toxic amyloid beta (Aβ) and tau tangles in their brain than those with positive attitudes. If we believe we're becoming frail, the world appears more daunting, we become more cautious and we start doing less. Lower engagement with life is a prime risk factor for Alzheimer's and, before we know it, we've created a self-fulfilling prophecy. Our beliefs provide our brain with a blueprint for how to operate and how to evolve with the passage of time.

'In 1968, researchers gave 386 healthy men and women with an average age of 36 a questionnaire similar to the one you just completed. Thirty-eight years later, 70% of the people who strongly agreed with the negative statements had suffered a heart attack, stroke or some other serious cardiovascular disease compared with only 15% of the people who didn't believe that things went downhill as they aged. This was after ruling out the effects of smoking, family history, obesity and other known risk factors for heart disease. If there was a drug that reduced heart disease by 55% — from 70% to 15% — we'd all be taking it! **Stamping out age-related negative stereotypes is the most powerful thing we can do to boost our health,** wellbeing and longevity.'

'How can people go about changing their beliefs when our culture is steeped in ageist propaganda?'

'We need to offer myth-busting education programs, positive role models and empowering personal experiences to the public,' Dr Mills replied confidently. 'In a simple experiment, participants aged between 61 and 99 played a computer game while positive age-related words — such as wise, experienced, insightful, sage — were flashed rapidly across the screen. It was too fast for them to be consciously aware of what they'd read but their brain registered the words nonetheless. After only four sessions, their physical wellbeing, mobility and perceptions of ageing all significantly improved — even more so than was seen in a comparable group of participants who'd been attending a six-month exercise program without any attempts to change their attitude. Of course, we can't flash subliminal suggestions across everyone's computer screens but the point of the experiment was proof of concept. We CAN improve our attitude, which in turn improves our health. Senior citizen education programs that counter misconceptions about ageing and present a more positive perspective lead to immediate improvements in tests of memory and thinking skills. Even more effective are programs that combine education with physical exercise. A group of seniors were taught that becoming sedentary was not an inevitable part of ageing and were shown how to challenge their limiting assumptions about getting old. They were essentially trained to use cognitive behaviour therapy (CBT) to nip their own ageist attitudes in the bud. They were also invited to participate in a physical exercise program that demonstrated they were capable of more than they realised. The result was not only a boost to their health and fitness but an overall increase in their daily activities and life satisfaction. We're a highly suggestible species. Health professionals could learn a lot from the advertising industry.

'Greater exposure to successful agers such as actors Judi Dench and acrobatic salsa dancer Paddy Jones — both in their mid-80s and both still acting and dancing respectively — also raises awareness about what's possible as we age. Another strategy to reduce ageism is facilitating intergenerational friendships. The old become more animated and the young learn that ageing can be fun. **The first step to ageing better is to feel better about ageing.'**

Pausing for breath, Dr Mills turned her computer screen towards me to reveal the title of a research paper published in the medical journal *PLOS One*, Negative Perceptions of Aging and Decline in Walking Speed: A Self-fulfilling Prophecy.

'Have you heard of the TUG Test?' she asked.

'Yes — the Timed Up and Go Test. It's a reliable test of balance, co-ordination and overall physical functioning. A person starts off seated in a chair and is asked to stand up, walk three metres, turn around, walk back and sit down again as quickly as possible. The average adult under 80 years of age with no illness or injuries takes less than 8 seconds. Healthy 80-plus-year-olds take up to 13 seconds. If a person needs longer than 14 seconds, it indicates a high risk of falls.'

'Precisely,' Dr Mills concurred. 'The TUG Test is also used to track people's health over time. Injuries aside, if an older person's walking speed declines over a two-year period, they have a 90% increased risk of dying compared with someone whose speed remains the same. They are also more likely to be hospitalised in the near future. This is because slowed walking reflects muscle wasting, increased inflammation or chronic disease, all of which hasten progression to Alzheimer's or death. The researchers in this paper,' she tapped her screen, 'found that older people with negative perceptions of ageing (that is, they largely agreed with the first 16 questionnaire statements) walked more slowly and declined more rapidly over a two-year period than people with optimistic perceptions of ageing. Apart from optimism being associated with managing stress more effectively, people who feel they have greater control over their health engage in more health-promoting behaviours, thus creating a self-fulfilling prophecy.

'The point I try to get across to all my patients,' she continued, 'is that if you believe a particular gene will seal your fate, it's more likely that it will. You'll unconsciously live in a way that turns your belief into reality. On the other hand, if you recognise that you can do something to influence the expression of your genes, you'll play a significant role in whether or not you develop a wide range of diseases including Alzheimer's. Some genes appear to be immutable but the majority, like APOE, are not. Most genes have on–off switches or at least dimmer switches that are influenced by how we live. **Our genes are impacted by what we eat, how much we exercise, the quality of our sleep, how we manage stress, the toxins we're exposed to and what we believe.** These are all becoming huge areas of research. Epigenetics is the study of gene modifications caused by environmental and lifestyle factors, while nutrigenomics looks specifically at the interaction between food and our genes. **Sugar has a particularly destructive effect on genes in our hippocampus** — the brain's learning and memory centre. Chemicals in broccoli, on the other hand, can turn on anti-cancer genes. Together with our genes, we co-create our destiny, whether we realise it or not. Live as though your choices and daily habits make a difference, because they do.'

'Do you offer specific dietary advice or particular forms of brain training for people with and without the APOE4 gene?'

'No. I encourage everyone to live in the healthiest way they possibly can. To date, the research on APOE4 carriers is too ambiguous and conflicting to allow us to draw many practical conclusions. All I can say is that **APOE4 carriers are less able to get away with smoking, being sedentary and sustaining a head injury.** Put another way, having an E4 gene makes smoking, sedentary living and head injuries all the worse for your brain. On the other hand, E4 carriers who exercise are able to prevent cognitive decline and improve their memory. Several studies have also found that **E4 carriers who consume any amount of alcohol — even as little as a few drinks a month — increase their risk of Alzheimer's.** The more they drink, the worse their memory and ability to learn. Meanwhile, non-E4 carriers can enjoy a few drinks a week with no apparent harm — but no more than one standard drink a day and preferably not every day. For some people, this motivates them to live better; for others, it causes resentment. Which brings me back to the point of this visit. How would you live differently if you discovered that you had an APOE4 gene?'

'After thinking it through, I realise that I wouldn't live any differently. I'm already a teetotaller so I wouldn't have to change anything in relation to drinking alcohol. Everything that improves brain health makes for a more fulfilling and joyful life so why wouldn't I strive for greater life fulfilment and more joy regardless of my gene status?'

'Why not indeed,' she smiled. 'One more recommendation for APOE4 carriers is to visit the website apoe4.info. It was created by people who carry the APOE4 allele and is dedicated to providing the most up-to-date information and support for fellow carriers. You can simply read the content or join a conversation. Apoe4.info is a caring, thoughtful and well-informed community that encourages questions and contributions from members and aims to inspire everyone to live in the healthiest possible way.'

'Thank you, I'll check them out … Dr Mills, would you yourself want to know if you had the APOE4 gene?' I wasn't sure if she'd be willing to give me an answer.

'Yes, I would,' she didn't hesitate.

'Why?'

'So that as soon as scientists discover something uniquely helpful for APOE4 carriers, I'll be ready to start doing it, eating it or taking it immediately. In the meantime, I know I can reduce my risk of Alzheimer's through an optimistic attitude, regular exercise, a whole food diet and ongoing mental stimulation.'

Before leaving, I made a final appointment to see Dr Mills to discuss my results. The next morning I went to have the blood test.

* * * * *

Fast forward three years. Researchers from Baylor College of Medicine in Houston, USA completed a study on over 300 APOE4 carriers who remained cognitively healthy and free of dementia despite their increased genetic risk of developing Alzheimer's. What was their secret? Physical exercise? A strong sense of meaning and purpose? A sugar-free diet? Zero alcohol consumption? All these things play a role. In addition, extensive genetic analyses uncovered 68 genes with protective effects against Alzheimer's. If an APOE4 carrier had a subset of these 68 genes (they didn't need to have all of them), they did not get Alzheimer's.

The same researchers also studied APOE2 carriers who — despite their *reduced* genetic risk of Alzheimer's — developed the disease. Examining the genes of these people revealed 148 previously unknown pro-Alzheimer's genes that overrode the protection conferred by the APOE2 gene. If an APOE2 carrier had a big enough dose of the 148 harmful genes, they lost the protection conferred by the E2 variant.

I could imagine Dr Mills nodding her head and saying, 'I told you that APOE is only part of the picture. There are many more genes involved in the development of Alzheimer's. Some are damaging, while others are beneficial. We simply haven't found them all yet.'

But we're getting there. In February 2021, a worldwide collaborative effort by 354 Alzheimer's geneticists identified 42 new gene regions that also contribute to developing Alzheimer's. The importance of these findings are manifold. Firstly, when we elucidate the functions of these genes we come closer to understanding the cause of Alzheimer's. When we know the cause, we are better able to find a cure. Secondly, knowledge of these genes could be used to calculate a genetic risk score that predicts a person's likelihood of developing Alzheimer's far better than having the APOE test alone. And different combinations of genes could mean different treatments for different people.

The more we discover about Alzheimer's, the more we realise it is multifactorial and individual. A person can acquire the disease through various pathways. What applies to one person may not apply to others. By the time this book is published, more genes and more causal factors may come to light.

Science is an ongoing process yielding ever-evolving answers. That's the nature of it. While it might be frustrating that health advice seems to be constantly changing, it actually means that science is doing what it was designed to do: continually adding to our understanding of ourselves and the world around us. As such, we need to be open to regularly updating our beliefs and our approach to healing. As new research comes to hand, I'll make it available at outwittingalzheimers.com.

I encourage you to sign up on the website for my free **Health-e-Bytes** (pronounced Healthy Bites) so you can have the information delivered to your inbox.

CHAPTER 14

Do you want cheese with your whine?

Two things define you. Your gratitude when you have nothing and your attitude when you have everything.

Author unknown

'I'll take your suitcase to the car,' Dad offered.

'Thanks, I really appreciate your help,' I replied as I tied my shoelaces.

I was about to drive to the Hunter Valley, 160 km north of Sydney, where I was speaking at a conference the following morning. Given the unremitting traffic, it could take up to three hours to get there. I was looking forward to catching up on podcasts as I made my way through sprawling vineyards and lush green fields to one of Australia's oldest wine-making regions.

I had prepared and labelled all of Dad's meals and left detailed instructions about what to eat, when to eat and how to heat up the food. Felix (my partner) would be visiting him during my 24-hour absence so I had no concerns about Dad's safety and wellbeing. The morning after my return, Dad and I were going on a week-long Probus excursion (more about this in the next chapter) so I'd also packed Dad's suitcase in preparation for the trip. The last thing I'd feel like doing when I got home was another stint in packing.

I arrived at the hotel without incident and went to retrieve my suitcase from the boot (trunk) of my car. I froze. *Surely not. No. It couldn't be. It had to be a bad dream. A very bad dream.*

The suitcase in my boot was not my suitcase. It was very similar to my suitcase but it wasn't mine. It was Dad's. I hadn't thought to check after he'd put the bag in my car. It had never occurred to me that he might take out the wrong piece of luggage.

I peered into the backseat in case he'd taken *both* suitcases to my car. I knew full well this hadn't happened, but I checked anyway. The backseat was bare. I wanted to burst into tears. I left Dad's suitcase in the car and went to check into my room. It was 9.45 pm.

'Would you like me to bring in your luggage?' asked one of the bubbly hotel staff.

'No, thank you.' I forced a smile.

On the way to my hotel room, I noticed a flyer about the local Chinese gardens. The caption under the photo was a proverb: *It is better to light a candle than to curse the darkness.* It was exactly what I needed to hear.

As soon as I was in my room, I made a list of what I was missing. The situation wasn't as dire as I'd first imagined. My phone, Mac, presentation props, toothbrush and lipstick were all in my bottomless handbag. I could sleep in the T-shirt I was wearing. I could wash my underwear in the shower and dry it with the hairdryer. But I had no clothes to wear to the conference. Tracksuit pants, crumpled T-shirt and sneakers would not qualify as business attire.

I was speaking at 11 am. Sound check was during the morning tea break at 10.30 am. If I could find a nearby ladies' boutique I might just manage to deck myself out in appropriate garb and get back in time to glide onto the stage.

I googled 'nearby clothes shop'. The local area was not exactly a shopper's Mecca (unless you were after a Semillon or Shiraz) and my only hope was Hunter Valley Gardens Shopping Village, less than 7 km away. I scrolled through the stores in anticipation. Christmas Shop, Toy Chest, Exclusive Diamond Company, Australian Alpaca Barn. Just what I needed: *Soft, lightweight and warm, Alpaca has air pockets along the shaft of the fibre, making it not only insulating but breathable. It is also guaranteed not to itch.*

Maybe next time.

I continued my search. Finally, a ladies' fashion store. I browsed their catalogue. Kaftans, jumpsuits, knits, sarongs, strapless minidresses, flowing florals and pretty polka dots. Not quite what I was after. A second women's clothing store popped up on my screen. This one had promise. Did they also sell shoes? Yes! It opened at 9 am. I'd make sure I was there at 8.45 am. I fell into a fitful sleep.

I didn't enjoy shopping at the best of times; this was the worst of times. However, I managed to buy what I needed, did some box breathing and arrived to meet the conference organiser five minutes before the sound check.

A decade later, I'm still wearing that outfit.

CHAPTER 15

Who gives a dam?

Courage is not the absence of fear, but rather the assessment that something else is more important than fear.

FRANKLIN D ROOSEVELT (1882–1945)

Probus is an association of retired and semi-retired men and women who meet on a regular basis to foster fun, friendship and stimulating social connections. They have monthly guest speakers (such as myself) and engage in activities that promote a healthy mind, active body and positive outlook. There are more than 4000 clubs worldwide. The atmosphere at their meetings is always buoyant and welcoming. Signing up Dad to be a member was a no-brainer.

Every year his local club organised a weeklong bus trip. Every year I'd seat Dad on the bus next to Irene and then drive ahead and meet them at their designated motel. Irene was Dad's companion while they were out during the day. I was Dad's anchor when they settled down at night. Dad needed me to oversee his medications and make sure he was showered, dressed and ready for action in the morning.

Our 2012 destination was Dartmouth in north-eastern Victoria — 633 km away. Population 45. Yes, forty-five. There was one motel and one pub. There had also better be a damn good reason for visiting. Of course there was: a great big dam. I braced myself for the seven-hour drive.

Shortly before reaching Albury, I noticed that I wouldn't have enough fuel for the last 100 km to Dartmouth. The situation wasn't urgent but I began scanning the road for service stations. There had been plenty all along the Hume Highway for the last 400 km, so I knew there was no need for concern.

From that point onwards, all petrol stations seemed to have been obliterated from the face of the earth. There was no shortage of fast-food outlets and factories but no hint of fuel. Before I knew it, I had bypassed the towns of Albury and Wodonga and was no longer on a main road. Should I turn back and drive to the centre of Wodonga or continue to the next town? Not wanting to keep Dad waiting, I kept going. It soon became apparent that I was driving through uninhabited countryside. There were no buildings and no mobile-phone coverage. My fuel gauge indicated empty and my stomach was churning. Never in my life had I run out of petrol and never in my life had it been more critical that I didn't run out of petrol. Without taking my foot off the accelerator, I studied the tourist map I'd unfolded on the passenger seat. I heaved a sigh of relief. The next town was Tallangatta and it was marked as having a petrol station. Soon I arrived at a fork in the road. The left fork would take me to Tallangatta, 20 km away. The right fork led to Dartmouth, 70 km away. Did I have enough fuel to reach Tallangatta? I had no choice but to try. There were no petrol stations in Dartmouth and, even if there were, I had no hope of reaching Dartmouth before I ran out.

Despite the nip in the evening air, I was perspiring profusely. I wasn't worried for myself but I knew my father would be distraught. I had no way of contacting him and I hadn't seen another car for a long time. It was 5.45 pm on Sunday evening.

I decided it was a good time to play a meditation CD. So what if I had to spend the night in my car in the middle of nowhere? So what if I had to walk 20 km to the nearest petrol station and lug the petrol back to my car? I might even get lucky and hitch a ride with another motorist, should one ever appear. All this I could cope with. It was my father's inevitable distress that concerned me.

I continued box breathing[4] while cursing myself for my stupidity. How could I have let this happen? Hello? Suddenly, there it was: the welcome sign to Tallangatta! I let out another huge sigh of

---

[4] See Chapter 11 'In search of keys' for an explanation of box breathing.

gratitude and scanned my surroundings for the promised fuel. I spotted the Caltex station on the right-hand side of the road and felt my car roll to a standstill just as it pulled up beside the fuel dispenser. I'd made it.

There was just one small problem. The place looked like a ghost town. The streets were lined with well-kept houses but there were no signs of life. And the petrol station was closed. This was eight years before anyone had ever heard of COVID-19, so the town was not in lockdown. But it might as well have been.

I got out of my car and squinted through the window above the counter. I could not see anyone inside. I tapped on the glass. No answer. I walked around the building. Nothing. I looked up and down the length of the deserted street. Darkness was fast encroaching. Just over a block away, a lone light spilled onto the pavement from a nondescript building. I walked towards it and arrived at a takeaway food store. It was open and there were half a dozen people inside. Progress.

I approached the fair-haired genial woman behind the counter. 'Hello, I'm wondering if you can help me …' I began.

'Sure can. You're out of petrol, right? The motel is around the corner,' she waved towards the back of the shop.

'Thank you, but I can't stay here. I have to reach Dartmouth tonight.'

'Good luck,' she exchanged a knowing look with a kindly-looking woman eating at the counter.

'Do you know who owns the petrol station?' I asked hopefully.

'Yes, I do. That's why I said good luck.'

'Oh, I see.' I didn't see. 'Do you know how I could contact them?' My optimism was beginning to wane.

She took me to the door of the shop and pointed to an elevated weatherboard house across the road. 'See that grey roof? That's Ray's house. He owns the Caltex. But I don't know if he's home and I don't know if he'd come out to give you petrol even if he was home. It's Sunday night, after all.'

I ran across the road and unlatched the vine-choked iron gate. The crunch of dry leaves under my feet betrayed my approach. A faint light outlined the front door. I could hear the TV. I gave the glass panel my friendliest knock. The volume of the broadcast became fainter but no one came to the door. I knocked again. I heard shuffling, then a brief pause before the door hesitantly opened. A chain meant that only one eye could peer out through the narrow gap.

'Hello, are you Ray?'

'Yes.'

'I'm sorry to disturb you on a Sunday evening but do you own the petrol station?'

'Yes, and it's closed.'

'I know it's a terrible inconvenience ...'

'Yes, it is.'

'But would it be possible ...'

'No, it wouldn't be possible. Good night,' he cut me off before shutting the door with a clunk.

No, it was definitely not a good night. I trudged back to my car. I gazed at the sky as though the solution might be encrypted in the stars. They were certainly more prominent than in the suburbs. The ghost of an idea emerged. I took out a copy of my book *In Search of My Father — Dementia is no match for a daughter's determination* and walked back to Ray's house. I never leave home without a stash of books. You never know who might want one.

I took a deep breath and knocked on Ray's door for the third time. I wasn't confident he'd open it again. This time the volume of the TV remained unchanged. Heavy footsteps advanced towards me. The same eye aligned itself in the gap. I didn't wait for his reprimand and there was no punctuation in my monologue.

'Ray, I completely understand why you'd be annoyed with me. I would never normally trouble a stranger on a Sunday evening but my father has dementia and he's waiting for me in Dartmouth and he'll be absolutely beside himself if I don't turn up and I'm unable to contact him and he won't know where his medications are and he's in danger of wandering out and getting lost and his agitation could trigger a heart attack and he'll be inconsolable even if he survives the heart attack and here's a book I've written to prove I'm telling you the truth.' I pushed the book through the gap in the door frame and heard it land on the floor with a thud. The door snapped shut.

I waited. The moon was slowly becoming engulfed by clouds. I was about to drag myself away, utterly crestfallen, when I heard the chain on the door slide open.

'My mother had dementia,' Ray's voice was nostalgic. 'The long goodbye — isn't that what they call it? You lose them twice. Once when they slip away mentally and then again when they slip away physically. Wait at the gate and I'll drive us both to the petrol station.'

'Oh, thank you!!'

Ray filled my tank while chatting about a book he'd started writing himself. 'It's a historical book. I want to tell the story of how this town was relocated from the other side of the river in the 1950s. Everything was moved eight kilometres to the west.'

'Why?'

'Power and water. The authorities decided to increase the capacity of Hume Dam. By 1961 the dam could hold more than six times the amount of water in Sydney Harbour.'

'How amazing.'

'Then in 2007, the water level of Hume Dam dropped to 1% and you could see a clear line where the original streets had run through the valley. Of course, the buildings had rotted and washed away after 50 years under water. There you go,' he closed my petrol cap, 'you'll get to your dad within the hour.'

When I arrived at Dartmouth Motor Inn, I could feel why the region was described as alpine. The bracing air smacked my cheeks the minute I stepped out of the car. All the action seemed to be happening in the heritage-listed tavern across the road, so I made my way towards the buzz. As soon as I burst through the dining room door, Irene spotted me. Her face lit up as she tapped Dad's shoulder and called out, 'She's here!' Everyone in the pub stood up and cheered.

CHAPTER 16

What's happening to the brain?

It is in vain to speak of cures, or think of remedies, until such time as we have considered of the causes.

ROBERT BURTON (1577–1640)

NOTE TO READER — This chapter deals with a very complex topic: what are the underlying causes of Alzheimer's? If you have never studied biology, you might feel overwhelmed by the unfamiliar terminology and intricate concepts despite my attempts to simplify things as much as possible. Do the best you can and revisit this chapter as you progress through the book. It doesn't get any harder than this.

Over the ensuing year, Jasmin and I met once a month to discuss all things Alzheimer's. I enjoyed her cannonade of questions.

'I understand the jigsaw puzzle analogy,' she began one afternoon. 'Many different things impact brain function — sleep, stress, diet, physical exercise and so on. But what is actually going on inside the brain of a person with Alzheimer's? What is causing the symptoms? Is it a case of losing brain cells? Or does the person still have all their brain cells but they're not functioning properly?'

'Both ... In Alzheimer's, communication between brain cells (neurons) is impaired and cells are dying off. Firstly, neurons cease to function properly, then their connections with other neurons disintegrate and subsequently the cells die. As a result, the brain starts to shrink. This is referred to as brain atrophy and it can be seen on CT and MRI scans. This is why Alzheimer's is described as a neurodegenerative disease — brain cells are degenerating.'

'What causes brain cells to malfunction in the first place?' Jasmin pursued.

'That's a very complicated and hotly debated subject. Even in the 21st century we don't have straightforward answers. Several interrelated processes are taking place. One contributing factor is reduced blood flow to the brain due to decades of high blood pressure, hardening of the arteries (arteriosclerosis) or a weakened heart. Hence, you'll often hear the phrase "what's good for the heart is good for the brain". When blood flow to the brain is compromised, the brain does not get its fair share of oxygen and therefore can't generate enough energy to carry out its tasks. This is known as the Vascular Hypothesis of Alzheimer's.

'Another thing that can happen is the brain becomes less capable of using glucose for fuel. This is referred to as impaired brain glucose metabolism or cerebral glucose hypo-metabolism. Glucose is one of the basic building blocks of all the carbohydrates we eat, i.e. fruit, vegetables and grains. After eating carbohydrates, blood glucose levels rise and the hormone insulin allows glucose to enter the cells of our brain and body to be used as fuel. Unfortunately, in some people, cells in specific regions of their brain lose the ability to take in glucose and to metabolise it for energy. This impairment starts to happen decades before the onset of Alzheimer's symptoms and gets progressively worse. This suggests that the brain can continue to operate on less fuel for many years but eventually it can no longer function properly.'

'If there are no early symptoms of a reduction in brain glucose utilisation, how do we know it's happening?' Jasmin asked.

'The rate at which the brain uses glucose is described as the cerebral metabolic rate of glucose consumption, abbreviated as CMRglc. It can be measured by a special type of scan called an FDG-PET. PET scans are very expensive so they're mainly used for research or specific diagnostic purposes. Personally, I'd be very interested in having a peek inside my brain to check if it's using glucose properly.'

The Vascular Hypothesis of Alzheimer's

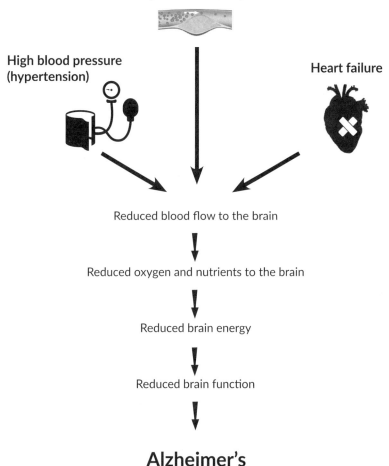

Hardening of the arteries
(arteriosclerosis)

High blood pressure
(hypertension)

Heart failure

Reduced blood flow to the brain

Reduced oxygen and nutrients to the brain

Reduced brain energy

Reduced brain function

Alzheimer's

Jasmin hesitated before countering, 'I was taught that Alzheimer's is due to the accumulation of amyloid beta (Aβ) plaques.'[5]

'Tell me what you've been taught about Aβ plaques,' I encouraged.

'Amyloid beta plaques are the hallmark of Alzheimer's because they're found in the brains of people with Alzheimer's. The plaques are made of clumps of related proteins. The proteins are collectively called amyloid beta hence the designation amyloid beta plaques. This is actually a misnomer. Amyloid derives from the Latin word *amylum* meaning "starch" and the Greek suffix *oid* meaning "like". The scientist Rudolf Virchow, who first saw amyloids under the microscope, mistakenly thought they were a type of carbohydrate so he named them "resembling starch". Now we know it's a stack of proteins. The more Aβ plaques scattered throughout a person's brain, the worse their symptoms.'

'You know your history,' I was impressed. 'What you've described is the Amyloid Hypothesis of Alzheimer's but **it doesn't always follow that more Aβ plaques equate to worse symptoms.**'

'Why not?'

'Amyloid beta plaques are a feature of Alzheimer's and in some people, the more plaques, the worse the dementia. However, there are people who lived to old age with all their mental faculties intact but when their brains were examined at autopsy, they were riddled with Aβ plaques. Yet they had no symptoms of Alzheimer's. Conversely, we've seen people with scant Aβ plaques in their brains who nonetheless had severe symptoms. So Aβ plaques are part of the story but not the whole story.

'Some scientists believe that it isn't Aβ plaques but rather, subtypes of Aβ proteins called Aβ oligomers (AβOs) that are toxic to neurons. AβOs are made during an intermediate step on the path to plaque formation. Meanwhile, a third group of scientists argue that Aβ proteins are in fact necessary for a healthy brain. However, when Aβ proteins undergo a change (they start misfolding) and begin to form plaques, it's the loss of functional Aβ proteins — not the

---

[5] Aβ plaques are also known as senile plaques or neuritic plaques.

accumulation of plaques — that most closely reflects cognitive impairment and symptoms of Alzheimer's.

'Therefore, even among scientists who subscribe to the Amyloid Hypothesis, there are conflicting ideas about how to cure Alzheimer's:
1. we have to rid the brain of Aβ plaques
2. we have to remove AβOs
3. we have to replenish functional Aβ proteins.'

'Regardless of whether we need to get rid of the Aβ plaques and oligomers or replenish the functional Aβ proteins, what causes things to go wrong with Aβ proteins in the first place?' Jasmin's curiosity was refreshing.

'When our brain is exposed to injury, infections, toxins, inflammation or glucose hypo-metabolism, it produces soluble Aβ proteins. One of the jobs of Aβ is to fight infections, clear away toxins and trigger damaged cells to self-destruct. This self-destruction or cell suicide is known as apoptosis.'

'Let me guess the origin of the word "apoptosis",' Jasmin jumped in. 'The Greek word *apo* means "from" or "away" and *ptosis* relates to "falling". So apoptosis suggests that cells are "falling away".'

'Spot on,' I smiled. 'Apoptosis is usually a natural self-protective mechanism because you don't want sick cells hanging around in your brain. But if your brain is exposed to repeated damage, it is constantly producing Aβ proteins. Eventually there are so many Aβ proteins floating around, they start misfolding and sticking together to form AβOs and plaques. The AβOs and plaques now surround healthy cells as well as sick cells and this can have many untoward consequences. Firstly, AβOs and plaques can interfere with the ability of cells to communicate with one another (known as synaptic dysfunction); secondly, plaques may start triggering healthy cells to self-destruct. So Aβ proteins begin by protecting the brain but, after a while, things get out of control.'

The Amyloid Hypothesis of Alzheimer's

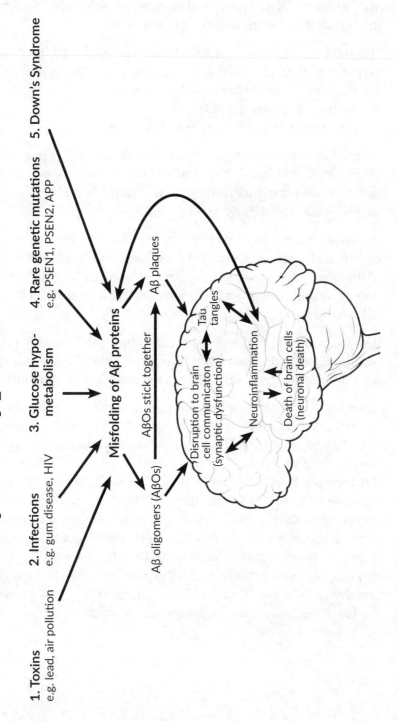

1. Toxins
e.g. lead, air pollution

2. Infections
e.g. gum disease, HIV

3. Glucose hypo-
metabolism

4. Rare genetic mutations
e.g. PSEN1, PSEN2, APP

5. Down's Syndrome

Misfolding of Aβ proteins

AβOs stick together

Aβ plaques

Aβ oligomers (AβOs)

Tau
tangles

Disruption to brain
cell communicaton
(synaptic dysfunction)

Neuroinflammation

Death of brain cells
(neuronal death)

Jasmin deliberated before responding. 'That explains why drugs that remove Aβ plaques from the brain don't alleviate the symptoms of Alzheimer's. Destroying Aβ doesn't address the root cause of the problem. We need to stop the injury, infection or inflammation that is producing Aβ in the first place.'

'Exactly,' I agreed. 'Hundreds of drug trials targeting Aβ plaques and AβOs have failed to improve any of the symptoms of Alzheimer's. Some scientists believe it's because the anti-amyloid drugs were given too late in the disease. They argue that if we can identify people who are starting to accumulate Aβ plaques but don't yet have symptoms, the medications might help.'

'Are you of that opinion?'

'No. I think the evidence points to Aβ proteins being the brain's way of responding to an insult or clearing out dysfunctional cells. Therefore, we need to discover the origin of the insult. I think glucose hypo-metabolism is one of the earliest signs of a brain in trouble but it also begs the question: why do brain cells lose their ability to use glucose for fuel?'

Jasmin suddenly had a light bulb moment. 'Problems with glucose in other parts of the body are associated with insulin resistance and type 2 diabetes. Even though most brain cells don't require insulin for glucose to enter, insulin has a number of regulatory roles in the brain. Therefore problems with insulin could lead to problems with cognition,' she proposed.

'Spot on again! It appears that in Alzheimer's, the brain's ability to use insulin has been compromised. That's why Alzheimer's is sometimes referred to as diabetes of the brain or type 3 diabetes. When scientists gave Alzheimer's patients an insulin nasal spray, their cognition temporarily improved. Trials of insulin nasal sprays are ongoing.

The bottom line is that anything that compromises the brain's supply of oxygen or interferes with the functions of insulin is going to hinder glucose metabolism. This also ties back to the Vascular Hypothesis of Alzheimer's: when our heart or blood vessels are not in optimal condition, we get less oxygen delivered to our brain.

'Likewise, type 1 and type 2 diabetes dramatically raise Alzheimer's risk. All these conditions eventually starve the brain of the elements it needs to create energy. Therefore, Alzheimer's prevention starts with keeping our heart healthy and our insulin working properly.'

'What causes things to go wrong with insulin?'

'The exact same things that cause heart problems:
1. **sugar** and **soft drinks**
2. **starches** (refined)
3. **seed oils** (e.g. sunflower, safflower, grape seed, canola, soybean)
4. **sedentary** living
5. **sleep** apnoea and **sleep** deprivation
6. **stress** (severe and chronic)
7. **smoking**.

'If we eliminated those seven things, we'd eliminate more than half of all cases of Alzheimer's — as well as most of the chronic diseases of our modern world. Being healthy isn't complicated. We, as a society, have made it complicated because we don't want to change how we live. If you educate all your patients about the **Seven S's**[6] and support them in making the necessary lifestyle adjustments, you'll be doing more to help people than any medication or high-tech procedure ever will.'

'What about the role of **inflammation**? Isn't inflammation getting the blame for just about everything these days? From arthritis, diabetes and heart disease to depression, anxiety and Alzheimer's?' Jasmin queried.

'Inflammation is the process by which our immune system deals with injury or infection in any part of the body. Immune cells travel to the site of the problem via the bloodstream and then release chemicals to destroy whatever is causing the damage. Immune cells are also responsible for cleaning up the ensuing debris and initiating repair of the tissues that have been affected. If you get a cut on your arm, you can see the process of inflammation taking place. The area becomes red, hot, sore and swollen before gradually healing over. If a person is immunocompromised and not able to mount a strong

---

[6] The Seven S's will be discussed in later chapters.

enough immune response, an infection could continue to spread and kill them. Therefore, acute inflammation is life-saving. In many instances we have antibiotics and antivirals to assist the process but the first step in dealing with infection or injury is inflammation.'

Jasmin nodded for me to continue.

'However, if the insult is ongoing or the immune system doesn't turn itself off when it's no longer needed, we get chronic inflammation. The consequences of chronic inflammation vary depending on the tissues involved. If it's happening in the walls of a coronary artery, it puts us at risk of atherosclerotic heart disease. If it's happening in a joint, we get rheumatoid arthritis. Therefore, it's true that inflammation is a component of many chronic diseases but it isn't the root cause. Once again, the Seven S's all drive chronic inflammation through various biochemical pathways.'

'How does chronic inflammation play out in the brain?'

'That requires a brief explanation of the two main types of cells found in the brain: neurons and glia. Neurons are responsible for the brain's functionality. Neurons have short branches called dendrites and long tails called axons. Neurons actually look like a human hand. Your fingers represent dendrites, your palm is the cell body, and your arm is like the axon. Dendrites receive information — in the form of chemical messengers called neurotransmitters — from other neurons. Axons transmit electrical signals along their length. When the electrical impulse reaches the end of the axon, it opens channels that allow neurotransmitters to exit into the space between neurons. The junction between neurons is called a synapse. When you see pictures of neurons, it looks as though the axon of one cell touches the dendrites of adjacent cells but that's not the case. The cells are separated by a minuscule space called a synaptic cleft. The neurotransmitter floats across the synaptic cleft to enter the dendrites of the apposing neuron. This is how neurons communicate with each other and produce all the complex functions we attribute to a healthy brain. These are the main cells that get destroyed in Alzheimer's.'

'Got it,' Jasmin affirmed. 'How are glia different from neurons?'

Schematic diagram of a brain cell (neuron)

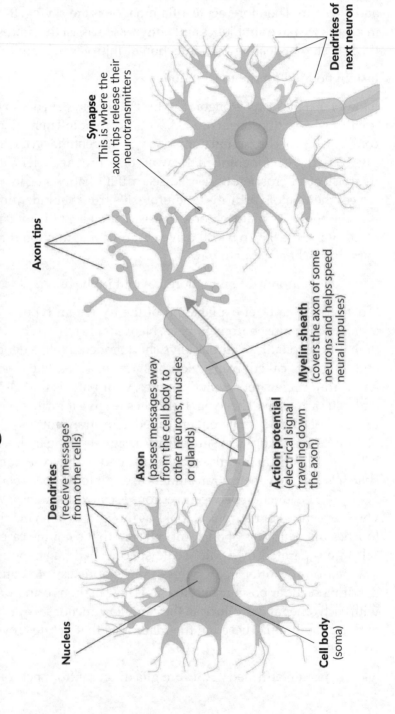

Dendrites of next neuron

Synapse
This is where the axon tips release their neurotransmitters

Axon tips

Myelin sheath
(covers the axon of some neurons and helps speed neural impulses)

Action potential
(electrical signal traveling down the axon)

Axon
(passes messages away from the cell body to other neurons, muscles or glands)

Dendrites
(receive messages from other cells)

Nucleus

Cell body
(soma)

'Glia are also referred to as glial cells or neuroglia. Since you seem to be interested in etymology, the name glia comes from the Greek word for glue because the cells were originally thought to hold the and they do a lot more than simply surround neurons and keep them in place.

'The different glial cells include astrocytes, oligodendrocytes, microglia and ependymocytes. They supply neurons with oxygen and nutrients, destroy pathogens, assist in transmission of information and dispose of dead neurons. Glia also remove toxins, waste products and excess Aβ from the brain.'

'You said earlier that Aβ proteins also remove toxins from the brain.'

'Yes, Aβ proteins and glia — in particular microglia — have overlapping functions. Microglia are the brain's immune cells. They circumnavigate neurons and are on the lookout for anything that might damage them such as toxins, bacteria or viruses. When microglia come into contact with a dangerous entity, they either engulf the hazard or release chemicals to destroy it. You'll recognise that this is the process of inflammation. What we find in some cases of Alzheimer's is that microglia become overactive — referred to as gliosis — and cause chronic inflammation.'

'What causes microglia to become overactive?'

'Cigarette smoking tops the list. NeuroAIDS is another cause. Or it might be that glucose hypo-metabolism or ongoing Aβ plaque formation fuels ongoing microglial activation, which fuels ongoing inflammation. Once again, it's difficult to pinpoint what happens first: hypo-metabolism, Aβ plaques or inflammation? It probably operates in all directions. Hypo-metabolism can trigger both Aβ plaque formation and inflammation just as Aβ plaques and inflammation can compromise the brain's ability to metabolise glucose. It's a self-perpetuating destructive spiral.'

'It certainly is! And what is neuroAIDS?' Jasmin cross-examined.

'Up to 25% of people with HIV develop symptoms of Alzheimer's. The condition is called neuroAIDS. The virus starts by infecting microglia and only later attacks neurons. This has led scientists to postulate whether other viruses or bacteria might also cause microglia to run amok.'

'What other viruses and bacteria?' Jasmin continued delving.

'Suspects include *Herpes simplex virus* (HSV-1) from cold sores and *Borrelia burgdorferi* which causes Lyme disease. Some researchers are also investigating whether mycotoxins made by moulds might provoke microglia to overreact.'

'But two-thirds of the world's population under the age of 50 carry HSV-1! I've had cold sores myself so does that mean I'm doomed?' Jasmin looked worried.

'No,' I dispelled her fears. 'It takes more than a handful of micro-organisms to set off the cascade that leads to Alzheimer's. It's a constant tug-of-war. One thing harms the brain, another thing protects it. We're back to the puzzle pieces. Keep adding protective pieces to minimise the chances of adversarial factors getting the upper hand.'

Jasmin continued probing. 'I've also heard that in addition to Aβ, there's another aberrant protein associated with Alzheimer's. It's called tau. Can you explain what that's about?'

'Yes, tau is an acronym for Tubulin Associated Unit and is found inside the neurons of people with Alzheimer's. In fact, **the presence of tau is more closely related to symptoms than the presence of Aβ plaques.'**

Jasmin interrupted to clarify. 'So you're saying that Aβ plaques build up *outside* neurons and tau builds up *inside* neurons?'

'Yes. In healthy brains, tau proteins help neurons transport molecules from one part of the cell to another via structures called microtubules. In the Alzheimer's brain, tau proteins combine with excessive amounts of phosphorus, which causes them to get tangled. They are then called hyper-phosphorylated tau tangles or neurofibrillary tangles or paired helical filaments. These are just three names for the same mess. This leads to the breakdown of microtubules, which means the neuron is unable to transport neurotransmitters to where they need to go. The result is disruption of activity inside brain cells and loss of communication between cells. Once again, cell death follows.

'Tau tangles also contribute to microglial activation and inflammation. Can you see how one thing leads to another? It's like a domino effect. Doctors have only recently been able to identify tau tangles in living patients by PET scan. In the past, tau tangles were only identified during post-mortem examination. And tau tangles are not only found in Alzheimer's disease — about 20 other brain diseases are associated with tau tangles. They're called tauopathies.'

'Are tau tangles found in everyone who has Alzheimer's or do some people get Alzheimer's without having tau tangles?'

'At this point in time, the consensus is that Alzheimer's involves both Aβ and tau. But most patients never have a PET scan to identify tau tangles so we don't know for certain. For decades, there's been a raging debate in the scientific community about what's more important in the development of Alzheimer's: Aβ or tau. The two camps are so fiercely divided, they've been labelled Baptists and Taoists. The biggest irony is that I think they're both wrong. Neither Aβ nor tau are the inciting event. Amyloid beta and tau are the brain's response to injury, infection, toxins or lack of energy.'

'That's very amusing,' Jasmin laughed. 'I suppose the name Baptist comes from the first three letters of beta amyloid protein?'

'Yes, very good.'

'What are you called if you believe that glucose hypo-metabolism is the first step in developing Alzheimer's?'

'You're designated as a member of the Mitochondrial Mafia!'

'Please explain!' Jasmin exclaimed.

'Mitochondria are referred to as the powerhouses of our cells because they're the site of energy production. They're found in every cell of our body except red blood cells. One of their many roles is to metabolise glucose. In other words, mitochondria convert glucose (from the food we eat) to a chemical called adenosine triphosphate (ATP). ATP is what provides us with energy. Cells that require a lot of energy, like brain, heart and muscle cells, contain thousands of mitochondria. Cells that don't require as much energy, such as skin cells, contain fewer mitochondria. Therefore, if mitochondria within brain cells are not functioning properly, what's the result?'

'Glucose hypo-metabolism!' Jasmin declared triumphantly.

'Correct.'

'Let me get this straight,' Jasmin continued. 'Brain glucose hypo-metabolism can have a number of causes:

1. Insufficient delivery of glucose or oxygen to our brain — because glucose and oxygen are the raw materials required to make energy. Hence the strong link between cardiovascular disease and Alzheimer's.
2. Problems with insulin utilisation — because insulin is an important regulatory protein in the brain. Hence type 2 diabetes more than doubles a person's risk of developing Alzheimer's.
3. Malfunctioning mitochondria — because mitochondria are where energy production takes place.'

'Great overview.'

'I understand that the Seven S's drive the first two factors but what gives rise to mitochondrial dysfunction?' Jasmin was indefatigable.

'I'll give you seven guesses.'

'The Seven S's!' she enthused.

'As I said earlier, being healthy involves a very simple strategy. Start by avoiding soft drinks, sugar, refined starches and seed oils. Include some daily physical exercise, good sleep and effective stress management and your brain and body will be bursting with energy and vitality. It's not necessarily easy, but it's definitely simple. At a later date, we can discuss the mechanisms through which the Seven S's cause so much havoc. Mitochondria can also malfunction because of rare genetic disorders or environmental toxins such as asbestos, industrial chemicals, air pollution and pharmaceuticals, but the Seven S's are by far the biggest culprits.'

'Let me recap everything from the start of our conversation,' Jasmin reflected. 'At least one of five processes is taking place in the brain of a person with Alzheimer's. In some people, all five things could be happening:

1. brain glucose hypo-metabolism leading to insufficient brain energy
2. accumulation of Aβ plaques or AβOs around brain cells
3. tau tangles disrupting brain cell function from inside cells
4. overactive microglia causing chronic inflammation
5. problems with mitochondria.

'Yes,' I confirmed. 'You've given an excellent rundown of the current theories on the underpinnings of Alzheimer's. Two other contributing factors are what's known as oxidative stress and a leaky blood-brain barrier (BBB) but we'll leave those for another conversation.'

'However, these processes are not the cause of Alzheimer's; they're our brain's response to toxins, infections, injury or lack of oxygen and nutrients,' Jasmin summarised.

'Exactly. And some people's brains can withstand more toxins and injury than others. Genes and gut bacteria both play an important role in our capacity to resist insults to our brain. I believe that Alzheimer's will turn out to be more than one disease. Even though symptoms appear to be similar, the underlying brain pathology may differ from one person to the next. Amyloid beta may play a significant role in some people but only a minimal role in others. Or the main problem might be insulin resistance or blood vessel damage. That's another reason why more than 99% of drugs developed to treat Alzheimer's have failed. A one-size-fits-all approach is not going to work because the cause of the disease differs between individuals and drug trials have not taken this into account.'

'So my role as a doctor will be to figure out what sets those damaging processes in motion for each individual patient.' Jasmin straightened her posture as if to rise to the challenge.

'Yes. Working out why someone might have developed Alzheimer's requires a lot of sleuthing. It's rarely due to one thing. It's always a combination of factors: genes, environment and lifestyle. And the mix of causative factors will be different from one person to the next. It's a never-ending detective story because no two patients will have the exact same set of triggers. Head trauma, heavy metals, excessive alcohol, chronic stress, sleep deprivation, poor diet, loneliness, lack of mental stimulation … the list of hazards goes on. Fortunately, so does the list of protective factors: staying socially connected, lifelong learning, volunteer work, dancing, singing, playing music, meditating … It's about balance. We live in a toxic world but our brain and body are equipped with a range of mechanisms to keep us healthy. It's only when our defences are overwhelmed that we get sick. What was the first thing you were taught in medical school?'

'First, do no harm,' Jasmin answered decisively.

'Never forget that. The first step is to avoid all the things we know are harmful to our brain. The second step is to do as many things as possible that stimulate the growth of new brain cells (known as neurogenesis) and strengthen the connections between them (synaptogenesis).'

'Will I find a comprehensive list of dos and don'ts in your book *In Search of My Father — Dementia is no match for a daughter's determination*?' Jasmin asked as she handed me a copy to sign.

'Yes, you will,' I smiled, 'and I expect that dementia is no match for a granddaughter's determination either.'

PART TWO

Obstacles or opportunities?

The most difficult thing is the decision to act. The rest is merely tenacity. The fears are paper tigers. You can do anything you decide to do. You can act to change and control your life; and the procedure, the process, is its own reward.

AMELIA MARY EARHART (1897–1937)

CHAPTER 17

Snore no more

Good decisions come from experience. Experience comes from making bad decisions.

MARK TWAIN (1835–1910)

Over one billion people worldwide suffer from Obstructive Sleep Apnoea (OSA). It occurs in about one in 10 women and one in four men. In Australia and other Western countries, the numbers are even higher. A recent Australian study found that 75% of over 65-year-olds were impacted by sleep apnoea. Our neighbour Jack was one of them. The bad news is that **OSA increases the risk of MCI (mild cognitive impairment) and Alzheimer's**. The good news is that OSA is treatable.

OSA is a condition in which a person stops breathing for up to 60 seconds many times — often hundreds of times[1] — throughout the night as they sleep. When we drift off to sleep, the muscles in our body start to relax. Usually, the muscles around our throat maintain enough tension to keep the airway open. In people with OSA, the muscles relax too much and thereby block air from entering the lungs. Sleeping on our back often makes the problem worse because the tongue can flop back and add to the obstruction. If the blockage is incomplete and allows a small amount of air to get through, it causes the tissues around the throat to vibrate and produce the characteristic sound of snoring. Partial blockage quickly leads to complete blockage and the result is a drop in blood oxygen levels. As soon as the brain senses it is not receiving enough oxygen, it jolts

---

[1] Hundreds of times is not an exaggeration.

the person awake so they start to breathe again. Within seconds, they go back to sleep and the cycle repeats itself. This is described as fragmented sleep. A person with OSA is often unaware that their sleep is disrupted. Their partner is usually ready to suffocate them with a pillow.[2]

Brain tissue analysis has revealed that sleep apnoea generates the same pattern of amyloid beta (Aβ) accumulation as seen in Alzheimer's. In mild sleep apnoea, Aβ plaques and tau tangles are found in outer layers of the brain near the hippocampus — exactly where they first appear in Alzheimer's. The more severe the sleep apnoea, the more Aβ plaques in the hippocampus. Why should this happen? One of the functions of deep slow-wave sleep is to clear the brain of toxins. **Sleep is by far our best form of detox.** Because sleep apnoea interrupts a person's sleep hundreds of times throughout the night, these people may not be reaching the deep stages of sleep needed to clear their brain of Aβ and tau.

Untreated OSA also contributes to obesity, type 2 diabetes, high blood pressure, heart attack, stroke and abnormal heart rhythms such as atrial fibrillation. All these factors further increase the risk of Alzheimer's. One could argue that OSA presents a chicken-and-egg scenario — for instance, obesity can lead to OSA just as OSA can lead to obesity — however, even in the absence of obesity, the more severe the sleep apnoea, the more likely that a person develops heart disease. This is due to OSA causing strain on the heart along with large changes in pressure within the chest.

How do you know if you have OSA? Doctors use two screening tests. Neither of these tests is definitive but they give you an idea of whether you might need a formal sleep study.

1. **The Epworth Sleepiness Scale (ESS)** — this comprises eight questions that assess the severity of daytime sleepiness. A licence is required to use the ESS but anyone can view the questions at: epworthsleepinessscale.com/about-the-ess.

---

[2] OSA can also occur in children, usually due to enlarged tonsils, adenoids or turbinates (bony structures in the nose). In addition to tiredness, sleep disruption can cause learning and behavioural problems. Tonsillectomy cures OSA in 80% to 90% of children.

A score of eight or more (out of 24) warrants a visit to your doctor. Depending on your symptoms and circumstances, a sleep study can be performed in a laboratory or in your own home.

2. **The STOP BANG Questionnaire** — this is a different set of eight questions that focus on biological factors that predispose a person to OSA. STOP BANG is an acronym for:
   (a) Do you **S**nore?
   (b) Do you feel **T**ired during the day?
   (c) Has anyone **O**bserved you gasping or choking in your sleep?
   (d) Do you have high blood **P**ressure?
   (e) Is your **B**MI (Body Mass Index) above 35? BMI = weight (in kg) divided by height (in metres) squared
   (f) Is your **A**ge over 50?
   (g) Is your **N**eck circumference over 40 cm (16 inches)?
   (h) Is your **G**ender male?

You can complete the questionnaire and receive an immediate result at: www.stopbang.ca/osa/screening.php

If you answer yes to three or more STOP BANG questions, I recommend a visit to your doctor for a more comprehensive medical check-up. Men over the age of 50 automatically score at least 2/8, so use your discretion about whether you feel your sleep needs attention.

Not everyone with OSA feels sluggish or inclined to nod off during a meeting but, if you do, your probability of developing cardiovascular disease goes up significantly.

Another disturbing finding is that people with untreated OSA have trouble remembering details of events from their own lives. This is known as impaired semantic autobiographical memory and it can make a person more vulnerable to depression — yet another risk factor for cardiovascular disease and Alzheimer's. Research suggests that **a person with OSA is three times more likely to develop depression** than a person who has consistent good quality sleep. Overall, one in five people with untreated OSA have depression and — like obesity — the relationship is bidirectional. OSA can lead to depression and depression can lead to OSA. Conversely, when people who suffer from both OSA and depression are treated for OSA alone, a third of them find that curing their sleep problems also cures their depression.

Hence OSA is not all doom and gloom. It's a medical story with a happy ending. There are numerous different treatment options, depending on the severity and specific nature of the obstruction.

Mild OSA can often be reversed with lifestyle measures such as:
- adjusting your sleep position
- reducing alcohol intake because alcohol contributes to excessive muscle relaxation
- weaning off sleeping tablets as these also cause excessive muscle relaxation
- shedding excess body fat.

Moderate to severe OSA is usually treated using a:
- CPAP machine (Continuous Positive Airway Pressure) or
- mandibular advancement device — custom-designed upper and lower mouth-guards that are fitted by a dentist and hold the jaw in a way that keeps the airways open.

Both of these treatments are only used at night so your daily life is not impacted. In fact, your daily life will dramatically improve as soon as you start getting regular refreshing sleep. Very rare cases of adult OSA require surgery. The Adelaide Institute for Sleep Health is also trialling a combination of two medications that keep the muscles in the throat active and thereby maintain an open airway.

Jack did not present with the common symptoms of daytime sleepiness, irritability, morning headaches or waking up with a dry mouth. His partner had a hearing impairment so she wasn't aware of him snorting, choking and gasping his way through the night. Instead, Jack was diagnosed with OSA after having two car accidents in the space of two months. In both cases, he'd had a micro-sleep at the wheel. His attitude to the whole thing was remarkable.

'It's the best thing that could have happened to me,' he announced one evening as we were both taking out our garbage bins.

'How so?' I was taken aback.

'It forced me to get my act together. My doctor says the two accidents saved my life in the long run. Luckily no one was hurt but I had to surrender my driver's licence until my OSA was fixed. I was given the option of using a CPAP machine for the rest of my life or, alternatively, losing weight, quitting smoking and cutting back on booze. I don't like anything touching my face so I had to tackle the lifestyle side of the equation. Plus, the money I saved by giving up cigs and alcohol made it a no brainer.'

'You've made a lot of changes in a short space of time.' I was in awe of his positive approach.

'Until now, I wasn't motivated to change because I wasn't in enough pain. Secretly, I was also scared I might be getting Alzheimer's because I was getting brain fog, but I didn't want to admit it to anyone, least of all to myself. My doctor kept giving me the usual reasons to improve my diet and give up my unhealthy habits, but the changes didn't seem worth the effort. I thought that life wouldn't be as enjoyable without a smoko and a drink with the boys. I was very wrong. Some of the boys have even followed suit. It simply took one of us to make the first move. In the past, my motto was "work hard, play hard" and if I died a few years younger, so be it — at least I'll have had a good time on the way to my funeral. The realisation that I could have killed someone was a big wake up call.'

'Unhealthy choices don't just lead to a shorter life, they lead to a more painful life,' I reinforced. 'However, because the aches and pains come on gradually, we don't notice our diminishing quality of life and we erroneously put it down to "simply getting old".'

'I'll never fall into that trap again!' Jack responded triumphantly. 'I can't believe how good I feel and how much better my brain is working. I haven't had this much energy for decades. I can work and play even harder now! I've just come to define "play" somewhat differently. And I don't have to take as many tablets for high blood pressure. My doctor says I might soon be off them altogether. Who'd have thought?'

'Fantastic work! When there is underlying OSA, heart problems are more difficult to treat. There is only so much that medicine can do. The rest is up to you and you certainly did it. Congratulations!'

CHAPTER 18

Blow it off

*Normality is a paved road. It's comfortable to walk
but no flowers grow on it.*

<small>Vincent Van Gogh (1853–1890)</small>

A few years before Dad showed any signs of cognitive decline, Mum started complaining about his snoring. He didn't want a sleep study and he wouldn't hear of going to bed with a CPAP machine. What to do? I diligently set about investigating solutions to snoring and discovered what I thought was a sure-fire winner. I broached the subject with my father.

'Dad, have you ever wanted to play the Didgeridoo?'

'The Didgeridoo?' he echoed in bewilderment.

'Yes — a long cylindrical wind instrument developed by First Nations Australians. It's traditionally a man's instrument — in some regions, women are not even allowed to touch it.'

'I know what a Didgeridoo is,' he replied matter-of-factly. 'What I'm trying to figure out is why you think I'd be interested in learning to play it.'

'Playing the Didgeridoo reduces snoring and daytime sleepiness in people with moderate to severe Obstructive Sleep Apnoea (OSA). I've heard you snoring from down the hallway and you frequently nod off in your armchair.'

'I pretend to fall asleep to stop you and your mother droning on. Oops, now I've blown that tactic,' he grinned mischievously.

'Why are women not allowed to play it?'

'I'm not sure. Different tribes have different laws. I've read that in some regions, it's believed that touching a Didgeridoo could render a woman infertile. Other tribes allow women to play the instrument in informal situations but only allow men to play the Didgeridoo in ceremonies. That's at least my understanding of it.'

'What kind of ceremony do you have in mind for me?' he posed charily.

'A better night's sleep!' I enthused.

'How can blowing into a hollow tree trunk stop a person from snoring?'

'In an experiment known as a randomised controlled trial (RCT), a group of men suffering from OSA were taught to play the Didgeridoo. They learnt specific lip techniques along with circular breathing and practised for 20 minutes a day, five days a week. After four months, their snoring and sleep apnoea improved as much as it did for people using CPAP machines. Playing the Didgeridoo strengthens the muscles of the upper airways and stops them collapsing when a person lies down to sleep. Not surprisingly, people enjoy playing the Didgeridoo a lot more than they enjoy wearing a mask when they sleep.'

'I will definitely NOT be wearing a mask when I sleep!' he declared.

'I know. That's why I'm suggesting a Didgeridoo.' I smiled at him hopefully. 'The Didgeridoo is a vastly under-utilised remedy for not only OSA but also asthma. Didgeridoo-playing doesn't completely cure asthma but it can improve symptoms and respiratory function. Not to mention the fun, satisfaction and cultural education that people derive from it.'

'I'm too busy to learn a musical instrument. Besides, it's the sort of thing a person should learn from a young age.'

'On the contrary. All the men in the OSA trial were over 50 years old. And learning a new instrument is one of the best ways to boost your brain and lower your risk of Alzheimer's.'

'Where are you going to find a Didgeridoo teacher?' he continued, casting about for excuses.

'It just so happens that Sydney Community College is offering Didgeridoo lessons for beginners. Or I could organise a teacher to come to our house and give you private lessons.' I had done my homework before broaching the subject.

'And where do you propose I get a Didgeridoo? There isn't any point in learning an instrument if you don't practise between lessons.'

'There are Didgeridoo-making workshops or I can buy you one for your birthday,' I grinned.

'But you're a woman — you aren't allowed to touch the thing!' he exclaimed triumphantly.

Touché. I put the subject to bed for another day.

CHAPTER 19

Let sleep be your medicine

The interval of a single night of sleep will greatly increase the strength of the memory.

MARCUS FABIUS QUINTILIANUS (CIRCA 35–100 CE)

What did Ronald Reagan and Margaret Thatcher have in common?

They both slept fewer than six hours per night and they both developed Alzheimer's.

Coincidence? Not according to a study published in the journal *Nature Communications* in April 2021. Researchers from London, Paris, Finland and The Netherlands analysed 25 years of data from 7959 men and women. Those who had six hours sleep or less per night in their 50s and 60s were 30% more likely to develop dementia in their 70s than those who slept seven or more hours per night. These people did not have obstructive sleep apnoea (OSA). They simply weren't getting enough sleep to maintain their brain.

Sleep is the most critical determinant of brain health at every age of our lives — newborn, adolescent or adult. Of course, genes, diet, exercise and a host of other lifestyle factors also impact our brain. But nothing trumps the power of sleep. I know a Trump who would disagree. Perhaps he carries one of a handful of genes that enable a person to sleep fewer than seven hours per night. However, these genes are exceedingly rare so I suspect he's just a sleep-deprived mortal like the rest of us.

We are all unique and so is our requirement for sleep. How many hours do you need to function at your best? Only you can answer this question based on your personal experience. At a minimum, you'll need seven hours per night. The range for healthy adults is seven to nine hours, depending on a complex interplay of genes, hormones and lifestyle factors. Women tend to need slightly more sleep than men. Adolescents need closer to nine and half hours per night.

If we don't get enough sleep, we are more prone to depression, anxiety, memory problems, over-eating and poor performance in mentally and physically demanding tasks. Your mother was right — if you want to do well in your exams, get a good night's sleep.

How does chronic lack of sleep lead to Alzheimer's? Once again, the key word is chronic. A few nights of poor sleep won't choke our brain with amyloid beta (Aβ) plaques. But decades of inadequate sleep quite likely will. During the day, our brain accumulates toxic waste products including Aβ. When we fall asleep, the brain switches on its waste removal apparatus called the glymphatic system. The process is ingenious. During sleep, neurons shrink to open up spaces between them. Cerebrospinal fluid (CSF) is then pumped along these spaces to collect waste that has built up between our brain cells. The waste products are, in turn, delivered to the bloodstream via glial cells and promptly flushed out.

A single night of insufficient or disrupted sleep is associated with a 10% increase in brain Aβ levels. As alarming as this is, if we get a good night of uninterrupted sleep the following evening, we can clear the excess Aβ. However, ongoing insufficient sleep leads to lasting increases in both Aβ plaques and tau tangles.

Sleep is also when the brain repairs DNA damage in neurons. Conversely, lack of sleep contributes to brain inflammation. The other mechanism by which insufficient or poor quality sleep leads to Alzheimer's is by driving up heart disease, stroke, high blood pressure, depression, type 2 diabetes and obesity, all of which independently bump up our risk of Alzheimer's. **Seven consecutive days of sleep deprivation push our blood sugar levels into the pre-diabetic range.** Not to mention we then feel too tired and unmotivated to engage in physical exercise and other brain-healthy habits.

To make matters worse, when a person develops Alzheimer's, the disease itself contributes to disrupted sleep and the situation becomes a self-perpetuating negative spiral. As with so many other factors linked to Alzheimer's, poor sleep and dementia have a bidirectional relationship.

Thus, sleep deprivation is the first domino that sets off a cascade of brain-eroding processes. Sleep is such a huge topic that I can't even begin to scratch the surface. My aim is to highlight sleep's pivotal role in mitigating Alzheimer's so that a good night's sleep becomes your number one priority. If you'd like to take a deep dive into all things sleep, I highly recommend the book *Why We Sleep* by Professor Matthew Walker.

Despite our best intentions, seven or more hours of shut-eye are not always easy to come by. A recent conversation with a 53-year-old patient, David (not his real name, of course), raised important issues relating to slumber. David was a lawyer who occasionally 'pulled an all-nighter' and worked an average of 70 hours per week. He exercised every second day and thrived on the stimulating nature of his work but was fearful of long-term negative health consequences.

'I saw you interviewed on TV about sleep deprivation being linked to Alzheimer's,' he began. 'But I'm convinced I won't get Alzheimer's.'

'How can you be so sure?' I challenged.

'Because I won't live long enough! Lack of sleep will lead to other diseases that will kill me first. Only the other day I heard that **the World Health Organisation (WHO) classifies shift work as a probable carcinogen.** Is that really true?'

'Yes,' I confirmed, 'particularly in relation to breast, prostate, colon and rectal cancers. But the problem isn't just shift work and cancer; **the risk of *all* diseases escalates with insufficient sleep,** whether or not you're a shift worker. Sleep deprivation decimates our immune system, plays havoc with our hormones, slows recovery from injuries, reduces sex drive and skyrockets mental illness. Just one night of insufficient sleep increases the reactivity of our amygdala — the part of our brain that regulates emotions. An over-reactive amygdala means we are quicker to feel angry, stressed, overwhelmed or just plain grumpy. Getting more sleep is the best way to improve our coping skills, no matter what life throws our way.'

'That explains a lot,' confessed David. 'I understand everything you're saying, but there's so much I have to do every day that I can't see how I can fit more sleep into my life.'

'Could you squeeze in an extra 10 or 15 minutes of sleep, either at night or in the morning?'

'That's hardly going to make a difference in *my* case.' He was visibly unimpressed.

'Oh, but it will. For a start, 10 minutes a day adds up to more than an hour more sleep every week. That doesn't sound like much in the short term but after a few months, you might be able to increase your sleep by another 10 minutes a day. More importantly, you're sending your brain the message that sleep is becoming a priority. The other factor you might like to consider is that if you get more sleep, you'll actually get more done because your brain will work more efficiently. Sleep deprivation dramatically reduces our productivity, patience and empathy but we're unaware of it because it happens night after night. We don't realise we're underperforming because we don't give ourselves the chance to have a good night of sleep and see the difference. Besides, sleep makes us a nicer person.'

'It doesn't help that I've chosen a career that rewards sacrificing sleep.'

'You've also chosen a career that has one of the highest rates of depression.'

'How do you change the culture of an entire profession?'

'Start a conversation, even with just one person. Someone has to be brave enough to take the first step. We'll never find solutions if we don't even raise the issues. I have another experiment for you to try. For one month — even just one week — prioritise getting seven plus hours of sleep every night and watch what happens. I guarantee people will start asking you what you're on. They'll get a shock when you answer "sleep"!'

'Hospitals are also notorious for having sleep-deprived staff, are they not?' David deflected his quandary back to me.

'Yes, they are and it can lead to fatal mistakes — literally. I agree that it's a huge societal problem. I'm extremely grateful that people are on hand 24/7 to treat medical emergencies, but the system could definitely be improved to allow doctors and nurses to get more sleep. More than anything, we need the willingness to change; the willingness to acknowledge that seven-plus hours of sleep are a non-negotiable biological imperative. Robbing ourselves of sleep is not a virtue; it's a disservice to ourselves and to everyone around us. That's not to say we should beat ourselves up about it. I know it's a challenge — especially if you have young children — but if we all got more sleep, we'd have fewer people in hospital in the first place!'

'It boils down to our values,' David observed. 'What do we, as a society, value? And what do I, as an individual, value?' He reflected for a moment before continuing, 'What do I want from life? Is getting ahead everything it's cracked up to be? And what does "getting ahead" actually mean? What exactly am I trading my health for? We tie so much of our self-esteem to what the world dictates we should achieve. If I were to turn up at work and suggest reducing my hours to look after my health, I'd be seen as weak and unambitious, even disloyal. You've prompted some tough decisions. And all I wanted was a script for sleeping pills,' he goaded.

'You must be joking! You've known me long enough to know that's not going to happen.'

'Are sleeping pills really that bad?'

'Is whacking you across the head with a cricket bat really that bad? Don't confuse being unconscious with being asleep. Sleeping pills knock you out but they do not give you good quality sleep. Sedatives inhibit essential restorative and memory-consolidating activities that take place in our brain while we sleep. And most sleeping pills are highly addictive. The Australian Sleep Association, along with the American Academy of Sleep Medicine, American College of Physicians and European Sleep Research Society, all unanimously advocate Cognitive Behaviour Therapy for Insomnia (CBT-I)[3] as the first line of treatment for people who have trouble falling or staying asleep. Sleeping pills were developed before we had elaborate polysomnography (PSG)[4] so we didn't realise they were highly disruptive to our natural sleep cycles.'

'What about over-the-counter sleeping aids?'

'They're unregulated so you can't be sure of what you're getting,' I cautioned. 'Plus, there isn't much evidence that they work. I wouldn't waste my money.'

'What about alcohol? I do enjoy an occasional nightcap,' he admitted.

'Unfortunately, your brain does not. Although alcohol helps people fall asleep, it causes what is known as rebound wakefulness four to five hours later. This means our heart rate increases and our sleep becomes shallow and fragmented. The other big problem with alcohol is that it disrupts a phase of sleep known as rapid eye movement (REM) or dream sleep. REM sleep is very important for our mental health and memory function. People are often not aware that alcohol has disturbed their sleep but they definitely won't be on top of their game the following day. This is not to say they have a hangover. It only takes one or two drinks to disrupt our sleep. Obviously, the more alcohol a person consumes before bed, the worse the quality of their sleep. Alcohol can also suppress breathing and precipitate OSA.'

'You're a bundle of bad news,' David chastised. 'So what are your top tips for falling asleep quickly and getting good quality sleep throughout the night? I wouldn't say I had insomnia but sometimes I struggle to fall asleep and then I worry that I won't get enough sleep, which makes it all the harder to fall asleep. I know that exposure

---

[3] CBT-I teaches lifelong skills for overcoming insomnia. It is much more effective than sleeping pills and can be learned online through sleep centres around the globe. You can also choose to work with a sleep therapist one-on-one.

[4] PSG is a comprehensive sleep study that records a person's brainwaves, breathing pattern, blood oxygen levels, heart rate, eye movements and leg twitching. It is used to assess sleep quality and diagnose sleep apnoea or other sleep disorders.

to blue light keeps us awake so I put all my devices on sleep mode to reduce blue light emissions in the evening.'

'Blocking blue light is a good first step but any light can delay sleep. A study published in the journal *Sleep Health* in April 2021 randomly assigned people to one of three groups. The first group had to spend one hour before bed using their phone with blue light-blocking night mode turned on. The second group used their phone without night mode. The third group were not allowed to use their phone at all for an hour before bed. Wrist accelerometers were used to track their sleep for seven nights. The results were disappointing: blue light blockers did not shorten the time it took to fall asleep. The people who didn't use their phone at all slept the best, while the two groups who used their phone, regardless of whether night mode was on or off, had the same result. It seems that any bright light suppresses production of the sleep-triggering hormone melatonin. In addition, the mental stimulation of using a device probably has a greater impact than whatever light it emits.'

'Is there any light at the end of the sleep tunnel?' he grinned at his own joke.

'Dim all the lights in your house and don't use any devices for at least an hour (preferably two) before bed. Make sure your bedroom is completely dark and develop a regular wind-down routine. We need to train our brain to anticipate sleep.'

'What would you suggest for an effective wind-down routine?'

'What do you find pleasant and relaxing? For some people it's listening to soft music, for others it's adding a few pieces to a jigsaw puzzle. Create a pre-sleep ritual that you look forward to. Light a few candles, brush and floss your teeth, mindfully put on your pyjamas, do some stretches or meditate for a few minutes. Or cuddle with your partner and reflect on what you both feel grateful for. It's also crucial that you dedicate your bedroom to nothing other than sleep and sex. The bedroom then becomes a trigger for your brain to switch to sleep mode.'

'What about reading a book in bed? That's something I enjoy.' David crossed his fingers.

'Only if it's a book that will help you fall asleep — not background reading for work or a subject that arouses you.'

'That means no checking soccer scores before bed?'

'Not if you care about the results. Speaking of soccer, did you know that Manchester United has a sleep coach?'

'A sleep coach? You mean someone who sings the team lullabies and tucks them in at night?' he smirked.

'No. Someone who trains them how to get good quality sleep to enhance their performance and reduce their risk of injuries. His name is Nick Littlehales and he provides sleep advice for many professional athletes. Research has shown that good sleep increases a person's aerobic capacity and maximal muscle strength. Sleep even affects our ability to perspire, which translates into greater athletic ability.'

'Amazing! What are Mr Littlehales's secrets to sensational sleep?'

'Exactly what every good sleep scientist will tell you. Apart from making your bedroom a sacred sleeping space and establishing a predictable wind-down routine, here is a checklist for you.' I handed David a document titled *Seven Secrets to Successful Sleep.*

1. Go to bed and get up at roughly the same time every day. This assists in programming our brain to fall asleep on cue.
2. Get at least 10 minutes of natural light — preferably sunshine — every day. The earlier in the day, the better. This helps regulate our circadian rhythm — our sleep–wake cycle, which is controlled by a tiny region of the brain called the suprachiasmatic nucleus (SCN).
3. Get at least 10 minutes of exercise every day at whatever level you can manage. If you can fit in more, by all means do so. But even 10 minutes of movement can make a positive difference to our sleep.
4. Avoid caffeine after 2 pm.
5. Keep the bedroom cool — below 19 degrees Celsius (67 Fahrenheit) is ideal. Our core body temperature plays a pivotal role in initiating sleep and keeping us asleep. A drop in body temperature helps

us fall asleep and a rise in body temperature helps us wake up. That's one of the reasons people enjoy a hot drink first thing in the morning. It isn't just the caffeine; it's the arousal brought on by a rise in our temperature.

6. Paradoxically, take a hot bath or shower 60 to 90 minutes before bed because your body temperature will drop when you get out. The trick is not to let your feet get cold. Cold extremities cause our blood vessels to constrict in order to keep the rest of our body warm. Conversely, warm feet make your blood vessels dilate so that we release heat through our skin and lower our core temperature.

7. Ideally, stop eating three hours before bed to avoid reflux, heartburn and the rise in body temperature that accompanies digestion. Sugary foods are particularly notorious in raising our core temperature.

'Sometimes I get so carried away with what I'm doing that I lose track of time and find it's later than I realised,' David frowned.

'Do you set an alarm to wake you up in the morning?'

'Yes.'

'What about setting an alarm to go to bed?'

'I never thought of that. Sure, that's an easy fix. And I don't have to worry about caffeine because it doesn't affect me. I can have a cup of coffee with dinner and still fall asleep without any trouble. It's a genetic thing, isn't it?'

'Yes, variations in a gene called CYP1A2 determine the speed at which an enzyme in our liver metabolises caffeine. However, even people who are fast metabolisers experience a reduction in sleep quality after an evening cup of coffee. You might not be aware of it because you fall asleep quickly, but caffeine produces shallow sleep. You're more easily roused and your capacity to reach the deeper stages of non-REM sleep is compromised. Even eating chocolate close to bedtime can disrupt a person's sleep.'

'Just when I thought I had something going for me, you go and ruin it,' he quipped.

I gave David an empathic smile.

'I presume that exercising shortly before bed is also not a good idea because I'll get hot and sweaty,' David continued.

'A walk or light stretching after dinner is fine. If you intend doing something more vigorous, I'd suggest leaving at least a two-hour window between exercise and sleep.'

'What about sex?'

'Sex releases a cocktail of hormones that make you feel relaxed and drowsy so you're good to go.'

'At last, some good news!'

'Above all, don't lie awake worrying if you're not able to fall asleep. If your mind is racing, turn on a dim light and write your thoughts down on paper. Then go back to bed and think about something that relaxes you and makes you feel good: walking in nature, swimming in the ocean, lying on the beach … whatever works best for you. Visualising pleasant scenes is surprisingly effective in helping us fall asleep.

'There are also many online resources that can help. The two I most highly recommend are:

1. Matthew Walker's Sleep Masterclass

2. Sleepschool.org — founded by sleep specialist Dr Guy Meadows. Sleep School's mission is "to create a world where everyone lives their best during the day by getting the best possible sleep at night, naturally". The Sleep School app provides a range of courses that target specific sleep problems.

'I have no affiliation with either of these individuals or organisations. My endorsement is on account of their evidence-based approach and patient satisfaction,' I assured him.

'I'll give it all a go,' David asserted, 'but on the nights when I really can't manage much sleep, is there anything I can do during the day to mitigate the damage and boost my performance?'

'I would suggest three things: drink more water than you usually would, have a nap if you can and take 40-second micro-breaks every 40 minutes.'

'More details please,' David enjoined.

'A study of 20 000 adults from the US and China found that those who slept less than six hours a night were up to 59% more likely to be dehydrated compared with people who slept eight hours per night.'

'Why is that?'

'While we sleep — and particularly after the first five hours or so — our body increases production of a hormone called vasopressin or antidiuretic hormone (ADH). As the name suggests, this hormone stops us making urine so that we don't get dehydrated overnight. If you wake up before you've had your quota of sleep, scientists postulate that you miss out on a portion of your vasopressin and therefore pass more water throughout a 24-hour period.'

'Fascinating! And what do you mean by a micro-break?'

'A micro-break lasts anything from 40 seconds to five minutes. It involves a change in focus and preferably time away from your desk and screen. Taking regular micro-breaks can lessen fatigue, improve concentration and reduce mistakes. Have a stretch or go for a short walk. Even if you can't move, looking at greenery, flowers or a rooftop garden is particularly effective. Viewing cityscapes is not as restorative as gazing at nature.'

'Can I look at a painting or does it have to be a real view of nature?'

'A live natural environment is ideal but a painting is a reasonable substitute. There are no rules about how you spend your 40 seconds. The key is to shift your attention from your work to something you perceive as pleasant.'

'How long should I nap if I get that luxury?'

'The jury is still out on the optimal length of napping. You'll find recommendations ranging from a few minutes to 90 minutes. It's likely that different people do better with different amounts at different times of day. Experiment and see what works best for you. Don't nap after 5 pm or you might have trouble falling asleep.'

'Do you really think if I chip away at getting more sleep, I can avert an early grave and get off the bullet train to Alzheimer's?' David asked in earnest.

'Absolutely! It's never too late to make a positive difference to our health. We're able to increase connections between brain cells no matter how old we are. By improving your sleep, you'll improve every aspect of your life — and you'll get more joy and satisfaction from everything you do. People have the mistaken belief that getting more sleep means missing out on life. On the contrary, **getting more sleep means getting *more* out of life.'**

David stood up to leave.

'Before you go, let me take your blood pressure.' I slipped his hand through the cuff. '132/84. A tad on the high side but it's an easy fix.'

'And what might that be?' David raised his eyebrows expectantly.

'Get a good night's sleep!'

CHAPTER 20

Philadelphia Rapper

*The best way to find yourself is to lose yourself
in the service of others.*

MAHATMA GANDHI (1869–1948)

Every Australian winter I took Dad to either Serbia or Los Angeles to visit relatives and friends. Although Sydney's temperature is mild by most people's standards, Dad had become extremely sensitive to the cold. Anything below 17 degrees Celsius (63 degrees Fahrenheit) and he was putting on his dressing gown over his jumper. Motivating him to be physically active was exacting at the best of times; in winter it was diabolical. Flying halfway across the world was a logical fix.

When we landed in Los Angeles on 13 June 2013, we were plunged into an unforeseen set of circumstances. It was the last time I booked a flight on the 13th.

Instead of our host Dean waiting for us at the airport, his next-door neighbour was holding a placard with our names on it. Where was Dean? In hospital recovering from triple bypass surgery! So it was straight from the airport to his bedside, where Dean lay weak and woeful. It wasn't the calm respite I had planned. However, Dean's plight unexpectedly ignited a new sense of purpose in Dad: to cheer up his longstanding friend.

For me, there was one complicating factor.

Halfway through our stay in the US, I'd registered to attend a conference in Philadelphia. During this time, Dad was supposed to be looked after by Dean and his wife Linda. Linda was barely managing with Dean and clearly not able to take on Dad as well. So I had to decide whether to cancel attending the conference or take Dad with me. Ambitiously, I decided to take Dad with me.

The first step was to find Dad last-minute seats on the same flights to Philadelphia that I was on. The second step was organising someone to care for him while I was at the conference. The third step was convincing Dad to spend four days with a complete stranger. Step three was by far the greatest challenge.

At 8 am on the first day of the conference, Dad and I waited in the lobby of the Marriott Hotel for the caregiver I had organised to take him sightseeing. Dad loved people-watching. Unfortunately, dementia had eroded some of his social inhibitions. He never did anything inappropriate but I had to guard against him asking young women why on earth they would cover up their lovely skin with a hideous tattoo. On the morning in question, a 20-something-year-old rapper caught Dad's attention. His vintage basketball jersey hung loosely over the back of his baggy jeans. At the front, it was strategically tucked into his jeans to reveal a designer belt. The tongues hung out of his bright red, high-top sneakers. As he meandered past reception it was evident that his arteries pulsed with music.

'That boy has a bird's nest under his cap,' Dad pointed at the dreadlocks.

'It's a particular hairstyle,' I started to explain but stopped mid-sentence as the young man approached us.

Flicking up his square-framed oversized black sunglasses, he leaned towards us to shake Dad's hand. 'You must be Ilija and Heleeena.'

What the …? I thought. A clairvoyant rapper. Only in America.

'I'm Drake. I'll be taking you out today.' He gave Dad a broad smile.

You've got to be kidding me. Dad looked to me for permission to reciprocate the handshake. I nodded as I tried to engage my prefrontal cortex to respond with good judgment and awareness of long-term consequences. Just because this young man didn't conform to my preconceived notion of Alzheimer's caregiver didn't mean he wouldn't provide Dad with appropriate supervision and support. I'd done my homework and he was from a reputable agency. Or was it a scam and he'd fleece our room as soon as I was safely behind conference doors? If it was a scam, they'd have sent a middle-aged woman with pinned-back hair wearing a pinafore so as not to arouse my suspicion. I was ashamed that my mistrust was based purely on his unanticipated appearance.

I took Drake the Rapper aside to ask him a few questions.

'Have you spent much time with people who have Alzheimer's?'

'Yes, I have, Ma'am. But if you know one person with Alzheimer's, you only know one person with Alzheimer's. Everyone is different.'

I was impressed with his response but he could have learnt it by rote.

'What made you want to work with people who have dementia?'

'My mother had early-onset Alzheimer's and died four years ago. I want to help others in the same boat. She had a rare gene called Presenilin-1. Anyone who carries the gene is destined to get Alzheimer's. I had a 50–50 chance of inheriting it from her so I took a genetic test.'

I caught my breath.

'I wanted to know whether I was going to go loco and die early. Thinking you have less time on the planet changes you. As it turns out, I didn't inherit the gene.'

I was duly humbled as I handed Drake our room key and wished them both an enjoyable day at the Philadelphia Art Gallery.

Dad returned with a swagger in his step. Drake had a new protégé.

Late afternoon on day four of our stay, Marriott management decided to pay us a visit. Was everything to our satisfaction? The *Do not disturb* sign was permanently taped to our door so they wanted to check if the room needed servicing? Thank you, no it did not.

I had three reasons for taping the *Do not disturb* sign to our door:

1. I had labelled all drawers, cupboards and towels so that Dad would be able to find his things. Unfamiliar surroundings overwhelmed him. I didn't want cleaning staff to wonder about the labels.
2. Everything needed to remain exactly the same from day to day otherwise Dad would become disoriented. I didn't want cleaning staff to inadvertently rearrange anything.
3. Whenever Dad was unable to find something (which happened several times a day), he would insist it had been stolen. If no one from housekeeping entered the room, it meant no one could be blamed for theft. I could then look for the item in peace.

I didn't think the *Do not disturb* sign would be of any concern to Marriott management. They should have appreciated the cost savings and environmental merits of not servicing our room. As it turns out, they were more than a little concerned.

Why was an elderly man going in and out of the hotel with a hip young black kid every day? On top of that, housekeeping were not able to enter the room. Would I care to explain? Luckily I never leave home without a stash of copies of *In Search of My Father* ...

CHAPTER 21

In search of an ostrich

Love, like strength and courage, is a strange thing. The more
we give, the more we find we have to give.

OLGA JACOBY (1874–1913)

'Wake up! Wake up! My South African ostrich skin belt with the Australian opal buckle has been stolen!' My father's panic-stricken voice broke my slumber.

I reached across to the bedside cabinet and fumbled around for my watch. It was 2.30 am. Exactly the same time as last night. Here we go again — the missing ostrich skin belt was turning into a replay of when Dad thought his car had been stolen.

'Dad it's okay. Your belt hasn't been stolen. We accidentally left it behind at Los Angeles airport.'

'Why would we have done that?' The light from the hallway exposed his bewilderment.

I repeated my answer for the fourth consecutive night. 'When we walked through the x-ray machines at Los Angeles airport, you had to remove everything metallic from your clothing. Your belt buckle is metallic so it had to be placed on the conveyor belt to pass through a separate machine. We were both tired and forgot to collect it on the other side.'

'That's very irresponsible. You should have had your wits about you. I'm old and I'm allowed to forget things. You're young. You have no excuse.'

'Let me take you back to bed and we'll talk about it in the morning. What are you doing rummaging around for your belt in the middle of the night?'

'I don't know.'

I waited until he'd fallen asleep and tiptoed back to my room.

Dad's South African ostrich skin belt with the Australian opal buckle was the bane of my life. I hadn't known such things existed until he started making a fuss about it a few years ago. We'd spent hours searching for it in every drawer, cupboard and tool-box (just in case) in every room of the house — to no avail. I was convinced it was a figment of Dad's grieving mind but he insisted that Mum had bought it for him while they'd been holidaying in California. Why would someone buy a South African ostrich skin belt with an Australian opal buckle in California? Far be it for me to question him. One day it miraculously appeared — neatly rolled inside a thermal sock — and, sure enough, there was a speckled blue-green opal embedded in the centre of the buckle. Who'd have thought? From then on, he wore the belt every day. 'Your mum bought it for me,' he reiterated whenever he threaded it through his trousers. Of course, he had to wear it on our trip to the US.

Now it was gone — sitting in a lost property kiosk at LA International. Or adorning someone else's dry-cleaned trousers. How was it that Dad forgot about everything except his South African ostrich skin belt with the Australian opal buckle? Just saying the words was a mammoth mouthful. I resolved to rectify the situation there and then. I looked up LAX Airport Lost and Found. Their hours of operation were 8:00 am to 3:00 pm Pacific Standard Time (PST). Given the time difference, ringing at 2.30 am Australian Eastern Standard Time (AEST) was perfect. Cheerful Charlie greeted me with the buoyancy of a radio announcer on his fifth cup of filtered coffee. He lyrically explained that I would need to search for my missing item through their online 'Visual lost and found inventory'. If I found my item, I would then have to submit a *Claim for a Specific Item*. If I didn't find my item, I would need to submit a *General Claim*. I thanked him for his assistance and went straight to the relevant page on their website. I was given three options:

1. for items left on aircraft, click *here*
2. for items left in taxis, buses, rental cars and public vehicles, click *here*
3. for items lost at LAX airport restaurants, stores, parking lots, sidewalks and security screening checkpoints, click *here*.

I clicked *here* relating to security screening.

I received an instantaneous response: *We found 579 unclaimed items.*

You're kidding me. But wait — I could narrow my search by date and category. I clicked on *Clothing*. No ostrich skin belt, with or without an Australian opal buckle. I clicked on *Watches and Jewellery*. No belt there either. I clicked on *Miscellaneous*. Still no belt. In desperation, I clicked on *Animals* followed by *Bags and Backpacks, Bicycles, Children's Items, Computers and Electronics and Mobile Devices* — just in case. No ostrich skin belt. I forlornly submitted a General Claim. I was informed that LAX Airport Lost and Found retained items for a maximum of 90 days. We had 82 days to play with.

Just as I was about to shut down my laptop, an advertisement for a Lost Property Service Agent popped up. For a small unspecified fee, I could engage a dedicated representative to look for my item. In my somnolent state, it was a tempting proposition. I continued reading. *Time is of the essence! Did you know that unrecovered valuable items are auctioned off by the airport for profit?*

No, I didn't know.

Don't be fooled by other online lost property services that charge extensive listing fees but don't actually assign anyone to do anything!

I didn't like the exclamation mark. How did I know these people weren't also going to charge me for doing nothing? The clincher was the extensive personal information they wanted. No thank you. Maybe it was a genuine service but I wasn't going to take the risk. I fell into a deep, long sleep.

The following morning, I threw myself into the task with renewed vigour. There was more than one way to skin an ostrich. Why not just buy a replacement? I typed *men's ostrich skin belt with opal buckle* into Google's search bar. I received 2 550 000 results in 0.54 seconds.

You're kidding me. I clicked on eBay. Much better — only 7302 results. I refined my search by adding *black*. This brought it down to 1860 contenders. Top of the list was *Men's black Billionaire Italian Couture ostrich belt with gold and silver tone for $1150 + $26.50 shipping.* That's not a typo. The price was one thousand one hundred and fifty dollars. I continued to add more filters such as price, theme and style. No luck on eBay.

Over the ensuing week, I worked my way down the list of ostrich skin belt suppliers including Amazon, Etsy, Gumtree and a myriad of niche outlets. In amongst the ostrich skin belts, I found ostrich eggs, ostrich feathers and ostrich feather dusters, pillows, jackets and trims, along with adult only content. Don't ask. The closest match to the buckle was a *vintage pair of brass-plated belt buckles opal inlaid.* I was running out of options. I was also running out of tolerance for fractured sleep.

I kept reassuring Dad that the Lost Property Team at Los Angeles airport were committed to finding his belt. However, they had 579 unclaimed items to sort through so we had to be patient.

'Someone in the team is probably wearing my belt with no intention of giving it back!' Dad lamented. 'A South African ostrich skin belt with an Australian opal buckle is not easy to come by,' he asserted.

Didn't I know it.

'Your mum bought the last two in the store,' he mused.

'Last TWO? What do you mean?' I almost shrieked.

'She bought one for me and one for our friend Dean. We were visiting Dean and his family in Los Angeles at the time.'

'Do you mean to say that Dean also has a South African ostrich skin belt with an Australian opal buckle?' I tried to sound nonchalant.

'Yes,' he affirmed.

'Is it exactly the same as yours or is it slightly different?'

'Exactly the same.'

I rang Dean as soon as the time difference allowed and Dad was out of earshot. After the usual niceties, I got straight to the point. 'This may seem like a strange question, but did Mum ever give you a South African ostrich skin belt with an Australian opal buckle?'

'As a matter of fact, she did.'

'Do you like it? How often do you wear it? Please be brutally honest. Is it your favourite belt? Do you absolutely love it? Or is it sitting in the back of a cupboard still in its original box?'

Dean hesitated. 'Why do you ask?'

'Did you know that Mum also bought Dad the same belt?'

'Yes, I remember how impressed he was.'

'Were you equally impressed? I won't take offence if you're not as enamoured as Dad.'

'It isn't that I don't like it,' Dean was choosing his words carefully, 'it's that I have so many other belts, I don't get around to wearing them all.'

'Have you ever worn the ostrich skin belt?' I persisted.

'Not recently,' he faltered. 'Why?'

I poured out Dad's story. Dean anticipated my request. 'Of course, I'd be happy to post you my belt. I'd love to be able to do something that would brighten your father's day. He's such a kind and generous soul.'

'I'll cover the cost of postage and send you something in return. What would brighten your day?' I was delirious with relief.

'You'll do nothing of the sort. Knowing that I've been able to help is all the thanks I need.'

When the package arrived I ripped open the padded envelope before Dad could see it was from Dean. 'Hey Dad, I think this is for you,' I called out to him.

'What new brain-boosting stunt are you going to subject me to *now?*' He eyed me suspiciously.

'This package just arrived from America — from Los Angeles. Go ahead and unwrap it.'

He peeled back the tissue paper to reveal a South African ostrich skin belt with an Australian opal buckle. 'My belt!' he exclaimed ecstatically. 'You'll have to write a letter to the Lost Property Team at Los Angeles airport apologising for my not trusting them.'

CHAPTER 22

The XX Factor

You have always had the power, my dear.
You just had to learn it for yourself.

THE WIZARD OF OZ by LYMAN FRANK BAUM (1856–1919)

'**W**hy is Alzheimer's more common in women than in men?' Jasmin didn't even wait to sit down before posing the question. **'Two-thirds of people diagnosed with Alzheimer's are women** but I can't find a clear explanation as to why.'

'The reasons for gender differences in Alzheimer's are extremely complicated,' I forewarned.

'Is there anything in Alzheimer's that's *not* complicated?' Jasmin started winding her ponytail around her index finger.

'No,' I smiled, '**and two-thirds of people caring for someone with Alzheimer's are also women.**'

'Well that explains it!' Jasmin pronounced facetiously. 'I was going to suggest that a drop in the hormone oestrogen at menopause might negatively impact brain function but now I think it's the stress of caring!'

'That isn't as farcical as it sounds. Both of your premises have merit so let's break them down. Firstly, oestrogen is not a single hormone but a family of related hormones that control the female reproductive system. The three main oestrogen hormones are oestrone (E1), oestradiol (E2) and oestriol (E3). The most abundant and potent oestrogen before menopause is oestradiol and it also has the greatest influence on brain function. During menopause, oestradiol levels plummet and the predominant circulating oestrogen becomes oestrone. A fourth oestrogen known as oestetrol (E4) is only produced during pregnancy. So I'll assume when you say oestrogen you're referring to the family of hormones, and when you want to single out a particular oestrogen, you'll use its specific name.'

'Yes,' Jasmin released her ponytail. 'From what I've learned so far, oestradiol seems to be a master regulator of not only brain metabolism but a wide range of biological processes involving the heart, liver, bones and immune system. Is that why women are at lower risk of heart disease than men *before* menopause and higher risk of osteoporosis *after* menopause?'

'Yes, on all counts — oestrogen is far more than just a group of sex hormones. Men also produce oestrogen but their dominant hormone is testosterone. After menopause, everything abruptly changes. This has led to the Oestrogen Hypothesis — a theory about why depletion of oestradiol might push a woman towards Alzheimer's. Of course, not all women experience cognitive decline after menopause so we need to look at the differences between those who do and those who don't.'

'Why is oestradiol so critical for brain health?'

'Oestradiol has multiple effects in many different regions of the brain. For a start, oestradiol facilitates glucose metabolism and mitochondrial function to ensure the brain has adequate energy. When oestradiol levels plummet, the brain has to use ketone bodies[5] instead of glucose for fuel. Astrocytes (a type of brain cell) make ketone bodies from fatty acids delivered to the brain via blood. However, if the brain can't get enough fatty acids from circulation, it starts to break down its own myelin. You'll recall that myelin is the fatty sheath that insulates axons to enable transmission of electrical impulses. Loss of myelin leads to loss of signalling between brain cells.'

'It sounds like menopause triggers the brain to start feeding on itself!' Jasmin exclaimed. 'Are you saying that after menopause, a woman's brain starts consuming its own tissue for fuel?'

---

[5] Ketone bodies are discussed in detail in Chapter 55 'Ketone crusade'.

'Yes, this may well be happening in a subgroup of women. Lack of oestradiol can put the brain into starvation mode. Some researchers suggest that symptoms of menopause, such as hot flushes, signify the brain's transition to using ketone bodies. When symptoms fade, it indicates the brain has adjusted to its new fuel source. The link with hot flushes is still only speculative but it's plausible.'

'I'm guessing that some women are able to make the switch to ketone bodies more quickly and efficiently than other women,' Jasmin concluded.

'Precisely.'

'And there are probably multiple — and as yet undetermined — reasons why.'

'You're a fast learner, Jasmin!'

'Is that what constitutes the Oestrogen Hypothesis? Loss of oestradiol drives the brain into an energy crisis that can compromise cognition later in life. Meanwhile, men don't undergo such dramatic hormonal changes with age because testosterone levels decline gradually and therefore give the brain time to adapt.'

'That's one component of the Oestrogen Hypothesis,' I agreed. 'Oestradiol also facilitates production of antioxidants, neuronal growth factors and clearance of brain toxins. When oestradiol declines, so do these protective functions. The result is increased accumulation of amyloid beta ($A\beta$) plaques and tau tangles — the hallmarks of Alzheimer's.'

'Nonetheless, not all women develop Alzheimer's. What's their secret?' Jasmin reflected.

'Why don't you try to work it out. From your understanding of Alzheimer's as a multifactorial disease, what would you predict might *worsen* brain function after menopause?'

Jasmin straightened her posture and resumed playing with her hair. 'Firstly, there could be a genetic component. I suspect that women who have at least one copy of the APOE4 gene might have more cognitive problems after menopause than women without an APOE4 gene.'

'Yes, women with one or two copies of the APOE4 gene are found to have less white matter and more Aβ plaques in their brain after menopause than women without an APOE4 gene.'

Jasmin was buoyed by the scientific support for her supposition. 'Pre-existing risk factors for Alzheimer's could also lead to menopause being the straw that breaks the camel's back — or in this case, brain,' she grinned at her own quip. 'Type 2 diabetes, high blood pressure, excess fat around the waist, poor sleep, chronic depression and ongoing stress would make the experience of menopause all the worse.'

'Absolutely,' I agreed. 'And what's more, menopause increases the risk of everything you listed. It's a two-way street. Even if a woman does not have any of the conditions you mentioned *before* menopause, a drop in oestradiol can precipitate type 2 diabetes, high blood pressure, increased visceral fat, sleep problems, depression and anxiety. It can also be a time of intensified psychosocial strain, such as having elderly parents who start needing more assistance. When you joked that being a caregiver impaired brain function, you were not far off the mark. The phenomenon is known as caregiver burden and it refers to family caregivers (as opposed to paid caregivers) having worse physical health, poorer quality sleep and greater stress than the rest of the population. Full-time family caregivers are also at higher risk of developing Alzheimer's themselves. Menopause + suboptimal physical health + psychological and emotional stress are a perfect storm for reduced brain function.'

'Does that mean women who go through menopause at an earlier age are at higher risk of Alzheimer's than women who have more years of oestradiol stimulating their brain?'

'Yes. **A little-known risk factor for Alzheimer's is premature surgical menopause.** Women who have their uterus removed (hysterectomy) or one or both ovaries excised (unilateral or bilateral oophorectomy) before they reach natural menopause increase their likelihood of Alzheimer's unless they take Menopausal Hormone Therapy (MRT)[6] immediately after their operation and at least until the age of 50.'

---

[6] Previously known as Hormone Replacement Therapy (HRT)

'I had no idea!' Jasmin's distress was palpable. 'I've never heard a gynaecologist mention Alzheimer's as a potential complication of hysterectomy or oophorectomy.'

'I suspect that Alzheimer's is a secondary consideration if you're facing a life-threatening cancer. Hysterectomy and oophorectomy are not undertaken lightly. The most common indications are malignant tumours or intractable pain and bleeding. Only after a person has solved the immediate, potentially fatal problem, do they have the headspace to think about averting cognitive decline.'

'I can understand why losing your ovaries can lead to loss of oestrogen production, but why hysterectomy? And I presume that removing both ovaries is more harmful than removing only one?'

'Yes, the extent of gynaecological surgery correlates with the extent of cognitive impairment. Having a hysterectomy alone is less damaging than having one or both ovaries removed. The worst-case scenario is having a hysterectomy *plus* bilateral oophorectomy. Removing both ovaries causes an abrupt cessation of oestrogen production and leads to the various brain changes we've just discussed. The ovaries also make progesterone and testosterone — two other hormones that contribute to a healthy brain. The good news is that if women are given oestrogen replacement, their cognition tends to be preserved. Therefore, loss of oestrogen — rather than other hormonal disturbances —seems to be the major problem. What's surprising is that removing just *one* ovary (unilateral oophorectomy) also precipitates worsening brain function. Contrary to the kidneys — where surgically removing one kidney (unilateral nephrectomy) will induce the remaining kidney to step up and do the work of both kidneys — the ovaries seem to operate differently. Surgically excising one ovary somehow disrupts the functioning of the other.'

'And yet women with only one ovary can still fall pregnant,' Jasmin interjected.

'Yes, the story of oophorectomy remains a mystery. The bottom line is we don't yet know how unilateral oophorectomy throws a spanner in the workings of the brain.'

'What about hysterectomy? Why would removing the uterus, while preserving the ovaries, interfere with brain function?'

'Most likely when the uterus is removed, there is disruption of blood supply to the ovaries, which might permanently hinder their hormone output. Once again, there is no clear explanation. The big lesson is that everything in our body is interconnected. And not surprisingly, the younger a woman is when she has surgery, the worse her long-term brain health is likely to be.'

'Is taking MHT 100% effective in ameliorating the damage inflicted by surgery?' Jasmin reiterated.

'Yes, that seems to be the case.'

'Does that mean all women should take MHT as soon as they enter menopause? If replacing oestradiol helps preserve brain function after surgical menopause, would it not also preserve brain function after natural menopause?'

'That's a very controversial topic. Numerous studies have tried to answer that question but the results have been disappointing and contradictory. In some instances, MHT for natural menopause has been linked to fewer cases of Alzheimer's and less brain shrinkage, while other research has pointed to the exact opposite: that MHT *doubles* the risk of Alzheimer's. This has led to the Critical Window Hypothesis — in other words, as long as hormone replacement is commenced within five years of menopause, there *may* be some brain-benefits. At the very least, there seems to be no harm. On the other hand, starting MHT more than 10 years *after* menopause seems to be counterproductive. This has led to yet another theory called the Healthy Cell Bias Hypothesis which states that if brain cells have not been exposed to oestradiol for over a decade, they lose their ability to respond to oestradiol in a favourable way. Hence MHT may actually cause harm.'

'This whole topic is overwhelming,' lamented Jasmin.

'And it gets even more complicated,' I empathised. 'Other variables that need to be taken into account include the following:
- APOE status — the jury is still out about whether women with an APOE4 gene respond better or worse to MHT. Once again, the research results are conflicting.

- If a woman is suffering debilitating symptoms of menopause that reduce her quality of life, MHT could improve her day-to-day functioning and indirectly reduce her risk of Alzheimer's.
- A woman's overall physical and mental health also mediate her response to MHT.
- Is there a history of breast cancer or other reasons that might preclude her from taking MHT?
- What type and form of oestradiol is most effective — pill, patch or gel?
- Does she need to take progesterone as well as oestradiol? For women with an intact uterus, oestrogen without progesterone can increase the risk of uterine cancer.
- What type and form of progesterone is most effective?
- If a woman starts taking MHT, how many years should she continue to take it?'

I paused to give Jasmin a chance to catch her breath. 'If you're looking to get into research, this is an area that will keep you busy for a very long time,' I encouraged.

'What if a woman has her uterus or ovaries removed *after* menopause? Does it still increase her risk of Alzheimer's?'

'No. Research suggests that after menopause, gynaecological surgery does not worsen brain function.'

Jasmin looked relieved. 'Is there anything else a woman needs to be aware of that puts her at increased risk of cognitive decline?'

'High blood pressure during pregnancy — known as pre-eclampsia — and gestational diabetes can both foreshadow heart disease and insulin resistance later in life, which in turn can lead to Alzheimer's or vascular dementia. If a woman has either pre-eclampsia or gestational diabetes, she needs to continue having her blood pressure and sugar levels checked after delivery.'

'I'd never have linked obstetric history to Alzheimer's,' Jasmin remarked. 'I'm beginning to see how everything in our lives has downstream consequences that can impact brain function decades later.'

'On a different but related note, women who sustain a head injury or concussion don't tend to recover as well as men. Women experience more severe symptoms, have more extensive brain damage and take longer to recuperate than men subjected to the same degree of trauma.'

'Why is that?' Jasmin asked.

'One possible reason is that men have stronger neck muscles than women. They're naturally more muscular and also more likely to do neck strengthening exercises as part of their training if they are professional football players. Consequently, when a man receives a blow to his head, his brain doesn't rattle around as much. Another factor affecting women could be damage to an area of the brain called the anterior pituitary gland which produces follicle stimulating hormone (FSH) and luteinising hormone (LH). These hormones influence oestrogen production. So, here again, we have evidence that oestrogen is critical for brain health.'

'This has long-term implications for women who suffer domestic violence, even after they escape the situation,' Jasmin noted with alarm.

'Yes, it certainly does. I find it terrifying that victims of domestic violence show the same degree of traumatic brain injury (TBI) and risk of chronic traumatic encephalopathy (CTE) as retired football players. A 10-year study found that two out of every five hospitalisations linked to family violence involved brain injuries.'

'And for every woman who shows up at hospital, how many are too afraid or unable to do so?' Jasmin posed.

'Even heading soccer balls is more dangerous for women than we ever realised. MRI scans of soccer players demonstrate that heading the ball causes five times more structural damage to brain cell fibres in female brains than in male brains. APOE4 carriers in particular should avoid any kind of head impact. Women + APOE4 leads to the worst outcomes after TBI. Personally, I think we need urgent research into the effects of heading at all levels of soccer. But that's a whole other subject.'

'Why is there a lack of awareness about these issues in the public arena? Someone needs to start a conversation. I know there are some voices out there, but they're still only a whisper. It needs to become a roar.'

'And I know just the person to raise the volume,' I prompted.

'Watch this space,' Jasmin resolved, 'but I need some good news for this story.'

'From the time we're born, women are the stronger sex in terms of biology. Girls are less likely to be born with congenital malformations such as tongue tie and clubfoot, and preterm baby girls are more likely to survive than preterm boys.'

'But women are more likely to suffer autoimmune diseases such as rheumatoid arthritis, lupus and multiple sclerosis,' Jasmin countered.

'That's because we have more reactive immune systems which means we're better at fighting infections and cancer. Melanoma kills twice as many young men as women, and 95% of people who reach the age of 110 are female. A woman's superior ability to survive prematurity, infections and cancer could also be the very reason she is more likely to get Alzheimer's. The men who were destined for Alzheimer's have already died from other causes. The men who last into old age are the truly hardy ones and are therefore more resistant to Alzheimer's. That's my personal hypothesis.'

'So what's a positive menopause message you can leave me with?' Jasmin asked sanguinely.

'Notwithstanding what I said earlier about avoiding head injury, women who engage in moderate to vigorous physical exercise, four or more times per week, have significantly fewer health problems than women who are sedentary. Exercise doesn't guarantee a disease-free life but it improves every aspect of physical, mental and emotional wellbeing to a far greater extent than most people realise. I know it's a challenge to fit exercise into our busy lives, but we always find time for what's most important to us. If you make the commitment, you'll make the time. The healthier you are *before* menopause, the healthier you're likely to stay *after* menopause.'

CHAPTER 23

Premonitions

We must go on because we can't turn back.

<small>FROM THE BOOK *TREASURE ISLAND* by ROBERT LOUIS STEVENSON (1850–1894)</small>

California, June 2014

With each passing year, Dad took a little longer to settle into our summer home in the United States. I'd rented a cosy two-bedroom house in a quiet tree-lined street in the friendly suburb of Pasadena. I found an Alzheimer's care-partner (the delightful Diana) to take him out twice a week so that I could have some time to myself. Dad and I took daily walks in the nearby park and once a week we went sightseeing with Dean and Linda. Each week's dinner conversation was a window into Dad's kaleidoscopic world.

Week One

'When are we going home?' Dad asked brusquely.

'When the weather warms up again in Sydney.'

'When will that be?'

'In two months.'

'That's too long! I want to go home. Everything in America is so complicated.'

'You'll get used to it. Meeting new people and having new experiences boosts your brain. If you find something complicated, it means you're stimulating the growth of new brain cells,' I enthused.

'What will I do with new brain cells at my age?'

'I'm sure you'll be able to put them to good use.'

Week Two

'When are we going home?'

'When the weather warms up again in Sydney.'

'Hasn't it warmed up yet?' he asked impatiently.

'No, not yet.'

'I have a premonition that I'm going to die soon. We'd better go back to Australia. You don't want to be carrying a dead body on the plane.'

'You look perfectly healthy to me. What makes you think you're going to die soon?'

'It's a premonition. Premonitions don't come with reasons.'

'I have a premonition that you're going to get fitter and healthier in America.'

'I don't believe your premonition.'

'I don't believe *your* premonition.'

Week Four

'When are we going home?'

'When the weather warms up again in Sydney.'

'When will that be?'

'In one month.'

'That's too soon! I want to stay. Everything in America is so beautiful.'

'Yes, it's a beautiful country.'

'When is Diana coming again?'

'Next week.'

'That's too long. Why can't she come sooner? Diana is so beautiful,' Dad gushed.

Week Six

'When are we going home?'

'When the weather warms up again in Sydney.'

'When will that be?'

'In two weeks.'

'That's too soon! I want to stay. Everything in America is so beautiful.'

'Australia is beautiful too.'

'When is Diana coming again?'

'Next week.'

'That's too long! Why can't she come sooner? Diana is so beautiful.'

'Yes, she is.'

'I have a premonition I'm going to get sick and not be able to fly on a plane.'

'You look perfectly healthy to me. What makes you think you're going to get sick?'

'It's a premonition. Premonitions don't come with reasons.'

'I have a premonition that you're going to remain as fit and healthy as ever.'

'I don't believe your premonition.'

'I don't believe *your* premonition.'

Week Seven

We'd just finished grocery shopping. The minute we stepped outside the store, Dad announced that he needed a toilet. We were 15 minutes' drive from home. 'Can you wait 15 minutes?' I asked hopefully.

'No. If you don't want to find me a toilet, I can go behind the row of shopping trolleys over there,' he suggested calmly.

'No, you won't!' I responded not so calmly.

I marched us back into the supermarket where I knew there were toilets adjacent to aisle 10. Job done, we walked outside again.

'Not so fast!' a strapping young security guard greeted us. 'Where do you think you're going with all those grocery items?'

'To the car,' I answered, mystified.

'Don't you think you should pay for them first?' propounded Mr Security Guard (who shall henceforth be referred to as Mr SG).

'I *have* paid for them,' I attested.

'Really? I just watched you walk out of the store without paying,' he admonished.

'That's because we paid for them earlier and then Dad realised he had to go to the toilet so we went back into the store.'

'And why wouldn't you have taken your bags to the car first?' asked Mr SG.

'Because I wasn't thinking.'

'Show me your receipt please.'

'I don't have one. I paid cash so I didn't take a receipt,' I regretted.

'Oh, that's a shame. Then how can I be sure you've paid for them?'

'What's a shame?' Dad interrupted. 'What's the problem?'

'Nothing. Everything's fine, Dad,' I reassured him before responding to Mr SG. 'The cashier will remember us.'

'Who was your cashier?'

We walked back to the row of cashiers. The cheerful young man who had served us was nowhere to be seen. 'I don't see our cashier,' I murmured.

'Oh, that's a shame. Then how will we ever know you've paid?'

'What's a shame?' Dad repeated. 'What's the problem?'

'Nothing. Everything's fine, Dad.'

'Then why aren't we going home?' he bemoaned. 'Lucky I went to the toilet. I certainly couldn't have held on for this long.'

'I'll find our cashier. He couldn't have just disappeared,' I turned my attention back to Mr SG.

After quizzing several of the other cashiers, we were eventually told that Mark (our cheerful cashier) finished his shift 10 minutes ago and had gone home for the night.

'Oh, that's a shame …' Mr SC began again.

'What's a shame? What's the problem?' repeated Dad.

I was ready to scream at both of them. Instead, I asked for the store manager to be paged, explained the situation to him, growled at Dad to stop chanting 'What's the problem?', waited while the manager rang Mark, snapped at Dad to stop chanting 'What's the problem?', endured suspicious glances from other shoppers, barked at Dad to stop chanting 'What's the problem?', continued waiting while Mr SG spoke to Mark in hushed tones, and finally walked outside to freedom after being told 'Yes, he remembers you'.

'Lucky I went to the toilet,' Dad reiterated when we got to the car.

CHAPTER 24

In search of meaning

*What do we live for, if it is not to make life
less difficult for each other?*

GEORGE ELIOT (1819–1880)

Back in Sydney

Dad and I had been volunteering with Meals on Wheels (MOW)
for four years when we received a notification that all volunteers
were required to complete a half day training in *Safe Food Handling
Essentials*.

'Of course I know how to handle food safely,' Dad rolled his eyes
with contempt as we drove to the course. 'If you drop food on the
floor, blow off the dirt. If it doesn't come off, tell people it's pepper,'
he smirked roguishly.

'Joan will be there,' I changed the subject.

He immediately brightened 'Jovial Joan! She's such a kind lady.'
Alliteration was Dad's way of trying to remember people's names.

We sat next to jovial Joan and waited for the training to begin. I
was soon feeling far from jovial. The trainer announced that at the
end of the course we'd need to complete a multiple-choice test. My
blood ran cold. Dad was fully capable of delivering meals in a safe
and responsible manner, plus I was always there to supervise him.
However, dementia had rendered his brain unequal to the task of
deciphering a multiple-choice test. The format of the test was the
problem. For Dad, having more than two options obfuscated any
options at all. What to do?

Dad stared blankly at the test paper when it was handed to him.

'Just write your name at the top,' I instructed. I answered the questions on my own paper as quickly as I could and then furtively looked around the room. My heart was beating so loudly I was certain everyone else could hear it. When the examiner's back was turned, I deftly swapped our papers.

'What …?' Dad started to ask. Jovial Joan gave us a startled look but said nothing. Had she noticed the switch?

'Shhh!' I whispered. 'People are trying to concentrate. Just wait quietly for a few minutes.' I lowered my head and raced through the questions on his paper.

'Does anyone need more time?' our examiner called out.

'One more minute please,' I sheepishly requested. 'I made a mistake and I need to correct it.'

There was a far-reaching reason I was so keen for Dad to be a Meals on Wheels volunteer: it gave him a sense of meaning and purpose. Meals on Wheels delivers more than meals to its clients and more than good feelings to its volunteers.

A study of seniors who received Meals on Wheels several days per week showed that it reduced feelings of isolation, loneliness, anxiety and depression. They also had fewer falls and better overall health than people receiving frozen meals once a week from an anonymous delivery truck. Even the briefest contact with someone who exchanges a few friendly words goes a long way to improving self-confidence and quality of life.

As for the effect on volunteers, contributing to others actually changes the structure of our brain.

A group of older women were invited to help primary school children with literacy. The women had functional MRI scans of their brains before and after six months of volunteering for 15 hours per week. The results were astounding. After half a year, volunteers not only performed better in memory tests, they exhibited increased activity in brain regions responsible for reasoning and problem-solving.

A four-year study of more than 6700 Americans aged over 51 showed that people who volunteered for 200 hours a year were 40% less likely to develop high blood pressure than those who didn't volunteer. Another study of 2000 Californians aged 55 and older found that volunteers were 44% less likely to die than non-volunteers during the four-year research period. Older adults who help to look after their grandchildren demonstrate sharper mental acuity than those who don't. And decades of scientific literature confirms that volunteering leads to less depression, fewer chronic illnesses and greater wellbeing. Even modest amounts — two to three hours of volunteering a month — can contribute to improvements in physical and mental wellbeing. The key is to do as much as makes you feel good without turning it into a chore. If you start feeling stressed, cut down. If you don't look forward to doing it, don't do it.

There are several interrelated and self-reinforcing mechanisms through which volunteering improves health:
- It stimulates production of feel-good neurotransmitters such as dopamine, serotonin and oxytocin.
- It promotes social connections and a sense of community.
- It may entail learning new skills or being more physically active.
- It increases feelings of usefulness, mastery and self-esteem.
- It gives people a greater sense of meaning and purpose.

Thus volunteering creates a positive domino effect in our lives. When we feel better, we do more and give more, and when we do more and give more, we feel better.

The *type* of volunteering also plays a role. Researchers have compared the effects of other-oriented versus self-oriented volunteering on a range of different health parameters. Other-oriented volunteering refers to activities that directly help another person and involve face-to-face interaction with the recipient of the assistance. Self-oriented volunteering involves behind-the-scenes work such as clerical and administrative tasks or volunteering for the purpose of skill acquisition, work experience or career advancement. While both forms of volunteering lead to better physical and mental health, other-oriented volunteering brings greater benefits in terms of life satisfaction, subjective wellbeing and a sense of belonging.

This distinction has inspired researchers to tackle the most tricky health topic of all: the effects of meaning and purpose.

There are many ways to define a sense of purpose:
- living in alignment with our values
- feeling that our life matters
- having a sense of direction
- working towards personally significant goals, regardless of how big or small
- doing work that we find meaningful and intrinsically rewarding
- doing what makes us happy
- following a passion
- engaging in random acts of kindness
- giving for the joy of giving
- having a sense of belonging or community
- experiencing 'flow'
- deriving joy from present-moment awareness
- knowing how to savour — a meal, a sunset, a warm breeze, a hot bath
- noticing beauty
- feeling gratitude and appreciation for what we have
- believing that what we do day-to-day is worthwhile and contributes something positive to the world — be it through art, agriculture, music, medicine, politics, plumbing, science, stonemasonry, teaching, writing, cooking, cleaning, child-rearing, cheerleading or anything in the service of others.

The medium doesn't matter. What matters is the meaning and satisfaction it gives us. Whether we're conscious of it or not, our deepest desire is to be of value to others and to bring good into the world. When we live in alignment with this yearning, we flourish; we are healthier, happier, sleep better and live longer.

Studies show that **a sense of purpose** lowers the risk of heart disease, stroke and depression. It improves blood sugar control in diabetes and aids recovery from addictions. And it **halves the likelihood of developing Alzheimer's.**

Analyses involving tens of thousands of people in the US and UK revealed that the higher a person's sense of purpose, the lower their risk of dying early. This was after ruling out the effects of education, smoking, exercise and depression. Purpose is an independent determinant of health and longevity. This concurs with Jewish psychiatrist Viktor Frankl's observation that Nazi concentration camp prisoners were more likely to survive if they could find meaning in their suffering and were driven to stay alive by a sense of purpose. Strength of purpose directly correlated with strength of body.

In 2017, Canadian researchers led by Nathan Lewis at Carleton University questioned 3500 people on their sense of purpose to investigate whether it affected brain performance. Those who felt more purposeful performed better in tests of memory and cognition. **Purpose protects against mental decline.**

How can this be? How can a feeling exert such a powerful influence on our fate? Scientists led by Steven Cole at the University of California set out to answer this question. Their findings attest to the mind–body connection on the deepest level. Having a strong sense of purpose switches on genes that lower inflammation and increase production of disease-fighting proteins. Focusing on things we find meaningful activates a region of the brain called the ventral striatum and reduces activity in the amygdala. This in turn lowers levels of the stress hormone cortisol. Purpose can also slow down ageing and shield our DNA from damage by strengthening what are known as telomeres — the caps on the ends of our chromosomes.

If I had to choose the most important piece in the brain-boosting puzzle, it would be cultivating a sense of purpose. All the other puzzle pieces link back to purpose. When we have purpose, we have more energy and greater life satisfaction. We're naturally inclined to help others. We're motivated to learn new things and we're proactive about staying healthy.

There are many ways to foster purpose in our lives. This is not about finding the purpose to one's life. Some people feel they have a specific reason for being in the world and they dedicate their life to it. Fantastic if this is you. For the rest of us, the purpose of life is to live — as fully, vibrantly and exuberantly as we are able. Each day can bring purpose in different ways. Choose anything from the foregoing list, become a volunteer, or simply go outside one evening and observe the waxing moon. **The very pursuit of purpose brings us purpose.**

'Congratulations!' beamed the receptionist at MOW as she handed Dad and me an envelope the following week. 'You both passed *Safe Food Handling Essentials* with flying colours.'

I framed Dad's *Certificate of Completion* and hung it next to his bedroom mirror.

SAFE FOOD HANDLING ESSENTIALS
(SKILLS AND KNOWLEDGE FOR FOOD HANDLERS (FSANZ STANDARD 3.2.2))

CERTIFICATE OF COMPLETION

Ilija Popovic

Has competently completed this training, which is based on:
The Requirements of Food Standards Australia New Zealand, Standard 3.2.2
(Knowledge and Skills of Food Handlers) including:

- Personal Hygiene and Food
- Food Contamination, Temperature and Bacteria Control
- Delivery, Storage and Service of Food
- Food Labeling, Ingredients and Allergens
- Facility Cleaning, Sanitising, Maintenance, Pest and Waste Management

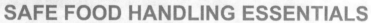

edible
solutions
1300 EDIBLE (334 253)

APPROVED: 13 / 11 / 2014

PART THREE

Let movement be your medicine

I am tomorrow, or some future day, what I establish today.
I am today what I established yesterday or some previous day.

JAMES JOYCE (1882–1941)

CHAPTER 25

No pain, more gain

Those who think they have no time for bodily exercise will sooner or later have to find time for illness.

EDWARD STANLEY (1779–1849)

Sea squirts are colourful marine creatures that begin their life resembling tadpoles. This early stage is referred to as their larval form. They have a tiny brain called a cerebral vesicle with organs that sense light and gravity, and a tail with a nerve cord that enables them to swim. As soon as the larvae find a suitable rock to call home, they attach their head to it and never move again. Lack of movement makes their brain redundant. The sea squirt then dismantles its brain and spinal cord and uses the tissues to develop new body parts. In colloquial terms, it eats its own brain. This is the ultimate example of 'use it or lose it'.

Notwithstanding that a human brain is infinitely more complex than that of a sea squirt, lack of physical movement also results in loss of brain tissue in humans. We were made to move. It's a modern societal phenomenon — not a biological imperative — to become less active as we age. In cultures that maintain their traditional way of life, older people stay physically active until their very last days. They don't go out of their way to exercise, they move in the course of their daily lives — planting crops, visiting neighbours and playing games. The only reason we need to find time to exercise is because modern living has engineered movement out of our lives.

It is well established that **physical exercise is one of the most powerful ways to protect our brain from Alzheimer's**. Brain scans reveal that amyloid beta (Aβ) plaques are associated with far fewer symptoms of Alzheimer's in people who are active. Let me repeat this because the implications are mind-bending (literally): if people are physically active, it buffers them against the damaging effects of Aβ. In addition, regular physical exercise leads to less brain Aβ in the first place, but if Aβ does start accumulating, physical exercise appears to render the Aβ less harmful. This is something that no drug to date has been able to achieve.

Here are the equations:
- Aβ + sedentary lifestyle = enhanced risk of Alzheimer's
- Aβ + regular physical exercise = a brain that is protected against Alzheimer's
- regular physical exercise = less Aβ in the first place.

Perhaps the most striking discovery is that **exercise can modify the impact of Alzheimer's-related genes**. People who are born with one or two copies of the APOE4 gene[1] (which is associated with a greater likelihood of developing Alzheimer's) nullify their increased risk if they exercise. **Movement really is medicine.**

Consider two more equations:
- APOE4 gene + sedentary lifestyle = increased risk for developing Alzheimer's
- APOE4 gene + regular physical exercise = NO increased risk for developing Alzheimer's.

This is great news and spawns a number of important questions:
1. What exactly do we mean by regular physical exercise?
2. Is physical exercise the same as physical activity?
3. How much exercise do we need to do? How often and for how long?
4. How intense does the exercise need to be?
5. What type of exercise is best for the brain?
6. Is walking better than weightlifting? Is cycling better than stretching?
7. Are 10,000 steps per day enough to ward off Alzheimer's?
8. How does exercise exert its manifold effects on the brain?

---

[1] For a detailed discussion of APOE genes, see Chapter 12 'To test or not to test?' and Chapter 13 'Genes are like teens'.

9. If you haven't exercised for decades, is it too late to start? Are you ever too old to exercise or past the point of being able to make a difference?
10. What if you're confined to a wheelchair?

These are questions that scientists all over the world are expeditiously tackling because the answers will transform our lives. I'll discuss our current state of knowledge pertaining to each question in the chapters that follow. Even though we don't know every detail, we know more than enough to begin boosting our brains through physical exercise. We can't let what we *don't* know stop us from putting into practice what we *do* know. So let's get started!

First and foremost, **ANY physical activity/exercise is better than NO physical activity/exercise.** The greatest gains occur when someone goes from doing nothing to doing something — even just a few minutes a day. The two most critical factors are:
1. Doing something you enjoy — viewing exercise as play, not work.
2. Doing something you can sustain on a regular basis — preferably daily or at least every other day.

Replace the mantra 'no pain, no gain' with the more helpful maxims 'no pain, *more* gain' and 'fun, not force'. If exercise is a stressful or negative experience, we produce excessive amounts of the hormone cortisol. High levels of cortisol impede neuroplasticity and block the brain-benefits of exercise. No pain really does mean more gain. Furthermore, if you don't enjoy something, you're unlikely to sustain it over the long term. Of course, any exercise imposes a degree of stress on the body. That's one of the reasons it strengthens our immune system and protects us from cancer and chronic diseases. But like any medicine, we need to get the dose right. So what is the optimal dose of exercise?

Researchers from the University of South Australia performed a series of experiments involving 128 people whose brains were monitored after different patterns of aerobic exercise (anything that raises our heart rate) on treadmills and stationary bikes. They found that:
• 25 minutes of walking, jogging or cycling at moderate intensity or
• 20 minutes of alternating high and low intensity — known as High Intensity Interval Training (HIIT)

produced equivalent brain-benefits. This supports the World Health Organisation (WHO) and most government recommendations that people need to engage in 30 minutes of moderate intensity aerobic exercise at least five days per week. How do we put these findings and recommendations into practice?

If you can only manage to walk to your front gate and back, do it. Don't think that it's too little to make a difference. It *will* make a difference. **Once you start, you'll have something to build on**. It might be one minute per day the first week, 90 seconds per day the second week and two minutes per day the third week. If you increase your exercise time by just 30 seconds a day each week, you'll reach the recommended **150 minutes per week** within 10 months. That means you can revolutionise your health and dramatically reduce your risk of Alzheimer's (and heart disease and diabetes and cancer) in just 10 months — starting with as little as one minute of exercise a day and increasing by a mere 30 seconds a day every week. This will get you to 21 and a half minutes per day, which adds up to 150 minutes per week. If Dad and I could do it, so can you. Even if you never reach 150 minutes of moderate intensity aerobic exercise per week, whatever you achieve will benefit your brain as well as your body.

What is meant by moderate intensity? The simplest way to gauge the intensity of physical exercise is by applying **The Talk Test**. Remember that intensity is relative. A walk around the block would be low intensity for an athlete but high intensity for a beginner. What matters is how *you* perceive the activity. Work to your level and you'll receive the promised benefits.

- If you can continue talking and singing while exercising, you are at low intensity.
- If you can talk but not sing, you are at moderate intensity.
- If you can only get a few words out before needing to catch your breath, you are exercising at high intensity.

If you like the idea of HIIT, alternate 30 seconds to a few minutes of high intensity walking, jogging, cycling, swimming, rowing, dancing, etc. with a few minutes of low to moderate intensity. Games like tennis, squash and soccer are a natural form of HIIT. Even just incorporating one bout of high intensity in the middle of a moderate intensity workout will give your brain and body an added boost. Many people find HIIT to be exhilarating and highly satisfying.

If you have a fitness tracker that measures your heart rate and oxygen consumption, by all means use it to determine your intensity. But you don't need fancy gadgets to get fit.

With respect to accomplishing 150 minutes of aerobic exercise per week, is it better to do:
- 50 minutes of exercise three times per week?
- 30 minutes of exercise five times per week?
- 21 and a half minutes of exercise seven days per week?

Research to date suggests that the three regimens are equally effective.

What about shorter bouts of exercise several times a day? It depends on the intensity. If you remain at moderate intensity, it takes a minimum of 10 minutes to trigger biochemical benefits. If you can push yourself to reach high intensity (after you've built up your fitness), doing HIIT or SIT (Sprint Interval Training) for only a few minutes will provide enormous boosts to your brain and body. Warning: SIT is definitely not for the faint-hearted (literally) and requires a well-defined and supervised approach until you really know what you're doing. It involves going all out (getting completely breathless) for 20 to 40 seconds and then walking or pedalling very slowly for several minutes until you get your breath back. This can be fatal if you're just starting out. Please consult your doctor as well as a personal trainer or exercise physiologist before you try SIT.

One morning, the delightful Melanie from Daughterly Care turned up shortly after I'd demonstrated HIIT and SIT to Dad. Daughterly Care is an in-home aged care provider servicing the Sydney metropolitan area. Melanie was Dad's surrogate daughter while I was at work. Her patience, sense of humour and penchant for practical jokes meant the two of them hit it off from day one. I felt completely at ease when I knew Dad was with Melanie.

'What have you been up to this morning?' she smiled at him disarmingly.

'My daughter and I did a SHIT together,' he replied earnestly.

Melanie's smile quickly metamorphosed into consternation. I wanted the floor to open up and swallow me.

'It's not the way it sounds,' I desperately tried to salvage the most embarrassing of moments. 'He's mixed up the terms HIIT and SIT.'

Melanie raised her eyebrows.

'HIIT stands for High Intensity Interval Training and SIT refers to Sprint Interval Training. Dad has mistakenly spliced the two acronyms together …' my voice trailed off.

'Don't worry, I'll get the full story out of your dad,' she winked at him as I scurried out of the house. But I digress …

Is 180 minutes per week better than 150 minutes? Probably. But don't sweat it (pun intended) if 150 minutes is as much as you can manage. We know that 150 minutes is boosting your brain. Do more if you want and if it brings you pleasure.

What about different types of exercise? Is aerobic exercise (the type of exercise I've been discussing so far) the only form of exercise that matters to our brain or is strength training equally important? Spoiler alert: strength training is equally important. **Strengthening our muscles strengthens our mind.** But don't panic — strength training is not as arduous or time-consuming as it sounds. More on this anon.

Is physical activity the same as physical exercise? What about stretching and toning?

The terms 'physical exercise' and 'physical activity' are often used interchangeably but they're not exactly the same.

Physical activity is anything we do that involves moving our body. It can be low, moderate or high intensity and includes walking, cycling, swimming, stair climbing, dancing, bowling, vacuuming, mopping, sweeping, raking, gardening, shovelling, dusting or picking up a child. Different types of physical activity engage different muscles, require different levels of exertion and confer different benefits. Variety is good for both brain and body. Over the course of a month, Dad and I managed to engage in all of the above — apart from picking up stray children. When people's physical activity was tracked continuously with an actigraph (a device that is similar to a fitness tracker or pedometer), those who moved at moderate intensity for more than 150 minutes per week scored higher in a range of cognitive tests than those who moved less vigorously and didn't reach the 150-minute mark. Therefore, even non-specific physical activity is beneficial for the brain. If you move furniture for a living, you can probably tick all the boxes in Chapter 33 'Your anti-Alzheimer's physical exercise plan'.

Physical exercise, on the other hand, is structured physical activity with the goal of improving health or aiding recovery from injury. Most of the research on brain health has focused on physical exercise rather than physical activity because exercise is more specific and easier to measure. The important thing is to understand the principles that underpin the brain-benefits of different types of movement. This will enable you to create an effective and varied program that best suits your likes and lifestyle.

There are four components of physical exercise, each of which plays a unique and synergistic role in keeping our brain at its best. The four components of exercise are:

1. **stamina** = aerobic or endurance training such as walking, running, cycling, rowing, swimming, ice skating, tennis, basketball, badminton, dancing and CrossFit. This list is far from exhaustive. The longer you can sustain an activity at a given intensity, the greater your stamina and cardiovascular fitness. Stamina is what most people are referring to when they use the word 'exercise'. It's what I've been writing about so far.

2. **strength** = lifting weights, carrying groceries, climbing stairs, pole dancing or performing exercises against resistance. The resistance can be provided by dumbells, machines, bands, walls or your own body weight, e.g. holding a squat or doing push-ups. Strength training is discussed in Chapters 27 and 28, 'Resistance is not futile' and 'Get a grip'.

3. **stability** = practising good balance and reducing the risk of falls. Discussed in Chapter 30 'Tip the balance'.

4. **stretching** = maintaining flexibility to reduce the risk of injury.

There are also five supporting factors that help you attain maximal benefit from whatever exercise you choose to do. These factors are:

1. **sit less** = avoid long hours of complete inactivity. Apart from sitting being dubbed 'the new smoking', prolonged sitting negates some of the benefits of exercise by stimulating production of inflammatory chemicals and switching off fat metabolism — even after an hour of moderate intensity running. Discussed in Chapter 26 'Jack-in-the-box'.

2. **step it up** = take as many steps as you can throughout the course of your day. Use the stairs instead of the escalator or elevator. Just because you've done your 50, 30 or 21 and a half minutes of aerobic exercise, doesn't mean you can stop moving for the rest of the day. Discussed in Chapter 29 'Step it up'.

3. **socialise** = when exercise is a social activity, it provides greater brain-benefits than exercising alone. It's also more enjoyable and we're more likely to keep our commitment to exercising because we don't like to let others down.

4. **smile** = make it fun. Engage in exercise that puts a smile, not a scowl, on your face.

5. **spend time outdoors** = if you can exercise in nature, you'll receive additional brain gains. Not only do you get all the health benefits of fresh air, sunlight, flora and salubrious microorganisms, it is often more challenging to exercise outdoors because you need to deal with uneven surfaces and wind resistance. Walking the dog, visiting your local botanical gardens or yoga in the park are all great options. Discussed in Chapter 76 'Have you tried forest bathing?'.

All the different components and supporting factors begin with the letter S so they're easy to remember. Many types of exercise such as dancing, cycling, CrossFit, martial arts, gym classes and yoga incorporate more than one component so you don't have to make time for four different training regimes. Or you might divide your weekly exercise schedule between the four components as follows:

- 150 minutes of moderate intensity aerobic exercise +
- two sessions of strength training for 20–40 minutes each +
- balance and stretching exercises for a few minutes at the end of your aerobic and strength training sessions. Alternatively, you

can take specific classes such as yoga and Pilates, either live or online. You can also practise balancing and stretching while watching TV or sitting at a desk (an excellent way to break up sitting time).

Don't be afraid to join a team sport or try something you've never done before. Learning new skills — whether it's dance steps or volleyball moves — is another powerful way to boost our brain. As for the five supporting factors, they're simply about making brain-boosting tweaks to our daily lives.

The various components and factors work together to help us live longer, stronger, healthier and happier. They are also critical to preventing Alzheimer's. Instead of viewing it as a chore, turn exercise into an exciting, enjoyable, fulfilling project. Chapter 33 'Your anti-Alzheimer's physical exercise plan' summarises what each component and factor entail. The rest of this chapter is dedicated to stamina.

Stamina is the component of exercise that has been researched the most extensively and is referred to as aerobic or cardiovascular fitness (CVF). A 44-year study of Swedish women found that the greater a woman's cardiovascular fitness in midlife, the lower her risk of Alzheimer's and other dementias as she aged. At the start of the study, CVF was assessed by how long a woman could pedal against increasing resistance on an exercise bike. Based on the results, the women were classified as having high, medium or low CVF. Forty-four years later, *those with the highest CVF were 11 times less likely to have dementia* than those with the lowest CVF! In addition, the few women with high CVF who developed dementia were nine and a half years older than the unfit women when symptoms appeared. So, if you're destined to get dementia despite your best efforts, exercise will delay the onset of the disease by almost 10 years!

Similar results were found by the Cooper Center Longitudinal Study in the US in which midlife CVF was tested in men using a treadmill. Twenty-four years later, those with high CVF were substantially less likely to have dementia. Countless other studies throughout the world support these findings.

Does this mean that if you weren't pounding the pavement or riding your bike in your 20s, 30s and 40s, you've missed the prevention boat? No! Countless experiments in which sedentary people were taught to safely exercise (known as intervention studies) demonstrated that **it's never too late to improve your brain function through physical movement.**

Researchers at the University of Texas Southwestern Medical Center recruited 30 people with an average age of 66 who had mild cognitive impairment (MCI = a precursor of Alzheimer's) and did no regular exercise. At the start of the study they underwent MRI brain scans and memory tests. They were then randomly assigned to an aerobic exercise group or a stretching and balance group. After 12 months of regular exercise, the aerobic group improved their memory scores by 47% while the stretching group showed only minimal improvement. This was supported by repeat MRI scans that demonstrated increased blood flow to areas of the brain associated with memory — the prefrontal and anterior cingulate cortex — in the aerobic group but not the stretching group. This is not to say that stretching has no value. Stretching nonetheless halted further deterioration but to *improve* memory — even after signs of decline — aerobic exercise is a must.

A similar study at the same university revealed that when sedentary 70-year-olds engaged in 30 minutes of aerobic exercise three times per week for 12 months, it slowed shrinkage of their hippocampus — another region of the brain critical to memory. Other studies have shown that **even just a half-hour walk a day — or every other day — keeps memory loss away.**

Meanwhile, researchers at the University of Wisconsin found that six months of moderate intensity aerobic exercise three times per week improved brain glucose metabolism and executive function (the ability to plan, problem-solve and follow instructions) in previously inactive people with a high risk of Alzheimer's due to family history and genetics.

Across the border at Canada's McMaster University, 95 healthy young male and female adults enhanced their memory after only six weeks of intensive daily aerobic exercise. Those who improved their CVF by the greatest degree also had the biggest increase in brain-derived neurotrophic factor (BDNF)—a protein that stimulates the growth of new brain cells and strengthens connections between them. Just as you're never too old or too ill to boost your brain, you're never too young or too healthy either.

You're also never too busy to exercise — as little as 10 minutes of exercise can give your brain an immediate boost. Researchers at Western University in Canada measured reaction times in healthy young adults during a mentally challenging eye movement task. They were then randomly asked to either sit and read a magazine or ride a stationary bike at moderate to vigorous intensity for 10 minutes. Immediately after they finished reading or exercising, their reaction times were retested. Those who had exercised performed the cognitive task with greater speed and accuracy than they had 10 minutes earlier. This translates into having sharper focus and better problem-solving skills. Those who had been reading showed no improvement. Thus 10 minutes of exercise will actually save you time because you'll get through your to-do list more quickly and efficiently.

I could fill this book with study after study confirming the same key messages:

- The earlier you incorporate regular aerobic exercise into your life, the lower your risk of developing any type of dementia, especially Alzheimer's and vascular dementia.
- It's never too late for exercise to boost brain function, even after you've started having memory problems.
- As little as 10 minutes of aerobic exercise makes a positive difference to your mind and mood.
- The best exercise for your brain is whatever you enjoy doing most.

What are you waiting for?

CHAPTER 26

Jack-in-the-box

Tell me and I forget, teach me and I remember,
involve me and I learn.

BENJAMIN FRANKLIN (1706–1790)

'My daughter always wanted a Jack-in-the-box,' Dad was solemnly telling Melanie. 'I searched all the toy shops but never found one. She's now wreaking her revenge.' Dad was referring to my prompting him to stand up every half hour.

Melanie had arrived to take him to our local Japanese gardens. She tilted her head in my direction, inviting me to explain.

'Prolonged sitting leads to brain atrophy,' I began.

'Brain what?' Dad interrupted.

'Atrophy. It means shrinkage or deterioration.'

'Then why didn't you say so in the first place? Melanie isn't impressed with your fancy medical terms,' he winked at her. 'How can sitting cause brain shrinkage? It sounds like nonsense.'

'Scientists who are much smarter than me have assessed that at least 20% of Alzheimer's cases are attributable to sedentary lifestyles. That means one in five cases of the disease are due to sitting down for too many hours a day. Mathematicians then calculated that if we all reduced sedentary habits by 25%, we could prevent more than one million cases of Alzheimer's globally. And exercising for at least 150 minutes per week — that's 30 minutes five days a week — can reduce the risk of Alzheimer's by 45%.'

'You didn't answer my question. **HOW can sitting cause brain shrinkage?**'

'High resolution MRI scans allow researchers to measure the thickness of a part of the brain called the medial temporal lobe (MTL). This area of the brain contains the hippocampus, which is critical for memory. If your hippocampus gets damaged you can't remember what you did or where you went from one day to the next. A study of men and women aged between 45 and 75 revealed that the more hours they spent sitting every day, the thinner their medial temporal lobe and the worse their memory.'

'You should have been a politician,' Dad pronounced. 'I'll give you one more chance to answer the question of HOW sitting can possibly make my brain shrink.'

'Sitting for long periods disrupts blood glucose regulation, reduces blood flow to the brain, raises blood pressure and promotes inflammation. All of these conditions are damaging to the brain.'

'I've heard that **sitting is the new smoking**,' Melanie corroborated.

'Yes, that's right. The more of our life we spend sitting, the shorter our predicted lifespan. When Harvard University researchers analysed the most common causes of death worldwide in the 21st century, they concluded that prolonged inactivity kills more than five million people every year. Not moving leads to damage and dysfunction on many levels. Sitting is also linked to depression, diabetes, obesity and heart disease, all of which further increase the risk of dementia.'

Dad suddenly became serious. 'So why do children spend most of their day sitting at a desk? Why do workplaces not encourage people to stand up?'

'They're very good questions, Dad. I think many people still aren't aware of the hazards of prolonged sitting, especially in relation to their brain. Or they believe that going to the gym for an hour after work reverses the harm caused by sitting.'

'You mean it doesn't?' Melanie's eyes widened. 'Are you saying that even if I go for an hour's walk or bike ride every day, my brain will still shrink if I sit for the rest of the day?'

'Yes. The latest research suggests that daily exercise can offset some — but not all — of the hazards of prolonged sitting. People who have desk jobs and take a daily walk, jog, cycle, swim or dance class have less brain shrinkage than people who sit and do no exercise. **Physical exercise builds brain as well as brawn**. However, if you want your brain to work at its best, break up your sitting in addition to doing regular exercise. Sitting makes us physically and mentally sluggish. Try the following experiment. When you know you'll be spending a long time at your desk, commit to standing for two minutes every 20 minutes. Set a timer so that you don't forget. At the end of the day, assess how you feel and how productive you've been. People are mentally sharper throughout the day if they interrupt their sitting time.'

'Does it matter how one sits? For example, the Japanese do a lot of kneeling. Is that any better than sitting in a chair?'

'Great question, Melanie, and yes, **how we sit makes a difference**. When we sit in a chair, we turn off the muscles in our core and legs which means we no longer need to provide those muscles with fuel. This leads to a build-up of fats — specifically triglycerides — in our blood because the fats aren't being used by our muscles. High levels of circulating triglycerides contribute to heart disease. On the other hand, when we kneel or squat, our muscles remain activated. When scientists gave people in the Hazda community of Tanzania wearable sensors, they found that squatting — their way of resting — generates up to 10 times more leg muscle activity than sitting in a chair. It also requires balance and flexibility. This coincided with low blood triglyceride levels and healthy blood vessels. Kneeling also requires more energy than sitting. The most interesting finding was that Hazda people don't spend more time running or walking than the average Westerner. The difference is that Hazda people don't have chairs and they spend their downtime squatting or kneeling.'

'But squatting and kneeling are uncomfortable. I doubt I'd last more than a few minutes,' Melanie lamented.

'I agree. Unless you've grown up practising those postures, they can be quite painful. I've been making an effort to kneel while I type. When I get sore I switch back to my standing desk.'

'What about bus drivers and judges who have no choice but to sit for prolonged periods?'

'If I were a judge, I'd periodically raise my heels and tense my quads and gluteal muscles. Bus drivers are in an even trickier situation.'

'How are you defining prolonged sitting? How much is too much?'

'More than four hours of non-stop sitting every day starts to increase our risk of chronic disease. The effect then becomes dose-dependent. Eight hours of sitting a day increases our risk of early death by 15%. Eleven hours of sitting a day increases our chance of dying prematurely by 40%. The younger you are when you adopt a sedentary lifestyle, the sooner you'll start having health problems. As Dad mentioned, it isn't good for children to be sitting either. But the good news is that you can stop the damage by standing up for two minutes every 20 to 30 minutes.'

'That's a lot of standing! It's a big cultural shift for organisations to adopt,' she reflected.

'Yes, it is. But if they're sold on the benefits, they'll make it happen. Standing up every half hour boosts concentration, creativity and efficiency. Counterintuitive as it sounds, people also report feeling less tired at the end of the day. It's because their brains are working better and their bodies aren't inflamed. In 2018, Apple CEO Tim Cook announced that everyone at the company's new headquarters would get a standing desk. Other big-name businesses are doing the same. If something is important enough — if decision-makers discover that it impacts the bottom line — they'll make the necessary changes. Standing up doesn't mean taking a two-minute work break three times an hour. You can continue reading, typing or talking on the phone. By all means have a stretch, do some squats or run on the spot if you want, but just getting up on your feet breaks the cycle. Surveys indicate that meetings are more effective if people stand rather than sit. Participants are more focused and engaged, and issues get resolved more quickly. Anyone who has ever run a standing meeting says they'd never go back to having chairs.'

'What about lying down? I don't mean when we go to sleep, but when we want to read or listen to music. Is lying any less of a health hazard than sitting?'

'If you're not activating your muscles, lying has a similar effect to sitting. People confined to bedrest lose bone and muscle and increase their risk of heart disease. That's why it's important to have a physiotherapist or whoever is looking after them to move their muscles while they're in bed.'

'I have a simple solution for all the workers,' Dad chimed in. 'A bell.'

'A bell?' I echoed.

'Yes,' he said. 'A bell needs to ring every half hour in every school, office, factory and courthouse. In every building in the world — even in libraries and churches. People would soon get used to it and no one would think twice about it.'

'What a great idea!' I enthused. 'If a bell signals everyone to stand up, no one feels self-conscious and no one stops working. We need an education campaign to get decision-makers onboard with it.'

'Aren't you supposed to be educating people?' he bantered, 'So get educating.'

'Well, you've certainly educated *me*!' Melanie affirmed. 'I'm going to buy my son a standing desk. He's studying law and spends all day sitting down. How expensive are they?'

'Mine was less than $80 but you can spend thousands. It depends on the features you're looking for.' I went to the study to bring her the small adjustable standing desk that cradled my laptop.

'You don't need to spend any money,' Dad declared. 'Just find a crate or sturdy box and turn it upside down on your existing desk.'

'It might not be the right height,' Melanie was contemplating Dad's suggestion.

'Bring me a saw and I'll cut the crate to whatever size you want,' Dad offered with a broad smile.

'How can I refuse that smile?' Melanie responded warmly. 'Let's you and I go to the Japanese gardens and see if we might pick up a crate along the way.'

* * * * *

Unfortunately, Dad remembered nothing of our conversation the following day. He was back to his sudoku in his comfortable armchair. I was back to finding excuses to get him on his feet.

Dad, can you check the mail please?

Dad, can you help me unload the dishwasher?

Dad, can you boil the kettle please?

Dad, let's throw some quoits.

Dad, can you help me sweep the floor?

Dad, can you bring me that book?

Dad, can you help me find my phone?

Dad, let's have a game of darts.

Dad, can you check the mail please?

Dad, can you help me unload the dishwasher?

Dad, can you boil the kettle please?

Memory loss sometimes had its advantages. I could cycle through the same set of excuses several times a day without him remembering. I sighed. I'd have given anything for him to catch me out.

CHAPTER 27

Resistance is not futile

Some men see things as they are and say 'Why?'
Others dream things that never were and say 'Why not?'

GEORGE BERNARD SHAW (1856–1950)

Late one autumn evening in November 2019, 82-year-old grandmother Willie Murphy was startled by a loud knock at the front door of her home in Rochester, New York. As she approached the door, the pounding escalated and a man called out to her, 'I'm sick, I'm sick. Please call an ambulance!'

She promptly dialled the police but before she could finish the call, the man broke down the door and started charging towards her. She immediately dropped the phone and did what any five-foot (1.5 metre), 105-pound (48 kg) octogenarian would do. She grabbed the nearest table and smashed it over his head. When he fell to the floor, she squirted a bottle of shampoo in his face and then jumped on him while jabbing him with a broom. By the time the ambulance arrived, he was definitely in need of their services.

What the young man hadn't anticipated was that Willie Murphy was an award-winning bodybuilder. In 2018 — at the age of 81 — she won all her events at the World Natural Powerlifting Federation (WNPF) Upstate New York Championships and in 2014 she was WNPF Lifter of the Year. She can deadlift 225 pounds (102 kg) — more than twice her weight — and her training includes one-arm push-ups, fingertip push-ups and one-arm pull-ups. When she started a decade ago, she could barely lift five pounds (2.3 kg). Today, she confidently shovels thick snow from her driveway in winter and is able to push her car if it gets stuck. She can also sprint 100 metres in 14 seconds. When she ran out of room for her trophies at home, she started displaying them at the YMCA where she trains. But it's not about the trophies, Willie beams. It's about inspiring women, seniors and people of colour, like herself, to take up exercise and take control of their health.

Seventy-seven-year-old Australian bodybuilder Janice Lorraine has the same attitude. At the age of 55 she noticed a frail old woman struggling to shuffle across a car park and decided she would not allow herself to go down the same path. She'd heard that resistance training was good for maintaining bone density and preventing osteoporosis so she ventured into the weightlifting room at her local gym and has never looked back. The grandmother of three has accrued 23 bodybuilding titles from around the world, was a contestant on *Australia's Got Talent* and plans to train for as long as she lives. Her aim is to show others what's possible and to encourage women of any age to live a life unbounded by stereotypes.

It isn't only older women who are breaking barriers and conventions. When Raymond Moon contracted polio as a child, doctors thought he would never walk again. Instead, at the age of 84 he became the world's oldest competing bodybuilder for which he was awarded the Guinness World Record in 2009. He achieved this after giving up decades of heavy drinking and cigar smoking. Age and past experiences do not have to limit us.

This is not to say we all need bulging biceps and palpable pecs. We simply need to maintain our strength and stop our muscles from wasting away. Why? If we don't use our muscles to lift, carry, push and pull, we start losing strength as early as our mid-30s. The medical term for loss of strength is dynapenia. It comes from the Greek words *dynamos* meaning 'power, force, ability' and *penia* meaning 'poverty'. This is usually, but not always, accompanied by loss of muscle — also from our 30s onwards — at a rate of 5% every decade and even more rapidly after the age of 70. The medical term for muscle loss is sarcopenia — from the Greek word *sark* meaning 'flesh'.

The good news is that neither dynapenia nor sarcopenia are inevitable if we continue to put our muscles to work. But what does brawn have to do with brain?

Most people are familiar with the gut brain connection: the ongoing two-way communication between our brain and our gut. It turns out there's also **a strong muscle–brain connection with ongoing communication between our muscles and our brain.** Thus, dynapenia has been linked to poorer cognition and larger amounts of amyloid beta (Aβ) in the brain while sarcopenia contributes to insulin resistance.

People with stronger leg muscles (quadriceps) score higher in a variety of tests that assess brain function. The same is found in people with stronger hand muscles. Fortunately, **after just three months of resistance training, weaker subjects not only became physically stronger, they improved their mental capabilities.** Reversing dynapenia and sarcopenia also reduces the risk of heart disease, stroke and type 2 diabetes, all of which are significant risk factors for Alzheimer's and vascular dementia.

Even a single bout of high intensity resistance training enhances our ability to process complex information and improves reaction time and accuracy in mentally challenging tasks. Before your next job interview or attempt at Ikea furniture assembly, you might like to pump some iron.

Does resistance training work for everyone? It certainly seems to. Researchers have tested male and female, young and old, healthy and frail — including people with mild cognitive impairment (MCI) and in early stages of dementia. The programs involved one to three 30-to-40-minute strength training sessions per week for a few months up to one year. All participants enhanced their executive functioning — reasoning, planning, problem-solving and memory. Those who did two sessions per week had greater improvements than those who only did one session per week. Those who did three sessions per week improved the most.

How do stronger muscles create a stronger mind? Putting our muscles to work (through both aerobic and resistance training) releases a cascade of proteins such as BDNF, IGF-1, VEGFA and

irisin.[2] These proteins travel to the brain where they stimulate:
- neurogenesis (growth of new brain cells)
- synaptogenesis (development of new connections between brain cells)
- angiogenesis (growth of new blood vessels in the brain)
- repair and survival of existing brain cells
- repair and strengthening of connections between brain cells
- removal of toxins, including $A\beta$ plaques
- enhanced insulin sensitivity.

In addition, physical exercise dampens down inflammation and improves brain glucose metabolism. This means the brain is better able to use glucose to carry out its various activities. As you'll recall from Chapter 16 'What's happening to the brain?' one of the problems in Alzheimer's is a decrease in the brain's ability to utilise glucose for fuel. This leads to progressive deterioration in many areas of the brain. **We don't get weak as we age. We age if we allow ourselves to get weak.**

Exercise even stimulates our liver to produce proteins that boost our brain. In a fascinating study by scientists at the University of California in San Francisco, older mice were given either a running wheel or nesting articles. Six weeks later, the exercising mice showed increased neurogenesis in their hippocampus accompanied by improvements in their memory, while the sedentary mice showed no increases in these areas. When the sedentary mice were then given blood transfusions from the exercising mice, they too grew new neurons in their hippocampus and performed better in tests of learning and memory without having to do any exercise themselves! When researchers examined the blood from exercising mice, they discovered that a protein made by the liver called Gpld1 was responsible for the brain-benefits. Turning their attention to humans, they found that Gpld1 is also found in the blood of physically active older adults. The more we

---

[2] BDNF stands for brain-derived neurotrophic factor.
IGF-1 stands for insulin-like growth factor 1.
VEGFA stands for vascular endothelial growth factor A.
These are the proteins that have been most studied in relation to the brain-benefits of exercise.
There are many more factors at play, but they are beyond the scope of this book.

study the link between physical exercise and brain health, the more brain-boosting pathways we uncover.

Phew! Who would have thought a bit of huffing and puffing (aerobic exercise) and grunting and groaning (resistance training) could have such far-reaching brain-benefits? Physical exercise not only protects our brain from decline, it actually increases the size of our prefrontal cortex and hippocampus (our memory and learning warehouse) — two key areas that are damaged in Alzheimer's. What were Dad and I waiting for?

At the age of 78, I bought him his first ever gym membership. 'You've got to be joking,' was his less than enthusiastic response.

'A gym is an adult playground,' I encouraged.

'I'd have thought "torture chamber" was a more accurate description.'

'Oh no, definitely not! A gym is where we wake up our muscles, learn new skills and simply have fun.'

'You have a warped sense of fun. Sometimes I wonder where I went wrong with you. Didn't I play enough games with you when you were a child? Don't you remember playing Monopoly, chess, backgammon, dominoes, ping pong and card games? I pushed you on swings, caught you at the bottom of slippery dips and built sandcastles with you at the beach. Didn't that teach you what constituted fun?'

'Fun comes in many forms. I don't see why playing with levers and pulleys at the gym is any less fun than bouncing on a seesaw. It's physically exhilarating. The problem with gyms is poor marketing. They should be advertised as places to play, not work. Who wants to have a workout after work? After a hard day at the office, most people want to relax and have fun, not do something because they "should". Moving our muscles is simultaneously relaxing and stimulating. It releases a cocktail of feel-good chemicals. Regrettably, our culture has created a negative mindset around gyms and exercise. Your response is very much the norm.'

'Moving our muscles is tiring,' he pronounced.

'Everything we do is potentially tiring. Life is tiring. But if you enjoy something, you don't notice that it's tiring. Let's see if we can find something at the gym that you'll enjoy. New experiences are exciting. If you don't find it fun, you don't have to keep going. I promise.'

CHAPTER 28

Get a grip

Hang on to your youthful enthusiasms — you'll be able to use them better when you're older.

SENECA (4 BCE – 65 CE)

'Can I interest you in a test of your handgrip strength?' invited the broad-shouldered, jaunty personal trainer at the entrance to our gym.

Definitely, I thought, this is exactly the information that Dad and I needed. Grip strength is a reflection of muscle strength in general and an undervalued tool for assessing a person's risk for future disease. **Low grip strength is consistently associated with poorer quality of life and a shorter life expectancy.** Besides, who was I to argue with Hercules?

'Why not?' I steered Dad towards him.

'I don't like tests,' Dad resisted.

'Hi, I'm Paul.' He tried to shake Dad's hand. It was before the days of COVID-19.

Dad reeled away from him. 'I'm not having him test my grip strength. He'll crush my hand!'

'I won't be using my hand to test you,' Paul laughed. 'I've got an instrument called a handgrip dynamometer. Let me show you.'

'Why? What's the point?' asked Dad.

'Handgrip strength indicates how strong the muscles in your hands, wrists and forearms are. You need those muscles to open jars, turn door handles and hold on to shopping bags and stair rails.'

'I can do all that already. I don't need a test to prove it,' Dad contended.

'I'm sure you can.' Hercules was unfazed.

'Be careful,' Dad warned me in Serbian. 'He's going to try and sell you something. He'll tell you that you're abnormally weak and then offer you some fancy jar-opening device. I wasn't born yesterday.'

Paul continued affably, impervious to Dad's disdain. 'Apart from being essential for everyday life — and assuming you haven't injured your hand recently — grip strength reflects your overall muscle strength and bone mineral density (BMD). If your grip is weak, I'd recommend you have a DEXA scan to test for osteoporosis. Studies that track people over many years show that poor grip strength is also predictive of a higher risk of dying from heart disease and cancer.'

'Why? What does the strength of my fingers have to do with the health of my heart?' Dad started to show a flicker of interest.

'When you activate your muscles, they send messages to different organs in your body to keep them in good working order. If you have weak muscles and need to undergo surgery for any reason, there's a greater chance you'll have complications and a slower recovery. Overall, stronger muscles mean life is more enjoyable because you're able to do more. Of course, you have to take into account a person's age, sex, height, weight and occupation. All those factors impact grip strength. There are tables that list what's optimal for your specific stage of life,' Paul clarified.

'You know your stuff.' I was impressed.

'I'm an exercise physiologist. I spend most of my time explaining to people why it's crucial to maintain muscle mass as we age. The World Health Organisation (WHO) and most governments include strength training in their physical activity guidelines. We need at least two sessions of muscle building per week on top of our 150 minutes of aerobic exercise. Unfortunately, the message hasn't yet taken hold with the general public.'

'Strength seems to be even more important than size,' I asserted. 'I think people need to be reassured that they don't need to bulk up to see benefits. If someone equates size with strength they may get discouraged if they don't see changes in the mirror. The best signs of improvement are getting out of a chair with greater ease or lifting progressively heavier weights. Being able to do push-ups is another coup.'

'Yes, push-ups are a great goal,' Paul nodded. 'A 10-year Harvard University study of over 1000 firefighters found that **men who were able to do 40 push-ups in one go had 96% lower risk of heart disease and stroke** compared with men who were unable to achieve 10 push-ups. It's a better predictor of cardiovascular health than treadmill tests.'

'There's no hope for me then,' Dad mused.

'Of course there is,' Paul encouraged. 'Start by doing push-ups against a wall. Let me show you.' Paul placed his palms on the nearest wall and proceeded to do a push-up by leaning forward at 45 degrees.

To my surprise, Dad imitated him.

'Excellent!' Paul praised.

Dad continued until he'd done 10 wall push-ups. 'Is that enough?' Dad looked triumphant.

'If you can do more than 10, you're on your way to reducing your risk of heart disease,' Paul affirmed. 'The Harvard study showed that as soon as you hit 11 non-stop push-ups you start to reduce your risk of cardiovascular disease. Over time it will get easier and you'll naturally want to try the floor. Begin on your knees and eventually progress to your toes.'

Dad did one more wall push-up.

'Great!' Paul grinned. 'Since you accomplished that so well, let me give you another way to bolster your heart. If you can **walk faster than one metre per second** — that's 360 metres in six minutes — you'll halve your risk of heart attack compared with people who are not able to walk as fast. Notwithstanding any injuries that limit mobility, of course.'

'We'll time ourselves on our next walk,' I committed.

'Getting stronger doesn't mean spending hours at the gym,' Paul continued. 'All you need is a few minutes at a time and something for your muscles to lift or push against. Hold a heavy object above your head and raise it up and down. Practise dips using a chair and do squats while watching TV. Hand weights and elastic exercise bands are also very effective — op shops, Gumtree and eBay are full of them.'

'Thank you for the excellent advice,' I was pleased we'd stopped to engage with Paul. 'You're probably familiar with the Health and Retirement Study in the US?' I asked.

'Refresh my memory,' he prompted.

'Nearly 14 000 people aged 50 or older had their handgrip strength and cognition monitored over an eight-year period. Every five kilograms less strength was associated with an incremental drop in mental functioning. It's one of many studies that all reach the same conclusion: **weak handgrip strength is a predictor of cognitive decline.** People who are physically stronger perform better in all tests of brain function — including memory, reaction speed and problem solving. Strength training also reduces depression and anxiety.'

'What's the biological mechanism that links handgrip strength to mental functioning?' I could see Paul joining the dots.

'Maintaining muscle mass protects against insulin resistance and improves the brain's ability to use glucose for energy. As we age, our brain becomes less efficient at metabolising glucose and this reduces overall brain function and speeds up cognitive decline in Alzheimer's. Conversely, strengthening our muscles increases production of neurotransmitters such as brain-derived neurotrophic factor (BDNF), which stimulates growth of new brain cells and strengthens connections between them. In addition, strength training two to three times a week is an established treatment for depression, and depression is a risk factor for Alzheimer's. So anything that improves mood will also improve mental functioning. Everything is interconnected.'

'On the flip side,' Paul added, 'once you start losing strength, it sets off a downward spiral. Mental decline means you're less able to perform daily tasks, which means you're less likely to use your muscles, which leads to further and further weakness.'

'Exactly,' I agreed.

'So who wants to go first?' Paul was ready with his dynamometer.

I turned to Dad. 'I'll go first,' I offered.

Paul placed the instrument in my left hand. 'We'll test both sides but we'll start with your left. No doubt your dominant hand will be stronger. The flat base of the dynamometer should rest on the heel of your hand. Curl your fingers around the lever. Let both your arms hang down against the side of your body. Now lift your left hand in front of you until your elbow is at 90 degrees. That's it. Keep it as close to a right angle as you can. When I count to three, squeeze as hard as you can for five seconds and don't move any other parts of your body. Are you ready?'

We repeated the test three times with each hand and then took an average reading. Dad followed suit. Our results were better than I'd anticipated. Dad was only slightly weaker than average for his age. Asking him to carry the groceries was worth the disdainful looks I frequently received from fellow shoppers. I knew they thought I was a lazy princess for allowing my elderly father to carry our bags. Little did they realise it was part of his weekly strength training.

'Well, that's our 40 minutes at the gym!' Dad declared. 'We can go home now. Thank you for the training, young man!'

CHAPTER 29

Step it up

*One never notices what has been done; one can only see
what remains to be done.*

MARIE CURIE (1867–1934)

'I'm really worried,' Melanie burst through the front gate. She had arrived to take Dad kite flying. He was still in his bedroom deciding which shoes to wear.

'What's happened?' I swung around to see her looking uncharacteristically distraught. She usually brought rays of sunshine with her.

'I've just done the Sit-Stand Test and I couldn't get up. Apparently it means I have a shortened life expectancy.'

'Nonsense!' I shook my head vigorously.

'It's true,' she insisted. 'Everyone in my Pilates class took the test. We were asked to sit down on the floor with our arms stretched out in front of our body and then get up again without using any support. If you needed to use your hands, forearms or knees to help you get up or down, you lost points. You weren't even allowed to put your hands on your knees. And if you were very wobbly, you lost half a point. The lower your score, the more likely you are to die at a younger age. It's based on the findings of a Brazilian study of over 2000 people.'

'Yes, I'm familiar with the research but it needs to be put into context. Firstly, everyone in the study was between 51 and 80 years old. In that age group, not being able to get up and down has different implications to what it means in a younger person like yourself. Basically the test — officially known as the Sitting-Rising Test or SRT for short — measures leg and core strength, balance, flexibility and co-ordination. In an older person, these factors are linked to being able to live independently and avoid falls, which makes the SRT a valuable predictor in the 50+ age group but not so much in a younger person. In addition, if an older person falls, they are much more likely to sustain a serious injury that threatens their life than if a younger person falls. Plus, a young person is less likely to break bones and more likely to make a full recovery if they do. Can you see how the implications are different depending on the age group in question? A low score could also mean arthritis, inner ear problems or a recent knee, hip or back injury.'

'But I haven't had any recent injuries,' she remained dubious.

'Did you try crossing your legs while you were doing the test? Some people find it easier that way — and yes, it's within the rules,' I assured her. 'You can also hold your arms out to your sides to help with balance.'

'OK, I'll try again another day,' she seemed to brighten up.

'You can also improve your score with a few simple exercises that strengthen the necessary muscles.'

'Such as?' She was bouncing back to her sunny self.

'Squats, lunges, push-ups and core work. Not surprisingly, people who practise yoga tend to do better in the SRT than people who don't. Another good exercise is to lie on your stomach with your arms straight out in front of you and your legs stretched out behind you. Look down so you aren't arching your neck or back and then simultaneously lift your opposite arm and leg off the floor for about 10 seconds before swapping sides. Do 10 repetitions on each side, three times a week and watch how you improve on the SRT. The real value of the SRT is to demonstrate the importance of engaging in all four components of physical exercise — strength training, stretching and balance, as well as aerobic activities like walking and cycling. Physical exercise is about being fit for life, not about being fit for show.'

'So attaining full marks in the SRT is still a worthwhile goal?'

'Yes, improving your strength, balance and co-ordination is a worthwhile goal. Just keep in mind that some people's bodies are constructed in a way that makes the SRT very challenging regardless of their level of fitness. Don't get deflated if you never achieve a specific target with respect to physical exercise. We need to **set our sights on progress, not perfection.'**

'I like to have something specific to aim for — such as walking 10 000 steps. I find it motivating.' Melanie admitted.

'Not everyone is motivated by the same thing. Some people love wearing a pedometer because it encourages them to take more steps. Other people say it takes the pleasure out of walking. Do what works for *you* and don't allow one measure of fitness to define you.'

'Your dad enjoys trying to outsmart the pedometer you gave him,' she divulged.

'I know,' I smiled. 'He waits until I leave the room and then gleefully sits in a chair and marches his feet up and down to increase his step count without actually walking. What he doesn't realise is that sitting and lifting his feet is better for his brain than sitting still. I'm happy to play along. It gives me a chance to say to him later, "Well done! You only need to walk a few more steps today before you reach … whatever the next multiple of 1000 happens to be. We might as well finish on a round number." I'll bet he does the same thing when he's sitting on a park bench with you.'

'Yes!' Melanie giggled. 'But aren't you trying to walk 10 000 steps per day? Isn't that the magic number?'

'Not necessarily. The notion of 10 000 daily steps originated from a marketing campaign, not a scientific study. Just prior to the 1964 Tokyo Olympics, a Japanese company created a pedometer called *Manpokei. Man* is the Japanese word for 10 000, *po* means step and *kei* means system. It was a catchy idea and it certainly caught on. Since then, researchers from around the globe have tried to determine the minimum number of steps that yield meaningful gains in health. It turns out the magic number might be 7500. But if you can do more, by all means do more.'

'Why 7500?' Melanie asked.

'A 2019 Harvard Medical School study of 16 700 women with an average age of 72 found that those who took at least 4400 steps per day were 41% less likely to die within the next four years than women who walked less than 2700 steps per day. The more steps they took, the lower their risk of dying until it levelled off at 7500 steps with a 65% reduced mortality rate. Both fast and slow walkers reaped the benefits of taking more steps — but faster is better.'

'That's such an encouraging message,' Melanie looked buoyant. 'I know people who think there's no point unless you reach 10 000 steps. In reality, it sounds like **every extra step is a positive step.**'

'Yes, definitely. A year later, a 10-year study of 4840 US men and women aged 40 years and over also showed that more daily steps translated into living longer. Those who walked 8000 steps were half as likely to die from heart disease, stroke, cancer or chronic diseases than those who walked 4000 steps. Those who achieved 12 000 daily steps dropped their risk of dying to one-third that of 4000-per-day steppers.'

'Why did the two studies show different results?' Melanie queried. 'Admittedly the outcomes are similar but they aren't the same.'

'It may be because participants in the latter study were younger and included men. Also they were followed for twice as many years as participants in the earlier group.'

'Do you prescribe walking to all your patients — assuming they are able to?'

'Yes, if they enjoy it. Any aerobic activity is beneficial. Walking is simply the most convenient. It's particularly important for people with diabetes and obesity. Researchers in Finland demonstrated that obese adults with pre-diabetes showed significant reductions in waist circumference and blood insulin levels when they increased their daily steps from 2800 to 6500. Once again, they did not need to reach 10 000 to substantially improve their health. Meanwhile, an Australian study confirmed that every additional 2000 daily steps improved blood sugar control in people at risk of diabetes.

Those who reach 10 000 daily steps can expect to see a threefold improvement in insulin function compared with people who only manage 3000 steps.'

'I'm assuming that all these steps count towards my 150 minutes of aerobic exercise per week?'

'Yes, of course. Having said that, don't feel compelled to stop moving after you've clocked up 150 minutes. Remember our chat about prolonged sitting? If you exercise for an hour every day but sit for your remaining waking hours, you won't get the full benefits of the exercise. Long periods of sitting switch off enzymes that break down body fat. You don't have to move constantly — just break up your sitting time. It isn't about calories, it's about biochemistry.'

'So where exactly do all these studies leave us in terms of a target number of daily steps?'

'There is no one size — or rather, step count — that fits all. Combining the available data delivers several key messages:
- Any number of daily steps is better than no steps.
- The more steps you take, the healthier you tend to be. That doesn't mean you have to hit 10 000 a day. Do as many as you enjoy. Rats forced to run on a wheel don't experience the same benefits as those who run the same amount by their own volition. **Fun brings more rewards than force.**
- Significant benefits start to accrue from about 5000 steps a day. **A great target is 7500 plus.**
- If you don't like counting steps, don't! Just aim to move for 150 minutes per week.'

CHAPTER 30

Tip the balance

Be kind, for everyone you meet is fighting a great battle.

PHILO OF ALEXANDRIA — ALSO CALLED PHILO JUDAEUS (BORN 25 BCE)

Try the following party trick — but only if you're sober. Find a space within reach of a wall or piece of sturdy furniture and stand unsupported on one leg. When you've established good balance, close your eyes. Does closing your eyes make it harder? When you've re-established your balance, keep your eyes closed and subtract 47 from 673. Continue subtracting 47 from your answer. Does doing arithmetic make it more difficult to balance?

Closing our eyes or attempting something mentally taxing makes it more challenging to balance. Why? For us to balance, our brain integrates constantly changing information from our joints, muscles, eyes and vestibular system (part of our inner ear). We tend to take our balance for granted but it's actually a complex undertaking. Adding another complex task such as arithmetic makes both tasks more effortful.

Poor balance can result from muscle weakness or unstable joints and increases the risk of having a fall. **Falls contribute to head injuries, which contribute to dementia.** Worldwide, falls are the second most common cause of accidental deaths after traffic accidents. Every year, one in three people aged 65 and over have a fall.

Being insecure on our feet is an underrated health hazard. Several studies have shown that 50-plus-year-olds who are unable to stand on one leg for 10 seconds (known as the 10-second one-legged stance or OLS) have a shorter life expectancy than those who can.

The most recent research followed 1702 Brazilian men and women aged 51 to 75 from the years 2008 to 2020. Those who could not complete the 10-second OLS had an 84% higher chance of dying from any cause during the course of the study.

Our mental health also affects our balance. Stress, anxiety, depression and schizophrenia have all been associated with alterations in posture and poorer balance. This is attributed to changes in an area of the brain called the cerebellum, which is responsible for controlling movement as well as regulating thoughts and emotions. Researchers are currently investigating whether improving balance might also improve mental health.

If regaining balance can strengthen multiple regions of the brain, could it also ameliorate the symptoms of Alzheimer's? As yet, we don't know, but the signs are promising. What we *do* know is that improving balance improves overall health, self-confidence and exercise capacity — all of which help to protect against Alzheimer's.

The biggest factors contributing to deteriorating balance are excessive sitting and lack of physical exercise — yet another example of 'use it or lose it'. With each generation, our balance is getting worse at a younger and younger age. Getting old per se does not lead to waning balance; more years of being sedentary is the biggest determinant. Declining balance then becomes a self-perpetuating negative spiral. Poor balance means we are less able to exercise, which means we are less able to maintain good balance.

Fortunately, this is another good news story: we can improve our balance at any age just as we can enhance our strength, flexibility and stamina. People who have specific neuromuscular problems may need to work with a physiotherapist or exercise physiologist. The rest of us can easily incorporate a variety of balance exercises throughout our day. Many of these focus on making our foot and toe muscles stronger. Knowing we have better balance reduces the fear of falling which, in turn, reduces the likelihood of falling. Balance drills — along with stretching and toning — are a good place to start if you haven't exercised in a long time. They are gentle ways of reacquainting your body with movement without risking a heart attack.

Here are some suggestions for improving balance:

- Practise standing on one leg. If you're wobbly, use a wall and progressively release your hold for longer periods of time.
- When you can stand for 30 seconds without support, close your eyes.
- When you can stand for 30 seconds with your eyes closed, increase the time to 60 seconds and challenge yourself with mental arithmetic.
- When you can balance on solid ground, try standing on a BOSU (half spherical exercise ball). BOSU stands for 'both sides up' and refers to the fact that you can use both sides — the dome and the platform. There are many ways to use a BOSU to improve balance as well as other components of fitness. Visit bosu.com for tips and training videos.
- Go barefoot whenever you're at home indoors.
- Go barefoot outdoors as long as you're not likely to step on something that could cause an injury.
- Walk heel-to-toe along a line on the floor.
- Rock forward and back between your toes and heels.
- Take 10 steps on your toes followed by 10 normal steps. Then take 10 steps on your heels followed by 10 normal steps. Keep alternating between toes and heels for a few minutes. You can do this around the house or whenever you go for a walk.
- Walk sideways and alternate crossing one foot in front of the other as you go.
- Calf raises[3] — aim for three sets of 10 or more throughout the day.
- Does your local park have a low balance beam or log you can practise walking on?

---

[3] A calf raise simply involves standing up straight and slowly raising your heels so that you're now on your toes. Hold for two to three seconds then lower your heels back to the ground. Repeat five to 10 times. You can do this while waiting in a queue, brushing your teeth or watching TV. If you want to increase the intensity, here are a few variations:

- hold a weight in each hand while you're doing the exercise
- stand on a step with your heels hanging off the end so that you can drop your heels lower than the rest of your foot
- stand on one foot at a time — this will give your balance an extra boost.

- Pick up a pen or marble with your toes.
- Take up tai chi, Pilates or yoga.

As with all things brain-boosting, make it enjoyable. **Find ways that feel good to move and improve.**

CHAPTER 31

Mind over muscle

The greatest revolution of our times is the discovery that human beings, by changing the inner attitudes of their minds, can change the outer aspects of their lives.

WILLIAM JAMES (1842–1910)

As the preceding chapters indicate, if there's one thing all scientists, researchers, epidemiologists, doctors, psychologists, chiropractors, naturopaths, dietitians, nutritionists, other health professionals and even food companies agree on, it's the brain and body benefits of physical exercise. But what if chronic pain, injury or illness restrict your mobility? Or you simply can't fit anything more into your busy day? Never fear, a solution is here!

Researchers from Edith Cowan University in Western Australia and Niigata University of Health and Welfare in Japan tested the arm strength of young sedentary individuals before assigning them to one of four groups. The first three groups did a single bicep curl for three SECONDS (not minutes, in case you thought it was a typo) five days a week for four weeks. The fourth group did no exercise and served as controls. Each of the three exercise groups performed a different type of bicep curl (elbow flexion and extension).

- Group 1 lifted the heaviest weight they could, by flexing their elbow to their shoulder (known as a maximal concentric curl).
- Group 2 lowered the heaviest weight they could, by extending their elbow towards their thigh (maximal eccentric curl).
- Group 3 held the weight stationary with their elbow at a 90-degree angle (maximal isometric curl).

Did three seconds of exercise a day for one month make any difference? To my astonishment, yes!

Group 1 improved their strength by 6.3%, Group 2 by 11.5% and Group 3 by 7.2%! The control group saw no changes. The key to getting stronger was using the maximum weight the participants could manage and making it a daily habit. So get the heaviest weight you can hold, place it next to your bed and perform a three-second eccentric curl every morning. Done and dusted. Although I haven't come across research testing other muscles for just three seconds, I see no reason why the same wouldn't apply to our legs, back and abdominals. That means you could exercise 10 muscle groups in half a minute. The excuse that 'I don't have time for exercise' doesn't hold weight anymore — pun intended!

In some cases, pain or injury can be so severe that even minimal physical exertion is out of the question. No problem! Professor Brian Clark and his team at Ohio University in the USA tested the arm strength of 29 volunteers before encasing their non-dominant wrist in a surgical cast for one month. Half (14) of the volunteers were then told to spend 11 minutes a day, five days a week, sitting completely still and imagining flexing their immobilised arm. The other 15 participants were not given any particular instructions. When the cast was removed four weeks later, both groups had lost arm strength but those who had been visualising themselves doing arm exercises were twice as strong as those who had done no mental exercises. In other words, those who had done nothing were 45% weaker than they'd been four weeks earlier, while the visualisers were only 25% weaker. How could this be?

Think of the brain as a puppeteer: our nerves as the strings and our muscles as puppets. Even though the participants were not able to physically move their arm, when they visualised flexing their wrist, their brain nonetheless sent electrical signals to their muscles — like a puppeteer pulling on the strings of a puppet that was fixed in place. This strengthened the neural pathways between the brain and muscles (known as neuromuscular pathways) and reduced the expected loss of power. **When we imagine doing something, we activate the same parts of our brain as if we are actually doing the**

thing. Thus the muscles in question continue to be stimulated and maintain a degree of strength, even if they are not able to visibly respond.

Another group of researchers from the Cleveland Clinic Foundation in Ohio randomly assigned healthy young adults to one of four groups:

- Group 1 were asked to repeatedly extend their little finger out from the side of their hand (known as finger abduction).
- Group 2 were asked to simply imagine doing the same exercise that Group 1 were doing.
- Group 3 were asked to imagine flexing their elbow (bicep curls).
- Group 4 were told to do nothing. They simply had their finger and bicep strength measured at the start and end of the study as did the other three groups.

The exercises (real or imagined) were undertaken for 15 minutes a day, five days a week for 12 weeks. What were the results?

- Group 1 (real finger abduction) increased their finger strength by 53%. No surprise — physical exercise is known to strengthen our muscles.
- Group 2 (imagined finger abduction) increased their finger strength by 35%. Big surprise as this group didn't move a muscle.
- Group 3 (imagined bicep curls) increased their bicep strength by 13.5%. Likewise, a surprisingly good result.
- Group 4 showed no change in strength. No surprise as this group did nothing.

When participants' brain activity was measured by EEG (electro-encephalogram), scientists saw that both real and imaginary exercise increased the electrical activity in brain regions responsible for movement. Greater brain activity translates into greater muscle activation, whether or not we actually move the muscles in question. Real exercise produces larger increases in strength than imagined exercise but an increase of 35% and 13.5% is still a substantial improvement.

In case you're concerned that visualisation only works for our upper limbs, scientists from the Department of Psychology at Bishop's University in Canada recruited 30 male university athletes (football, rugby and basketball players) and assigned 10 people to each of three groups.

- Group 1 used weight machines to physically train their hip flexors for 15 minutes a day, five days a week.
- Group 2 visualised training their hip flexors for 15 minutes a day, five days a week.
- Group 3 did no hip flexor training.

Hip strength in all three groups was measured before and after two weeks of training. The results will not surprise you.

- Group 1 (physical training) increased their hip strength by 28%.
- Group 2 (imaginary training) increased their hip strength by 24%.
- Group 3 showed no change in strength.

The most remarkable finding in this study is that both physical and mental training also produced similar decreases in heart rate and blood pressure! This suggests that imagining yourself exercising can improve the health of your heart!

Hundreds of other studies have shown wide-ranging benefits of visualisation. Here's another party trick. Invite someone into a dimly lit room (I suggest you do this with a friend and not a stranger) and ask them to keep their eyes open while imagining being outside in bright sunlight. As they imagine bright sunlight, you will see their pupils constrict even though they're in a darkened room. Conversely if you're standing in bright light and ask them to imagine a black screen, their pupils will dilate. This is another example of the brain instructing a part of the body — in this case our eyes — what to do based on an image held in our mind. The reason this occurs is because our brain is wired to make predictions about what we're about to encounter. We know that when we go outdoors on a sunny day, the light will be bright so our brain constricts our pupils in preparation for the glare, even if the glare is only imagined. This is enormously empowering because it means **our thoughts can influence our bodily functions.**

Another example is the experience of jet lag. It's generally believed that the severity and duration of jet lag is determined by the direction of travel and number of time zones a person crosses. German researchers led by Eva Winnebeck gave 90 fledgling travellers, aged between 18 and 34, questionnaires about their expectations of jet lag prior to commencing a long-haul flight. The scientists chose people with little prior experience of long-distance travel so that participants would not be able to draw on previous episodes of jet lag. After crossing at least three time zones, the travellers were asked to provide details of any jet lag symptoms. It turned out that time zones and direction of travel had NO bearing on jet lag symptoms. Instead, the greatest predictor of severe and long-lasting jet lag was a person's pre-travel expectation that they would suffer jet lag!

This experiment is reminiscent of studies demonstrating that people with **negative views of ageing had a higher likelihood of developing heart disease and dementia** (see Chapter 13 'Genes are like teens').

One of the most exciting applications of visualisation is assisting people in recovering from a stroke. A 2015 study of 29 stroke patients asked half (14) of them to visualise exercising their affected arm for 10 minutes a day, five days a week, for two weeks, in addition to conventional rehab. The other 15 patients received the same rehab without any visualisation exercises. After only two weeks, the mental practice group demonstrated significantly greater improvements in arm function and ability to carry out daily tasks than the group who had only received conventional rehab. Dozens of similar studies have yielded the same results: **mental practice is an effective treatment for stroke, sports injuries and muscle wasting,** especially in combination with physical exercise.

It's important to note there are two types of visualisation:
1. Internal Mental Imagery (IMI) — also known as first-person imagery or first-person visual imagery or kinaesthetic imagery (I don't know why there are so many names for the same thing)
2. External Mental Imagery (EMI) — also known as third-person visual imagery.

In IMI, a person imagines themselves performing the exercise from within their body and conjures up the feeling of doing the task. In EMI, a person sees themselves performing the task as though watching themselves on a screen or in a mirror. IMI produces greater bodily responses such as muscle activation and changes in heart rate, breathing rate and blood pressure than does EMI. Consequently, IMI yields more powerful results in terms of strength gains and real-world functional improvements. Thus, when you visualise, feel yourself performing the exercise rather than watching yourself from a distance.

There are many other practical applications of visualisation discussed in my two previous books, *In Search of My Father* and *NeuroSlimming*. See:

- *In Search of My Father*, Part IV, the chapters 'Imagination' and 'Perfect Practice'
- *NeuroSlimming*, Part IV, Mission 12: Imagination sparks creation.

CHAPTER 32

In search of the dog

Dogs never talk about themselves but listen to you while you talk about yourself and keep up an appearance of being interested in the conversation.

JEROME K JEROME (1859–1927)

'Wake up! Wake up! The dog's been stolen!' My father's panic-stricken voice broke my slumber.

I reached across to the bedside cabinet and fumbled around for my watch. It was 4.15 am. Exactly the same time as last night. Déjà vu stolen car and stolen ostrich skin belt.

'Dad it's okay. The dog hasn't been stolen. She's gone to live on a farm.'

'Why? What happened?' The light from the hallway exposed his bewilderment.

I repeated my answer for the fourth consecutive night. 'Our dog, Rosie, needed more space to run around. Our small backyard wasn't the best home for her.'

'What? No! How come I don't remember?'

'You don't remember because you're half asleep. Let me take you back to bed and we'll talk about it in the morning. What are you doing up at this hour anyway?'

'I don't know.'

I waited until he'd fallen asleep and tiptoed back to my room.

Rosie was a Kelpie Border Collie Cross. Dad had chosen her name. Shortly before our trip to Belgrade via Los Angeles (exploits of which are in the prequel, *In Search of My Father*), we were asked if we'd like to provide a loving home for a newborn puppy. The timing was perfect as the puppy needed two to three months to be weaned. I jumped at the opportunity.

Animal Assisted Therapy (AAT) and Animal Assisted Activities (AAA) can improve symptoms and quality of life for people with all types of dementia including Alzheimer's. The animals most studied are dogs, cats, fish, horses and guinea pigs and the benefits are far-reaching for the person with dementia as well as their care-partners. Of course, one needs to ascertain that the recipient of AAT is not afraid of animals and has no allergies or medical conditions that preclude them from interacting with pets.

Contraindications aside, **the presence of an animal can trigger an automatic relaxation response and help to reduce agitation, anxiety and fear.** The calming, non-judgmental companionship of a dog or cat spreads joy and unconditional love to its fellow residents and decreases loneliness and social isolation. Stroking a dog or cat provides much-needed tactile stimulation and releases the hormone oxytocin. Oxytocin lowers feelings of stress, enhances mood and makes us feel more connected to each other, not just to the animal. This enables people with dementia — as well as children with autism — to become more engaged in social interactions.

Research has found that AAT can even lower blood pressure and alleviate physical pain, thus improving heart health and subjective wellbeing. Remarkably, **animal companionship can reduce the need for a wide range of medications** including analgesics, anti-hypertensives (drugs that lower blood pressure), anxiolytics (drugs that lower anxiety) and antipsychotics. This is not to suggest that pets can replace pills, but pets might reduce the frequency and dosage of pills required.

Specifically in relation to dementia, a well-trained animal in a person's home or residential care facility has been shown to:
- increase physical activity through walking the dog or even just getting up to pat it

- relieve agitation, restlessness and disorientation
- reduce anxious outbursts
- enhance memory and communication
- improve appetite and encourage better eating.

How can the presence of an animal have such profoundly positive effects on a person with dementia? How can a dog, let alone a fish, prompt nursing home residents to eat better? There are many different mechanisms at play. By reducing stress, there is immediate improvement in brain function, energy levels and sleep quality. Regaining a sense of meaning, connection and relevance delivers huge psychological, emotional and physical benefits. Increased social engagement sets off another cascade of positive behaviours and one thing bolsters another to create a self-perpetuating uplifting spiral.

If I were to take off my scientific hat, I'd say that something deeper is also transpiring: the magic of pure, genuine, non-judgemental connection with another living being; the perception of not being alone. The spark of one life can reignite another.

One assisted living facility in Canberra, Australia, called RSL LifeCare Sir Leslie Morshead Manor, has purchased several pets — including a cavoodle puppy called Edie and two fluffy rabbits — for the enjoyment of all residents. People can also apply to bring their own pets, one of whom is a cheeky cockatiel (a medium-sized parrot) that perches on its owner's shoulder. Another feature that provided an unexpected benefit for residents is the onsite creche provided for the staff's children. Every morning, five little post-people, complete with postman's hat, deliver mail to their surrogate grandparents. Animals and children bring spontaneous fun to any situation and remind us to live in the moment. Morshead Manor is a beautiful example of re-imagining aged care to enable more joy for residents and workers alike.

As for re-imagining our life with Rosie, what I didn't realise was that Animal Assisted Therapy was not the same as randomly acquiring a pet. You need an animal with a suitable temperament that has been trained to support the recipient's specific needs and interests. A hyperactive Kelpie Border Collie Cross with boundless energy was not an ideal choice for an 80-year-old man with Alzheimer's.

Even so, Rosie evoked happy memories from Dad's childhood and captured his attention longer than any other activity. I was also pleased he didn't notice the incidental exercise he was getting whenever he bent down to attach her lead, throw a ball or top up her water. Studies have found that playing with dogs improves an older person's balance and lessens their risk of falls by sharpening their co-ordination and increasing their range of movement. I also assigned Dad the responsibility of brushing, bathing and feeding her, which allowed him to maintain a sense of contribution and importance. No longer was he simply the recipient of my care; he was essential in providing care for Rosie. It didn't matter that many a morning I needed to remind him to feed her.

One afternoon while Dad and I were being dragged along behind her (a skateboard would have been helpful), Rosie suddenly froze, stared ahead and toppled over. Dad and I looked at each other and back at Rosie. She didn't move.

'You've killed the dog!' Dad cried out. 'I told you that you were overdoing it with the exercise. I'll be next!'

'Don't be ridiculous. Rosie was bred to run around a paddock and work all day long. She's a high-energy animal. This is nothing for her.'

'Then why does she look dead?'

'I don't know. Maybe she's playing.' I knew nothing about dogs until Rosie arrived and I was finding myself on a steep learning curve.

Almost as abruptly as she'd fallen, Rosie shook herself awake and tried to get up on splayed, unsteady legs.

'See, she's fine,' I ventured.

Rosie staggered forward for a few steps before toppling over again.

'She doesn't look fine to me,' Dad challenged.

A few seconds later, Rosie wobbled up again. She appeared limp and exhausted.

'Do something,' commanded Dad. 'You're a doctor.'

'Yes, and Rosie needs a vet,' I contended as I picked her up to carry her home. She was heavier than she looked. An abandoned shopping trolley and a blanket would have been welcome.

'If she were human, what would you diagnose?' Dad persisted.

'I don't know. Syncope? Stroke? Heart attack? Hypoglycaemia? Vertigo? Epilepsy?'

It turned out — after several such episodes and visits to the vet — that Rosie had idiopathic epilepsy. The term *idiopathic* means the cause is unknown. I hadn't known that dogs could get epilepsy. I didn't know I'd have to keep a seizure diary to record dates, times, duration, affected body parts, potential triggers and related behaviours. I didn't know there were multiple medications to treat canine epilepsy and I didn't know how Dad would cope if Rosie had a seizure when I wasn't home. Between seizures, she was as frisky as ever. After a few months on medication, the seizures seemed to subside, by which time Rosie had dug up our entire garden. When she burrowed under the fence to start on the neighbour's lawn, our perceptive neighbour suggested we take Rosie to live on his friend's farm. The farmer's family would manage her epilepsy and she'd be free to run and dig to her heart's content. We could call in to see Rosie whenever we wanted. Sad as we were to let her go, it was the kindest option for everyone, especially Rosie. The children at the farm loved her and we loved visiting them. It provided Dad with an exciting weekly excursion.

Meanwhile, I decided that offering Dad a pot plant might be a wiser undertaking than a pet. In an experiment at an aged care home in Connecticut, 47 residents all occupying the same floor were asked if they would like a pot plant in their room (referred to as the Choice Group). They were informed that the plant would be theirs to keep and look after. They all accepted the responsibility and were allowed to choose which type of plant they wanted. In addition, the residents were given options about where and when to accept visitors, which days to see movies and what activities they preferred. They were also encouraged to provide feedback about all aspects of their living arrangements.

A second floor of 44 residents (the Non-Choice Group) — who were similar in age, health status and demographics — were also given a pot plant but were not asked which type of plant they wanted and were told that staff would look after it. They were offered all the same activities as the Choice Group but without the option of time and place. The differences seemed inconsequential but the short- and long-term impacts were astounding.

Eighteen months later, the residents who were given choices and responsibilities were more active, mentally sharp and happier than the residents in the Non-Choice group. Ninety-three per cent of the Choice Group had measurable improvements in their physical and mental health and only half as many of them had died as in the Non-Choice Group! Most of the residents in the Non-Choice Group who were still alive had become increasingly debilitated. The implications of the experiment are groundbreaking. **There is no medication more powerful than empowering people.**

Subsequent studies have revealed that whenever people are allowed to make choices or feel they have a degree of control — regardless of the context — their stress goes down and their performance goes up. In hospital settings, giving patients choices in relation to their care, not only lowers anxiety, it improves their prognosis and reduces the need for painkillers.

Having a sense of agency is critical to every aspect of our wellbeing. If we are unable to exert any influence on our day-to-day experiences, what point is there to life? If all our choices are taken away from us, we feel diminished and incompetent. Our self-esteem crumbles and every part of us shrinks — our brain, body and sense of self. We attempt less, do less and become less. It's a deadly downward spiral.

Being offered choices — no matter how seemingly small — makes us feel valued. It communicates that our opinions matter and we have something to contribute. When a person loses an aspect of their physical or mental functioning, it's essential to provide them with opportunities to continue making decisions. When a person develops dementia, we fear for their safety and sometimes overcompensate by doing too much for them. A care-partner's most important role is relentlessly supporting their loved one's self-efficacy; tirelessly seeking out ways to allow choices. Do you want a bowl of cherries or strawberries? Do you want to eat now or later? Do you want to sit in the living room or the garden? Do you want to listen to the radio or read a magazine?

The more reasons a person has to maintain their mental faculties, the longer their mental faculties will last. Even when someone with Alzheimer's loses their capacity to respond verbally, we still need to ask them about their preferences and opinions. Then watch closely for a flicker of response. Their reaction may be imperceptible, but giving them our undivided attention and demonstrating a desire to understand will nonetheless make a positive difference.

In 2017, with self-efficacy as the goal, the University of Melbourne teamed up with Vision Australia and Dementia Australia to retrain 20 Labrador guide dogs to assist people with younger-onset dementia (also called early-onset dementia) in maintaining independence and self-confidence. Younger-onset dementia accounts for 5–10% of dementias and can occur in people as young as 30 or 40 years of age.

The dogs were taught to recognise their owner's emotional state, voice quality and signs of distress and to help them if they got lost. The dogs were also trained to prompt the person to go to the dining table at mealtimes and to bring them their medication box. When the person was outside their home, the dog provided a sense of security in unfamiliar surroundings. If the person woke up during the night and became disorientated or confused, the dog was taught to get a family member for assistance. Care-partners, as well as people with dementia, reported feeling more in control of their lives. All this was in addition to the companionship, comfort, laughter and sense of purpose that a loving pet can bestow.

Some of the dementia participants disclosed that they preferred to reveal their emotions to their dog rather than burden their family and friends. The dog also provided a common interest and cheerful topic of conversation, which helped everyone stay meaningfully connected.

Dogs are always in the present moment. For a person with advanced dementia, the present is all they have. I believe this is one of the reasons that people with dementia are able to connect with canines. Rosie taught me the gift of simply paying attention and being with someone in the here and now.

Another way that dogs are helping humans with dementia is through stem cell research. Dogs can develop Canine Cognitive Dysfunction (CCD) which is similar to human Alzheimer's disease. Symptoms of CCD include failing to recognise their owners, staring blankly at walls, getting lost around the house and becoming incontinent. Just as with humans, the brain of a dog shows a build-up of amyloid beta (Aβ) and extensive destruction of neurons. At the University of Sydney Brain and Mind Centre, scientist have achieved a world first by reversing CCD using stem cell therapy.

One of their earliest patients was a 13-year-old Cocker Spaniel called Timmy. Timmy could no longer use the dog door or remember how to climb onto a bed. He spent hours barking at nothing. Timmy was confirmed to have CCD using the Canine Cognitive Dysfunction Rating Scale (CCDR). Researchers then removed a small piece of skin from his abdomen and used it to grow half a million stem cells in the lab. A month later, the cells were transplanted into a region of Timmy's brain called the hippocampus (the memory centre). The goal was neuro-regeneration — the regrowth of healthy brain cells.

Three months later, Timmy's owners reported that he was able to recognise them, could find his way home and was no longer incontinent. When he was retested using the CCDR scale, his score indicated that he no longer had dementia.

This is an incredibly exciting breakthrough. Researchers are optimistic that the treatment could also be effective in humans. For now, the trial — called DOGS+CELLS — is still only focusing on dogs. If you think your dog has CCD and you'd like to know more about the trial, please visit: rng.org.au/dogs-cells-trial-cell-therapy-for-the-reversal-of-canine-cognitive-dysfunction/ This study has been approved by the University of Sydney Animal Ethics Committee.

If you have a friendly pet with a gentle temperament and would like to bring smiles to residents in aged care, consider contacting your local facility and offering to visit them whenever you are able.

CHAPTER 33

Your anti-Alzheimer's exercise plan

I attribute my success to this — I never gave or took any excuse.

FLORENCE NIGHTINGALE (1820–1910)

Based on the latest available scientific evidence, the exercise plan shown on the following pages gives you an excellent chance of outwitting Alzheimer's. If you can practise all of these, you'll more than halve your risk of Alzheimer's and provide inspiration to everyone around you.

If you don't have time for everything, focus on aerobic and resistance training as they confer greater brain-benefits than stretching and toning.

The goal is not perfection; **the goal is progress.** Do whatever you can manage. Every bit of exercise is a boost to your brain and body.

If you make exercise a **social** or **outdoor** activity, your brain will receive an added boost — think of it as two brain-boosters for the price of one. Or three for the price of one if you exercise outdoors in company.

Likewise, if the exercise challenges your co-ordination or involves learning new skills, it will stimulate more parts of your brain.

The **American College of Sports Medicine** (acsm.org) has developed a seven-minute high-intensity exercise program that combines aerobic and strength training for all the major muscle groups — legs, hips, back, abdomen, chest, shoulders and arms. This is a great option when you're short on time. You can download a PDF free of charge from the website. Use the search bar to type in: *seven minute circuit.*

Type of exercise	Purpose	Intensity
Aerobic or endurance training, e.g. walking, jogging, cycling, swimming, Zumba and all forms of dancing	To improve **stamina** and cardiovascular fitness.	Moderate intensity as defined by The Talk Test or HIIT
Resistance or weight training, e.g. Pump classes, circuit machines, free weights, pole dancing, yoga and using your own body weight	To improve **strength** + increase muscle and bone mass. This reduces frailty and risk of fractures and translates into increased independence as we age.	Slowly build up your strength with progressively heavier weights and greater resistance.
Stretching, toning, balance and core work, e.g. yoga, Pilates, tai chi, qi gong, dancing	To improve flexibility and stability. This translates into reduced risk of falls and injuries.	Never stretch to the point of pain or discomfort. Gently and slowly improve your flexibility over time.
Avoid prolonged **sitting** time	To reduce inflammation, boost fat burning and improve all aspects of brain and body function.	Simply stand up.
Step it up — take as many steps as you can throughout the day	To remind you that even if you engage in regular physical exercise, it is counterproductive to be sedentary for the rest of the day.	Walk at your own pace but the faster the better.

Always consult your doctor before embarking on any physical exercise program. Even if you haven't exercised for decades, it's never too late to start.

Duration	Frequency	Goals
50 minutes or 30 minutes or 22 minutes	3 times per week or 5 times per week or 7 days per week	To have fun + if you're over the age of 65, try to walk 360 metres in under 6 minutes. If you're younger, aim to be able to walk faster than this.
20 to 40 minutes	At least 2 times per week	To have fun + be able to do 40 non-stop push-ups + try to sit down and stand up from a chair or floor without using your hands. This requires strong knees and leg muscles as well as balance and co-ordination. Use this as a way of tracking your progress rather than predicting your longevity.
Anything from 6 to 60 minutes. Find short routines online, join a class or incorporate this into your aerobic and resistance training	At least once per week	To have fun + be able to stand on one leg with your eyes closed for at least 30 seconds.
2 minutes	Every 20 to 30 minutes	To feel restless after 30 minutes of sitting so that standing up every half hour becomes a natural habit.
However long you like	Daily	To have fun + take at least 5000 steps per day with the aim of 7500 for added benefit + don't stop at 7500 if you'd like to do more! This can count towards your weekly 150 minutes of aerobic exercise. Try to achieve moderate intensity as defined by The Talk Test.

PART FOUR

Let food be your medicine

Everyone, at some time or another, sits down to a banquet of consequences.

ROBERT LOUIS STEVENSON (1850–1894)

CHAPTER 34

The best diet for our brain

Simplicity is the ultimate sophistication.

Leonardo da Vinci (1452–1519)

The most common question I'm asked is: 'What's the best diet for our brain?'

My answer: eat real, whole, unadulterated food.

That's it.

It doesn't need to be any more complicated than that.

Until it does.

Humans have made such a polluted mess of the planet that it's debatable whether real, whole, unadulterated food exists anymore. Pesticides, radiation, air pollution, bioaccumulation of heavy metals in marine life, contaminated and demineralised soils, deforestation, genetic modifications, selective breeding, overcrowded pens, feeding antibiotics and hormones to livestock, slaughtering animals in a state of stress, ultra-processing and many other detrimental practices have resulted in food that is vastly different to that of our ancestors. A pessimist would throw their arms up in despair and lament, 'Why bother even trying to make healthy choices when everything is toxic to one degree or another? I might as well eat anything I want.' The optimist realises that all foods sit on a toxic spectrum and it's in our power to make the best possible food choices we can, given the world we currently live in.

What, then, are the best possible choices? The science of nutrition has become an overwhelming quagmire of confusion and contradictions. No one seems to agree about anything. A food that is demonised by one researcher is heralded as a superfood by the next. How can we make sense of the conflicting dietary advice we're constantly bombarded with?

Several reasons account for the contradictions:

1. We are *not* what we eat. We are what our brain, body and microbiota (gut bacteria) do with what we eat. Our individual differences — determined by our genes, environment, in-utero influences, life circumstances, physical activity, state of health, sleeping habits, drug use, daily stresses and countless other factors — influence our responses to specific foods and patterns of eating. Some people need to consume more of a particular nutrient than others. Some individuals are gluten- or lactose-intolerant; some people have a drop-down menu of food allergies. Some people thrive on a vegetarian diet while others need meat every day. A one-size-fits-all approach simply doesn't work. It's little wonder that studies yield conflicting results. The good news is that health practitioners are slowly adopting the concept of 'precision nutrition' — tailoring their advice to match each individual's unique dietary requirements.

2. All foods consist of a mixture of nutrients, i.e. proteins, fats, carbohydrates, vitamins, minerals and trace elements. Proteins, fats and carbohydrates are known as macronutrients because we eat them in large quantities. Vitamins, minerals and trace elements are designated as micronutrients because we need them in much smaller amounts. Macro- and micronutrients do not operate in isolation. They exert different effects on our bodily processes depending on how they are combined. Food is greater than the sum of its individual nutrients and a meal is greater than the sum of its individual foods. Therefore, to study one food or nutrient in isolation is misleading because we rarely eat one food or nutrient in isolation. If you hear that food X or vitamin Y can improve memory, it immediately begs the questions: in what context?

A useful analogy is that of an orchestra. Think of each individual food as a musician, and the meal as an ensemble. A violinist playing a solo delivers a different musical experience to when the violinist is part of an orchestra. The same goes with food. A food eaten on its own is absorbed to a different extent and exerts different effects compared with when the same food is eaten in combination with other foods. Therefore, if you read that a particular food delivers specific health benefits, you need to know how the food was prepared, what other foods were part of the meal and what other variables in a person's life might have influenced the results.

3. Industry-funded research. Multibillion-dollar food companies pay scientists to design studies in such a way as to mask the harmful effects of their products. For example, a study that examines the effects of a particular product over a period of hours or days can yield a different picture to research that follows consumption over several years. Drinking a sugar-sweetened soft drink raises blood pressure, uric acid and triglyceride levels within four hours of ingestion. This fact is deliberately omitted. Twenty-four hours later, blood tests return to normal. This is the result that gets published. Furthermore, if a person consumes soft drinks and sugary foods every day, blood pressure, uric acid and triglyceride levels stay elevated. These are the first steps towards developing type 2 diabetes, heart disease, gout and Alzheimer's. Soft drink companies choose only to report the effects of a single soft drink 24 hours after consumption in healthy people. The immediate and cumulative effects are not mentioned. The processed food industry controls information by controlling the scientists who do the research. It is the indubitable goal of the processed food industry to confuse the public.

4. The only person who will ever truly know what is best for you is YOU. Medical tests can provide some guidance but you will ultimately need to embark on your own personal journey of trial and course-correction to discover a way of eating that brings you the greatest health, vitality, mental clarity and joy. Just because a specific way of eating makes one person feel fabulous doesn't mean the exact same foods will make *you* feel fabulous. It depends on a range of biological, environmental and lifestyle factors that scientists are still unravelling.

5. Our dietary requirements can change throughout our lives. **A brain-healthy diet for someone with no predisposing factors or**

symptoms of Alzheimer's differs from a brain-healthy diet for someone who has started to experience mental decline. This is a critical distinction. A person with Alzheimer's needs to eat in a way that will rescue their brain from ongoing deterioration. This requires specific dietary modifications that will be discussed in later chapters.

Notwithstanding our individual differences, **two fundamental principles** apply to everyone at every age. These are the cornerstones of healthy eating in the modern world:

1. Eat real, whole, unadulterated food (henceforth abbreviated to real food). This includes any or all of the following and will be based on your values, food intolerances, insulin sensitivity,[1] personal preferences and where you live: fresh vegetables, fresh fruit (NOT juices), fish, meat, offal, eggs, poultry, dairy, nuts, seeds, legumes and healthy fats.[2] Even though real food is not as untainted as it once was, it is still infinitely better for our brain and body than commercially processed food.[3] Other than cooking or fermenting, the less a food has been changed from its natural state, the healthier it is likely to be. Always choose the least processed food that is available to you and that you can afford. If you eat beef, opt for grass-fed. If you eat poultry and eggs, opt for free-range and hormone-free.

2. Avoid industrially processed food (which I refer to as fake food). Fake food includes not only junk food and fast food but also most store-bought cakes, sweets, pastries, pies, biscuits, ice creams, crackers, breads, chips, dips, sauces, dressings, soups, soft drinks, cordials, juices, breakfast cereals and ready-made meals. Avoiding fake food is not as straightforward as it sounds. Many foods marketed as 'real', 'whole', 'natural', 'healthy' and 'organic' are anything but healthy. Grocery stores and food outlets are crammed with so much fake food that when we see something remotely resembling

---

[1] Insulin sensitivity and insulin resistance are discussed in the chapters 'Sweet talk', 'Carb correction' and 'Insulin overhaul'.

[2] Healthy fats are discussed in the chapters 'What the fat is going on?', 'The fat is in the fire' and 'The fat hits the fan'.

[3] Processed food and different types of processing are discussed in detail in Chapter 38 'What happens when we don't like the answer?'

real food, we mistakenly believe that it's nutritious. Far from it. The chapter 'What happens when we don't like the answer?' will guide you through the minefield of processed food and its health implications. A list of ingredients to exclude from a brain-healthy diet can be found in Chapter 39 'The Noxious List'.

In summary, **the foundations for a brain-healthy diet** are to eat food that is:

From the land
From the sea
From the sky
Or from a tree.

Not from a packet
Not from a tin;
If it comes in a box
Toss it in the bin!

Of course, it is more
Nuanced than this,
But if in doubt,
Give the product a miss!

If you do nothing more than adopt the above principles — and memorise the poem — your physical and mental health will inevitably improve.

Now that you have the big picture, are you ready to delve into the details?

CHAPTER 35

Does what we eat really matter?

Repetition does not transform a lie into a truth.

Franklin D Roosevelt (1882–1945)

The next most common questions I'm asked are: 'How important is food for brain health? Does what we eat really make a difference?'

My answer: How important is it to use the right fuel for your car?

Real food is absolutely critical to brain health. The brain is our hungriest organ. Even though it constitutes less than 2% of our body weight, it uses more than 20% of our daily calories — and the quality of those calories matters enormously. **Every meal is an opportunity to heal.** Everything we put into our mouth has an impact on our brain. (As does everything that comes out of our mouth — see Chapter 13 'Genes are like teens'.)

Our brain uses the breakdown products of food to:
- provide it with energy
- build and maintain its structural components
- neutralise toxins
- make neurotransmitters, hormones, enzymes and transport molecules to carry out its many and varied daily tasks.

Food even interacts with our DNA — our genetic material — and can influence whether specific genes are turned on or off. This is known as nutrigenomics. The partnership between our genes and our food plays an important role in our physical and mental health.

Not eating all the nutrients that our brain needs to maintain its structure and functioning interferes with how our brain cells operate and communicate. Over time this predisposes people to depression, anxiety, ADHD, Alzheimer's and other neurodegenerative diseases. All the nutrients essential for optimal brain health can be found in foods provided by nature, i.e. real whole food: vegetables, fruit, fish, meat, offal, eggs, poultry, dairy, nuts, seeds and legumes. You don't need to eat every one of these foods to obtain all your essential nutrients. Your personal values and food tolerances will guide you. The point is that you don't need to take supplements or vitamin pills to stay healthy. Supplements are only necessary if you're found to be deficient in a specific vitamin, mineral or trace element, relative to your body's requirements. The Greek physician Hippocrates was onto something when he counselled 'Let food be your medicine'. **Eliminating fake food frequently eliminates the need for medication** but ALWAYS consult your doctor before stopping any drugs that you've been prescribed.

Conversely, **eating more than we need accelerates brain ageing.** Consistent over-consumption causes:
- chronic inflammation (the body's defence against damage or infection)
- build-up of toxic molecules
- insulin resistance (especially if the excess comes from sugar and refined carbohydrates)
- brain shrinkage.

The larger a person's waist circumference, the smaller a person's brain. This is not to advocate crash dieting or going hungry. It's to advocate eating when you're hungry and stopping when you're satisfied. Goldilocks was a guru: not too much and not too little. Eating fake food dramatically increases over-consumption because commercially made products are low in satiating ingredients such as protein, fibre and healthy fats and low in vitamins and minerals. In other words, we need to consume more of these products to feel full and to reach our requirement of essential nutrients. People automatically eat fewer calories when they switch to real food because their body obtains what it needs from smaller quantities of food.

The concept of a brain-healthy diet is actually redundant because there is no distinction between a brain-healthy diet, heart-healthy diet, gut-healthy diet, liver-healthy diet or foot-healthy diet. What is healthy for one organ is healthy for all organs. Of course, different organs vary in their requirements for specific nutrients, and the cells in each organ have designated receptors to absorb what they need. In addition, the nutrients we ingest interact with each other to keep our metabolic processes finely tuned. A healthy diet for the brain is a healthy diet, full stop.

Another redundancy in our vernacular is the concept of superfoods. **There is NO single superfood for the brain** or any other organ. Foods act synergistically to provide optimal benefits. All real foods are superfoods and nature has built-in checks and balances to moderate our intake. For example, dark leafy green vegetables are low in calories and we can eat a big plateful before we feel full. This is an indication that we can safely consume them in large quantities. Starchy vegetables such as corn and potatoes fill us up much more quickly. This suggests that we don't need to eat them in large quantities. The OPPOSITE is true when it comes to fake foods: the easier they are to eat and the more addictive we find them, the lower their nutritional value.

What about people who subsist on processed food but nonetheless appear to be in good health? Our resistance to toxins sits on a continuum. Some people are highly sensitive to pesticides, food colourings or flavourings while other people notice few, if any, symptoms from food additives — at least in the short term. Of course, all toxins need to be avoided as much as possible, but many people are lulled into a false sense of security because they don't experience immediate negative effects after eating fake food. The damage inflicted by fake food can be so insidious that we don't notice the gradual decline in our energy, mood and mental acuity until we hit a crisis point. Sadly, we tend not to attribute our health problems to fake food because we've been brainwashed into believing that poor health is simply a consequence of 'getting old'. This is the biggest fallacy and tragedy of our modern lives: that we expect our health to decline as we age. This self-fulfilling mindset needs to change. **Start thinking *bolder* not older and *wellderly*, not elderly.**

It is NOT ageing per se that causes physical and mental decline. It's the increasing number of years that our brain and body have been bombarded with a poor diet and stressful, sleep-deprived, sedentary living. Ageing does not need to be synonymous with illness, aches and pains. What we do with each year of life has a greater impact than the number of years we've been alive. The reason our health follows a downward trajectory is self-evident: fake food is EVERYWHERE and EVERYONE is exposed to it. If we're all subjected to an onslaught of dietary toxins, of course we're all going to get sick. We all have the potential for vibrant wellbeing at every stage of our lives. It's tragic that so many people never discover their full physical and mental capabilities because they're being quashed by fake food.

Even though I don't like to single out specific foods (because all real food provides a range of beneficial nutrients), you can use the acronym **BRAIN FOODS** to remind you of particularly powerful brain foods.

B = berries and broccoli

R = radish and **rucola** (a green leafy vegetable that also goes by the names rocket and arugula)

A = avocado and **anchovies**

I = iodine (a mineral found in seaweed, seafood, eggs and iodised salt) and **insalata** (the Italian word for salad)

N = nuts with **nothing** added — i.e. raw and unsalted. If you like them roasted, put them in a low-temperature oven or pan fry for a few minutes. If you buy roasted nuts they will most likely be drenched in unhealthy oils and excessive salt.

F = fermented foods, e.g. sauerkraut, kimchi, kefir, yoghurt (unsweetened, of course)

O = olive oil

O = onions

D = D vitamins from oily fish (see **SMASH** list), mushrooms and 10–15 minutes of sunshine (without sunscreen) per day

S = salmon and **sardines**

Use the acronym **SMASH** to remind you of seafoods that are rich in brain-boosting omega-3 fatty acids and lowest in heavy metals:

S = salmon[4]
M = mackerel[5]
A = anchovies
S = sardines
H = herring

Use the acronym **STINK BOMBS** to remind you of seafoods and meats to avoid because of mercury contamination, additives or overfishing.

S = **shark** (also known as flake)
T = **tile fish**
I = **in danger** because of overfishing, e.g. bluefin tuna
N = **nitrites** and **nitrates** used in some brands of smoked salmon as well as cured meats such as bacon, salami, pancetta, pastrami and pepperoni. Find a butcher who will tell you how their meats are cured.
K = **King mackerel**

B = **basa**
O = **orange roughy**
M = **marlin**
B = **bottom feeding fish,** e.g. sole and catfish
S = **swordfish**

Fish and seafood that don't appear in the above lists fall somewhere in between in terms of omega-3 content and mercury levels.

---

[4] I am proudly Australian, but I will not eat farmed Tasmanian Atlantic salmon because of the industry's destructive environmental practices and resultant deformed, diseased and dyed salmon. Tasmanian Atlantic salmon are devoid of omega-3 fatty acids and swim in a soup of sewage and ammonia, being fed the macerated remains of battery hens, antibiotics, carcinogenic pesticides and synthetic pink astaxanthin dye (otherwise the salmon would be grey and alert us to the fact that something was wrong). I found it hard to believe the industry could be allowed to run rogue until I read Richard Flanagan's chilling exposé, *Toxic: The Rotting Underbelly of the Tasmanian Salmon Industry.* I highly recommend the book to anyone who cares about what they eat and how it impacts the lives of Tasmanians. Seek out wild-caught Alaskan or New Zealand salmon instead. The only way to change the industry (and it can be done) is to stop buying their junk fish.

[5] There are several different types of mackerel. All are rich in omega-3 fatty acids, but King mackerel has high levels of mercury and is not recommended. Smaller mackerel such as Atlantic mackerel are safer.

Unless you have gut issues or require a low FODMAP diet to heal your digestive tract, aim for at least 30 grams of fibre every day (50 grams would be even better). Obtain the fibre from food sources, not supplements. Our ancestors probably ate close to 100 grams of fibre a day but this is far too ambitious in today's world — our gut would literally explode! Visit winningatslimming.com/resources for a list of fibre-rich foods.

Not only does what we eat matter, so does how, why and when[6] we eat. During each meal, bring your attention to your body and become aware of how different foods make you feel. You are your own best guide to the foods your body needs at any given time.

Make meal preparation as enjoyable as possible. My grandmother used to say that cooking was the best form of self-defence. Learning to cook turns you into your own pharmacist because food has medicinal properties. Yes, we lead insanely busy lives but we always find time for what's most important to us. Preparing meals from scratch doesn't have to be complicated or time-consuming. If we make it a priority and plan ahead, cooking fresh, wholesome, healing meals soon becomes a habit that fits seamlessly into our day.

Make eating as enjoyable as possible. When you eat, don't multitask. Pay attention to each mouthful. We don't overeat because something tastes too good. We overeat if we don't taste things enough. When we're fully focused on the flavour, texture and aroma, we find ourselves feeling satisfied with much smaller portions.

If you struggle with emotional eating, binge eating, food addictions or excess body fat, I encourage you to read my book *NeuroSlimming — Let your brain change your body*. The book will enable you to heal your relationship with food and attain your ideal healthy body weight without dieting or deprivation.

Ultimately, **nothing tastes as good as healthy feels.**

---

[6] When to eat is discussed in Chapter 50 'Fast to last'

CHAPTER 36

Broccoli just got even better

To affect the quality of the day, that is the highest of arts.

HENRY DAVID THOREAU (1817–1862)

'What's so good about broccoli?' Dad was pushing it around his plate.

'Everything!' I exclaimed. 'For a start, it's one of the top anti-cancer and anti-Alzheimer's foods. Plus, one cup of raw broccoli delivers your daily dose of vitamin C.'

'I could eat an orange instead,' he proposed brightly.

'Yes, you could. But broccoli provides more than just vitamin C. It also contains vitamins A, K and folate, as well as minerals, antioxidants and fibre. And it has more protein than most other vegetables.'

'I could eat meat for protein.'

'Yes, you could and you frequently do. But broccoli also feeds your good gut bacteria and helps keep you regular.' I broke off as I saw Melanie walking through the front gate. 'Sorry we're running late,' I apologised. 'We're still finishing lunch.'

'No problem,' she smiled warmly. 'It looks delicious.'

'By all means have it,' Dad pushed his plate towards her.

'Oh no thank you, I've already had lunch.' She watched as he cut the broccoli into smaller and smaller pieces.

'The more finely you chop your broccoli and the more times you chew it, the healthier it becomes,' I explained.

'The more finely you chop your broccoli, the less you taste it,' Dad countered.

'How does chopping and chewing make broccoli healthier?' asked Melanie.

'One of broccoli's biggest health benefits comes from a compound called **sulforaphane**. Sulforaphane is produced only when the plant is injured — for instance, by an insect trying to eat it or by a human cutting and chewing it.'

'What's so good about something I can't even pronounce?' Dad was unimpressed.

'For insects, sulforaphane is bad news because it acts like a pesticide, and that's precisely why broccoli produces it: to ward off predators. That's also why chopping and chewing can make vegetables taste more bitter. Insects find bitterness offputting but, for humans, sulforaphane is what's known as a genetic modulator. That means it interacts with our genes to create powerful antioxidants and trigger chemical reactions that help fight cancer, diabetes, autoimmune diseases and dementia. It also improves liver and gut function.

'Sulforaphane is an incredible compound. Mice that were fed sulforaphane along with a high sugar diet gained 15% less weight and had 20% less fat around their internal organs compared with mice that were not given sulforaphane along with their fat-inducing diets.'

Melanie looked alarmed as Dad started burying his broccoli under mustard powder.

'Mustard powder increases the production of sulforaphane,' I clarified.

'Mustard powder hides the taste of broccoli,' Dad grinned triumphantly.

'Cooking interferes with the production of sulforaphane,' I continued. 'Sulforaphane is made when two other chemicals in broccoli — glucoraphanin and myrosinase — come into contact with each other. However, the enzyme myrosinase is destroyed by high temperatures and that's where mustard comes into the picture. Mustard seeds are also a source of myrosinase, so by adding it back to your cooked broccoli, you restore its ability to produce sulforaphane.'

'What if you don't like mustard?' Melanie looked disappointed.

'Instead of mustard you can have your broccoli with raw red radishes, raw cabbage, raw watercress or half a teaspoon of horseradish or wasabi. All these foods also contain myrosinase.'

'Your Dad is using mustard powder rather than mustard. Is that because mustard isn't as potent in terms of myrosinase?'

'Yes. Mustard seeds and mustard powder contain higher concentrations of myrosinase because mustard also includes water, vinegar, salt, spices, lemon juice or wine, and sometimes the liquids are heated. I suspect that adding mustard is still beneficial but not to the same extent as the raw seeds or powder.'

'Does the same apply to other cruciferous vegetables like cauliflower and Brussels sprouts?' she asked.

'Yes. We add mustard powder after cooking all the vegetables in the cruciferous family: kale, bok choy, cabbage, turnips and broccolini.'

Dad winced skittishly as I listed each vegetable.

'What about frozen vegetables?'

'Unfortunately, the processing and cooking that often occurs before vegetables are frozen destroys the myrosinase. Once again, the answer is to add mustard powder — or your preferred source of myrosinase — just before eating.'

'What's the best source of sulforaphane? What will give me the biggest bang for my buck?' Melanie was on a roll.

'Broccoli sprouts — they contain up to a hundred times more sulforaphane than mature broccoli. The sprouts don't have all the other nutrients found in broccoli but if it's just sulforaphane you're after, eat the sprouts — raw of course.'

'I've never even heard of them. Where can I buy them?' Melanie inquired eagerly.

'Grow your own. It will cost a lot less and yield a lot more. All you need is broccoli seeds and a sprouting jar and they'll be ready to eat in a few days. You can store them in the fridge and sprinkle them on anything. They're particularly good on salads.'

'Maybe your dad can help me buy some broccoli seeds this afternoon?'

'Excellent idea!' I encouraged.

'And one more question: cooking also destroys vitamin C, doesn't it?' noted Melanie.

'Yes. Vitamin C is a fragile vitamin. It's destroyed not only by heat but also by oxygen. Don't cut up your fruit and vegetables until you're ready to eat them. As long as the skin is intact, vitamin C is protected from air. As for cooking, how much vitamin C is lost depends on the vegetable and the way it's cooked. Boiling is the worst thing you can do because vitamin C leaks out into the water. As a general rule, use the lowest temperature for the shortest amount of time with the smallest amount of water. Lightly steaming is usually the best way to go. Another trick is to add foods that are rich in vitamin C to casseroles so the vitamin C escapes into the sauce.'

'And now it's time for us to escape!' Dad beckoned Melanie.

'Have fun!' I waved them off.

Enticing Dad to eat vegetables was a major enterprise. It took several years of experimentation and groundwork before I finally found a guru who had the answers: Mary Poppins.

Dad loved Julie Andrews. He'd seen every movie she ever made, dozens of times. His favourites were *Mary Poppins* and *The Sound of Music*. One harrowing day when Dad could not be coaxed into eating, I resorted to familiar melodies. I found myself singing along with Mary Poppins's *A Spoonful of Sugar* and substituting a few of the lyrics …

A Spoonful of **Mustard**

In every **meal that we must eat**
There **needs to be a healthy treat**
You find the fun and snap!
The **meal's** *a game*
And every **vegetable** *you* **chew**
Becomes a **part** *of* **you**
Your brain! Your knee! Your fine anatomy — and

A spoonful of **mustard** *helps the* **broccoli** *go down*
The **broccoli** *go down-wown*
The **broccoli** *go down*
Just a spoonful of **mustard** *helps the* **broccoli** *go down*
In a most delightful way

Our brain needs lots of leafy greens
As well as cabbage, kale and beans
And Brussels sprouts and cauliflower too
They are delicious raw or cooked
The taste and crunch will get you hooked
The more you chew the healthier for you

For the rest of my amended lyrics, see the **Song** section at the end of this book.

CHAPTER 37

Food for thought

*How much more grievous are the consequences of anger
than the causes of it.*

MARCUS AURELIUS (121–180 CE)

L ate evening on Monday 11 May 2020, I was driving north along
the Pacific Highway towards the Gold Coast. I was approaching
the tiny riverside town of Woodburn — population 740. It was a
tranquil, treelined collection of cosy cottages and friendly eateries,
where I could stretch my legs and inhale the crisp night air before
tackling the final 90 minutes to home. Just before reaching the town,
a long snake of stationary cars forced me to a standstill. Why was
no one moving? There must be roadworks ahead. I'd be on my
way again in a few minutes. I waited. Fifteen minutes. Nothing. I
got out of my car and started walking towards the impasse. I was
intercepted by a paramedic.

'What's going on?' I enquired.

'There's been an accident. The highway will be blocked in both
directions for at least another seven hours.'

'Seven hours!' I gasped. 'That sounds like a terrible accident. Do
you need an extra pair of medical hands?'

'Unfortunately, it's too late for that. Two men began arguing in the
middle of the road after a minor ding. It escalated to a physical
altercation. While one of their partners was screaming at them to
break it up, a B-double truck hurtled around the bend and couldn't
slam on its brakes fast enough to avoid running over them. Both

men died instantly. The truck driver is in shock. It's a horrific scene.'

A wave of nausea swept over me. 'Oh, that's such a tragedy. A needless tragedy.'

'Yep. And it's going to take all night to clean up the debris and reopen the road. I suggest you either find a motel room or take the inland route that runs parallel to this highway. It's called Summerland Way. Unfortunately, both options entail driving more than an hour back to Grafton. It's the only access to Summerland Way and it's the closest place you'll find accommodation — unless you want to stay here and sleep in your car like the drivers in front of you. I'm sorry I don't have better news.'

I robotically did a U-turn and headed back to Grafton. From Grafton it would take another three hours to arrive home. By then it would be two o'clock in the morning. I wasn't going to last. On reaching Grafton I pulled up in front of the first motel. It was 11.30 pm and the reception area was deserted. I picked up the phone beside the door and gave my apology to the languid voice that answered. 'I'm sorry for disturbing you. There's been an accident on the highway and I'm unable to get home. May I have a room for the night please?'

'Sorry, it's too late. I can't come down and give you a room at this hour.'

I drove to the next motel. The night manager must have read from the same script. I rang three more hotels and received three more rejections. The backseat of my car was beginning to look inviting. Should I give it one last shot? I parked in front of a bright white sign that read *Grafton Lodge Motel*. Hesitantly I rang the phone number attached to the front door. As with the other motels, my call jolted the proprietor awake. 'Of course I'll come down and give you a room. What an awful thing to experience. Just give me a minute to change out of my pyjamas.'

'Thank you so much!' I was flooded with relief.

'Think nothing of it. You must be traumatised. Anyone in my position would offer you a bed.'

Michelle glided down the stairs and handed me a carton of milk.

'You might like a warm cuppa to settle you down.'

I fell into a deep sleep as soon as my head hit the pillow.

The next morning, I set out for home via Summerland Way. Even if the highway had been cleared, I didn't want to drive through the site of the crash. I found the incident deeply disturbing on many levels. Most of all, the unnecessary waste of life. The paramedic had referred to the inciting event as 'a minor ding'. If only the two men could have focused on the bigger picture: no one had been hurt and both of their cars were still roadworthy. They could have simply exchanged insurance details and continued on their way. Instead, they'd opted to fight over the minutiae. It had cost them their lives and irrevocably changed the lives of their loved ones.

It occurred to me that this tragic incident was a striking reflection of our approach to food. Bear with me while I reconcile the seemingly incongruous analogy. Dietary advice is a barrage of contradictions. Scientists, health professionals and consumers are constantly arguing over carbohydrates, fats, proteins, superfoods and supplements. An excerpt from *NeuroSlimming — Let your brain change your body* summarises the quandary:

Should we be eating low fat, low carb, low salt or low calorie?

High protein, high alkaline, high fibre or high folate?

Low cholesterol, low saturated fat, low omega-6 or low trans fat?

Low GI, non-GM or rich in antioxidants?

Sugar-free, wheat-free, gluten-free or dairy-free?

Yeast-free, grain-free, additive-free or preservative-free?

Paleo, keto, vegan or vegetarian?

Probiotic, macrobiotic, organic or Mediterranean?

Should we be juicing, fasting, supplementing or detoxing?

Food-combining, food-refining, food-fermenting or food-lamenting?

And do we need to know our genome, biochemistry, body type or blood type?

Whomever you ask these questions will give you a different answer. Even among exponents of the same diet, you'll never get complete consensus. This nutritional bickering mirrors the two men arguing about a ding. It wasn't the ding — the minor details — that killed them. It was the massive big truck.

In our food analogy, the hurtling truck is processed food or what I refer to as fake food: junk food, fast food, snack food, convenience food, frozen meals and soft drinks. That's what's making us sick. As long as we stick to real food, we'll work out the minutiae as we go. Whether it's via heart disease, type 2 diabetes, cancer, depression or dementia — **industrially processed food is the killer**.

CHAPTER 38

What happens when we don't like the answer?

I have just three things to teach: simplicity, patience, compassion. These three are your greatest treasures.

LAO TZU (CIRCA 5TH CENTURY BCE)

Lao Tzu's three treasures are the keys to healthy eating. How so?

Our way of eating has become so far removed from what nature intended, we've lost touch with what constitutes real food. Many people confidently announce that they do not eat processed food. They never dine at fast-food chains and they avoid lollies and chips (crisps). On further questioning, it becomes apparent that many people are unaware of what processed food actually means. Do you eat breakfast cereals, muesli bars, ice cream, biscuits, muffins, dips, savoury crackers, packet soups or instant noodles? Do you cook with bottled pasta sauces and pestos? Do you use store-bought ketchup, gravy or salad dressings? Have you ever heated up a ready-made frozen meal? Do you drink fruit juice? If you answered yes to any of these questions then you eat processed food.

Getting clear on the definition of real versus fake food is essential to understanding what constitutes a healthy diet. Get ready to never again be confused about what to eat.

Real foods are edible, life-sustaining substances supplied by nature that provide our body with energy and raw materials for optimal functioning, growth and repair. Examples are vegetables, nuts, seeds, legumes, fruit, fish, meat, offal, eggs, dairy and poultry. The qualification is that these foods must not have been changed from their original form (other than pasteurised, salted or fermented) or had anything added to them. Pesticides are unavoidable unless you grow your own produce. Even organic farming employs organic pesticides. Be stringent about washing all your fruit and vegetables. Some of these foods can be eaten raw while others require cooking.

In contrast, toxins are substances that erode our health and damage our organs, whether immediately or over a period of weeks, months or years. Heavily processed foods — by virtue of their disease-causing ingredients and methods of production — are actually toxins and have no place in our diet.

The reason the food industry gets away with marketing toxic substances as foods is that they don't kill us straight away. It can take decades of eating sugar, refined starches, hydrogenated fats and artificial additives for symptoms to appear. Furthermore, symptoms such as fatigue, brain fog and malaise are often brushed off as 'getting old' or 'just part of life'. This is the great tragedy of our time.

We've forgotten what it means to be truly healthy. We've forgotten that being healthy doesn't just mean being free of overt disease. We've forgotten how great it's possible to feel in our body.

Being healthy means having vibrant energy, vitality and mental resilience, well into old age. Processed foods are thwarting the human race from expressing our full potential. How? And what exactly do we mean by processed food. Does the degree of processing matter? Yes, definitely.

Processed food is a broad term encompassing any food that has been changed from its original form using mechanical, chemical or biological methods for one of several reasons:
- to make it easier, or indeed possible, to eat, e.g. cooking meat or grinding grains
- to extend its shelf-life, e.g. fermenting, salting, freezing or canning
- to make it quicker or more convenient to prepare
- to make it more tempting and even addictive, e.g. industrially produced snack foods such as sweets, biscuits, lollies, chips and crackers.

Therefore, not all forms of processing render food detrimental to health. It depends on how and to what extent a food is processed. In 2010, researchers at the University of Sao Paulo, Brazil, developed a food classification system called NOVA. This system allocates all foods and food products into one of four groups based on the nature, extent and purpose of processing. The four groups are:

1. **unprocessed or minimally processed food** — the processes permitted in this category include chilling, crushing, grinding, drying, juicing, pasteurising and cooking
2. **processed culinary ingredients** such as oils, butter, lard, sugar and salt
3. **processed foods** — these are made by combining Group 1 foods with Group 2 ingredients, e.g. bread, cheese, beer and wine
4. **ultra-processed foods** — these contain little if any Group 1 foods and are created through multiple industrial processes using artificial ingredients, colourings, flavourings and emulsifiers.

You can find a more detailed explanation of the NOVA system at: educhange.com/wp-content/uploads/2018/09/NOVA-Classification -Reference-Sheet.pdf

I'm sorry, but I think the NOVA classification system is of little use. It's a poor guide to healthy eating. Why? Because although Group 1 foods are obviously healthier than Group 4 products (I can't bring myself to label anything in Group 4 as food), several foods in Group 1 such as fruit juice and dried fruit contain far too much sugar to be considered healthy. More on this in Chapter 40 'Sweet talk' and Chapter 42 'Carb correction'. Examining the items listed in Group 2, sugar is blatantly toxic while 'oils' does not differentiate between harmful seed oils — such as soybean oil and corn oil — and healthy oils — such as olive oil and avocado oil. More on oils in chapters 44–46, 'What the fat is going on?', 'The fat is in the fire' and 'The fat hits the fan'. Meanwhile, the products in Group 3 sit on a huge spectrum from downright noxious to comparatively nutritious.

I mention the NOVA system in case you come across it and consider using it to guide your food choices. Don't. To be fair, the NOVA system is a start, but the categories are too broad and imprecise to be of practical value.

To address the shortcomings of NOVA, the Pan-American Health Organisation (PAHO) has developed a tool called the Nutrient Profile Model (NPM), which identifies unhealthy processed food products based on their sugar, fat and salt content. The purpose of NPM is to help governments recognise which products cause the greatest ill-health. This knowledge will facilitate regulatory strategies and public policies to discourage the consumption of these products. Of course, the success of the NPM is based on governments taking notice of the recommendations and acting on them. At least it's a clear acknowledgement by health authorities that ultra-processed foods are a big health hazard and I applaud every step in the right direction. The person who moves mountains begins by carrying away small stones.

You can watch a video explaining how the NPM tool works at: paho.org/en/nutrient-profile-model

Where does this leave individual consumers — you and me? The most useful way to classify food processing and identify harmful products is to employ the following four categories:
1. primary processing
2. secondary processing
3. tertiary processing
4. ultra-processing.

Primary processing makes raw ingredients edible or prevents bacterial contamination. This includes shelling nuts, deboning meat, pasteurising milk, soaking beans and boiling potatoes. Clearly this level of processing improves the nutritional value of food.

Secondary processing means making food from raw ingredients. Home cooking and baking bread are examples of secondary processing. Whether this form of processing is healthy or unhealthy depends on the ingredients and the cooking method. Deep-frying in cottonseed oil renders anything unhealthy. Lightly steaming vegetables and drizzling them with olive oil can enhance nutritional density and increase vitamin absorption.

Tertiary processing is the commercial production of ready-to-eat meals, sauces, salad dressings, dips, muffins and pastries. These are often referred to as convenience foods. This is where food is not only stripped of many of its health-giving properties, it actually becomes toxic. How? By removing fibre and water, containing little to no protein, and adding sugar, refined starches, hydrogenated fats and a string of artificial substances.

Ultra-processing is a method of creating edible substances that mimic food in terms of taste and texture but which actually contain very little, if any, real food ingredients. Ultra-processed 'food' is a carefully contrived concoction of cheap industrial chemicals, fillers, flavourings, colourings, stabilisers, emulsifiers and additives. It includes soft drinks, junk food, fast food and snacks such as lollies, sweets, chips and crackers. Junk food is an oxymoron because junk food is simply junk. Some convenience foods also fall into the ultra-processed category. These so-called 'foods' are deliberately engineered to make them more-ish and addictive. Every mouthful of ultra-processed concoction is literally a nail in our coffin. The governments of Brazil, Uruguay, Ecuador and Peru have recognised this in their national dietary guidelines and advise people to avoid ultra-processed food altogether. When will other governments have the courage to follow South America's example? **Due to its economic power, the food industry holds most governments to ransom.** That means we — the consumer — have to bring about change through the power of our purchasing choices.

If we were to eliminate all tertiary and ultra-processed food from our lives, many chronic diseases — including Alzheimer's — would virtually disappear.

Whenever I use the terms 'processed food' or 'fake food' I'm referring to products made by the food industry via tertiary and ultra-processing.

Most people know that a burger and fries from a fast-food chain aren't a top nutritional choice. But few people are truly cognisant of the extent to which these foods are toxic. The food industry's multi-billion-dollar marketing campaigns have brainwashed us into believing their products are safe 'in moderation'; that we deserve a 'treat'; that fizzy drinks put fizz into our lives. The truth is that fizzy drinks make our organs — especially our brain — fizzle out.

What constitutes moderation? Would you consume floor polish in moderation just because you enjoyed the taste? Is it a treat to visit the dentist for a filling or tooth extraction?

Even more alarming is that many healthy-looking products on grocery store shelves are little more than poisons in pretty packaging: sugar-laden breakfast cereals, baked goods, frozen meals, sauces and salad dressings. Yes, it depends on the ingredients, but most packaged foods are a health hazard to a greater or lesser extent. It isn't just a matter of processed foods providing excess calories. The ingredients and chemicals in processed foods cause all our organs to malfunction over time.

How do we determine whether a processed food is harmful?

Always read the nutrition panel on the back of the product. Don't believe anything written on the front. Memorise the following mantra: **front is fiction; back is fact.** If a product contains any of the following ingredients (**The Noxious List**), it is eroding our health by interfering with the functioning of our cells, organs and gut bacteria:
* trans fats
* hydrogenated, partially hydrogenated or inter-esterified fats and oils
* vegetable oils (which are in fact industrially processed seed oils)
* margarine and shortening
* sugar (in its many guises)
* emulsifiers, thickeners and bulking agents
* anti-foaming and anti-caking agents
* foaming, gelling, glazing and carbonating agents
* artificial flavourings and flavour enhancers
* colourings
* chemicals identified by numbers
* white, bleached or refined wheat flour.

The more of these ingredients that a product contains, the more harmful it is. One dose won't give you diabetes or dementia but several decades of doses quite likely will. Therein lies the problem — delayed harm. Because we don't experience immediate ill-health, we convince ourselves that 'it won't happen to me'. And because these products are so heavily and unscrupulously marketed, we are lulled into believing 'they can't be that bad'. **The world has been brainwashed into consuming toxins as treats.** The inevitable consequence is a pandemic of chronic diseases including Alzheimer's.

A seven-year French study of 44 551 adults aged 45 years and older showed that eating 10% more ultra-processed food led to a 14% increased risk of dying from cancer or heart disease.

In September 2019, *Annals of Internal Medicine* documented the case of a 19-year-old boy in the United Kingdom who consumed a diet of white bread, chips and sausages from the time he started secondary school. Over the ensuing six years he developed irreversible hearing loss and blindness due to nutritional optic neuropathy (NON). It's heartbreaking that this was totally preventable if only he had eaten real food. In another instance, a 34-year-old New Zealand woman died in December 2018 after she had an epileptic seizure induced by drinking three litres of soft drink in one day. Our threshold for experiencing harm varies. But sooner or later, toxic ingredients overwhelm our body's capacity to compensate.

There are several mechanisms by which ultra-processed foods cause mental and physical illness.

- Sugars, refined starches and vegetable oils (seed oils) promote widespread inflammation and insulin resistance. These two states — inflammation and insulin resistance — are the basis of high blood pressure, heart disease, stroke, type 2 diabetes, obesity, depression, gout, rheumatoid arthritis, fatty liver disease, polycystic ovarian syndrome (PCOS), many autoimmune diseases and Alzheimer's.
- In addition, when vegetable oils are heated, they produce toxic chemicals called aldehydes that increase the risk of cancer and Alzheimer's.
- Additives, including emulsifiers, preservatives and artificial sweeteners, disrupt our gut microbiota (the millions of bacteria, viruses and fungi that reside in our gut and play a major role in keeping us healthy).
- Eating ultra-processed food means we are not consuming sufficient protein, vitamins, minerals and fibre. Even if packaged

food is fortified with vitamins and minerals, it doesn't come close to the variety and quantity of nutrients contained in real food. It isn't just the vitamins and minerals in real food that makes them healthy; it's how they're combined in their natural state within the entire food.

- Ultra-processed food promotes overeating and leads to obesity. Midlife visceral obesity doubles the risk of Alzheimer's.

The seminal point is that all real food diets — be they low carb, high fat, Mediterranean, vegan, vegetarian, paleo or keto — have one thing in common: elimination of processed foods. That's why they all lead to improvements in health. First and foremost, it is because of what people are NOT eating.

A word of warning. Just because a product is labelled 'vegan', 'keto', 'gluten-free' or 'rich in vitamin C', don't assume that it's healthy. Remember: **front is fiction; back is fact.** Check the ingredients. If a healthy-sounding product contains sugar, vegetable oils or anything else on **The Noxious List,** leave it out of your shopping bag. Similarly, just because an actor, athlete, influencer or celebrity endorses a product, doesn't mean it's healthy. They are paid to say positive things about it. They may genuinely believe it's the secret to their success, but unless they have a science degree and have done a lot of reading, they are basing their recommendations on food industry claims, not on an understanding of the science.

An experiment published in the journal *Cell Metabolism* in July 2019 showed that ultra-processed food drives people to eat more calories and to gain body fat. Twenty adults (10 males and 10 females) were confined to a research clinic for 28 days. For the first 14 days, half of the participants were offered only real food and for the subsequent 14 days they were offered only ultra-processed food. The remaining half of the participants received the same foods in reverse order: ultra-processed food followed by real food.

Participants were given three meals a day and were instructed to eat as much or as little as they wanted. The composition of the real food and ultra-processed meals was the same in terms of proteins, fats, carbohydrates, fibre, sugar and salt. The differences lay in the foods that provided the proteins, fats, carbs, etc. The real food buffet only offered real food sources of proteins, fats and carbs. The ultra-processed buffet only offered ultra-processed sources of proteins, fats and carbs. Did the source of the nutrients make a difference? Very much so. When participants were on the ultra-processed diet, they consumed 500 more calories per day and quickly gained fat around their abdomen. Why?

Ultra-processed food is full of refined starches, vegetable oils, sugars and chemicals. When our body doesn't receive the nutrients it needs, it drives us to eat more and store the excess calories as body fat. Ultra-processed food ingredients also drive up insulin resistance and put our body in a state of chronic inflammation.

Interestingly, the increase in calories came from consuming more carbohydrates and fats but not from consuming more protein. People's protein intake was remarkably stable regardless of which diet they were on. This is one of many studies that supports the Protein Leverage Hypothesis. Each person needs to consume a certain amount of protein for optimal functioning. Until we reach our protein target for the day, we continue to feel hungry and we keep eating. Ultra-processed food is low in protein so we need to consume more of it to hit our protein target. Other reasons that we over-consume ultra-processed food include the following:

- It contains little, if any, fibre.
- It is deficient in vitamins and minerals so our body is under-nourished despite being overfed.
- It is deliberately formulated to be more-ish and addictive.

How do you calculate your personal protein target? Our protein needs vary according to age, gender, genetics and activity level. Too little protein leads to stunted growth and infertility. Too much protein accelerates ageing. Aim for at least 1.2 grams of protein (preferably 1.5 grams) per kilogram of your optimal body weight per day (up to 2 grams per day if you do a lot of strength training). In other words, if you weigh 100 kg but you know that your healthy weight is 80 kg, aim for 96 grams of protein over the course of the day. **Our body's ability to use proteins diminishes with age so we need to eat more, not less, protein in our senior years.** In reality, we don't need complicated formulas to figure out what to eat. Every animal — from locusts to baboons — has its own specific protein requirement and manages to hit the exact mark by following its instincts. Humans have the same innate food wisdom. Our bodies will guide us to eat precisely what we need — as long as we eat real food. Unnatural, ultra-processed ingredients hijack our brain and disrupt our capacity to self-regulate our eating. It's important to include sources of protein with every meal: meat, fish, poultry, soy, eggs, nuts, seeds or dairy.

Visit <u>winningatslimming.com/resources</u> for a list of protein-rich foods and how much protein they contain.

In January 2020, the journal *Nutrients* published a review of 61 studies on the relationship between adult mental health and fruit and vegetable intake. The studies covered depression, anxiety, attempted suicide, stress, sleep quality and optimism. The results were conclusive: higher intake of fresh whole fruits and vegetables — particularly green leafy vegetables, berries and citrus fruits — protected against depression and negative psychological states, and promoted higher levels of optimism and self-efficacy.

Of particular note is a 2017 study called the SMILES trial, devised by Professor Felice Jacka, director of the Food and Mood Centre at Deakin University in Melbourne, Australia. Sixty-seven participants with moderate to severe depression were randomly assigned to receive either dietary advice or social support for 12 weeks. The diet group were instructed to follow a modified Mediterranean diet consisting of vegetables, nuts, legumes, fish, whole grains, fresh fruit and extra virgin olive oil. The social support group were not given any dietary advice. After three months, one-third of participants following the Mediterranean diet were in remission compared with only 8% of the social support group. Those who improved their diet the most had the greatest reduction in symptoms of depression.

Even young people are not immune to the damaging effects of fake food. We are never 'young enough to get away with it'. Poor diet contributes to depression and poor mental functioning at any age. In March 2018, the University of Tasmania published a study showing that tertiary and ultra-processed food increases the risk of depression in adolescents. The diets of 847 teenagers were scrupulously examined and the correlation was indisputable: the higher their consumption of processed food — not merely junk food but any packaged foods and ready-made meals — the greater the likelihood of depression, anxiety, obesity, markers of inflammation and insulin resistance — a harbinger of impending chronic diseases such as type 2 diabetes. Chronic depression, anxiety, excess visceral fat, inflammation, insulin resistance and type 2 diabetes all increase the risk of Alzheimer's disease. Our diet can trigger a domino effect from an early age. Conversely, the more real foods the adolescents ate, the better their mental health.

An earlier study published in September 2011 in *PLOS One* tracked the diets and mental health of 3040 Australian adolescents aged 11 to 18 years for two years. The results were also clear-cut: more processed food and less real food led to poorer psychological functioning. When diet improved, so did mental health. A third study in the *Australian and New Zealand Journal of Psychiatry* examined 7114 adolescents aged 10 to 14 years and confirmed once again that higher consumption of processed food led to higher rates of depression. **Food and mood are intimately connected.**

Specifically in relation to dementia, **the more ultra-processed food a person consumes, the greater their risk of Alzheimer's and vascular dementia**, and the faster their rate of cognitive decline.

Seventy-two thousand and eighty-three men and women from the UK Biobank (a large database of health information from half a million people living in the UK) were assessed on their ultra-processed food (UPF) consumption and tracked for 10 years. The mean age of participants was 61.6 years and none of them had dementia at the start of the study. Over the course of a decade, for every 10% increase in UPF, the likelihood of developing any kind of dementia rose by 25%. Those who ate the most UPF had 50% higher risk of dementia than those who ate the least. The researchers concluded that in addition to the product ingredients being toxic, molecules from packaging leached into the food and also eroded memory and thinking skills. The good news is that the reverse is equally true: replacing UPF with real food is associated with lower risk of dementia. The study was published in the *American Academy of Neurology* in July 2022.

Also in July 2022, The Brazilian Longitudinal Study of Adult Health (ELSA-Brasil) presented at the Alzheimer's Association International Conference (AAIC) found that consumption of UPF dramatically speeds up cognitive decline. Ten thousand seven hundred and seventy-five adults with a mean age of 50.6 years were followed for eight years. Adjusting for the effects of socio-economic and lifestyle factors, people who consumed more than 20% of their daily calories from UPF had 28% faster rate of cognitive decline than those eating less UPF. Twenty per cent equates to roughly 400 Calories per day, which is only 75 grams of potato chips (crisps) OR four Tim Tam biscuits OR one large muffin.

How many more people need to fall into the abyss of depression or dementia before we stop promoting poisons as pleasure? Time and time again, worldwide research yields the same simple message: **eat real, whole, unadulterated food and avoid processed food**.

The food industry banks on safety in numbers. If everyone around us is consuming their products, surely they can't be that bad? Yes, they can. Do you remember the days when we were ignorant of the hazards of smoking? Even doctors were advertising their preferred brand of cigarettes. The food industry is even more powerful than the tobacco industry. If all the world's scientists, doctors, nutritionists and health professionals spoke out against processed food, they would still be drowned out by the clamour of food companies. Alarmingly, even health professionals have been duped into believing that small amounts of processed food won't do any harm. True. Small amounts — as in a few times a year — won't do any harm. But how many people consume processed food less than five times a year?

We are currently living in an age of unprecedented scientific and technological advancement. Modern medicine is truly extraordinary. We've mapped the entire human genome. We've synthesised hormones. We've implanted embryos. We've transplanted hearts — as well as livers, lungs, kidneys and pancreases.

Yet we're getting sicker, fatter and more depressed by the day. And we're getting sicker and sicker at a younger and younger age. We're experiencing an explosive increase in chronic diseases: asthma, autism, allergies, arthritis, Alzheimer's, obesity, cancer, heart disease, depression and diabetes. The list goes on. How can this be? With all the incredible progress in science and medicine, it doesn't make sense that we're getting sicker, not healthier. What's the explanation?

We're poisoning ourselves. Little by little. Every day. A donut here, a pretzel there, a dollop of mayonnaise,[7] a squirt of tomato sauce. Over the course of a lifetime, it adds up to a big toxic load and our organs eventually malfunction.

Of course, processed foods aren't the only health hazards in our lives. Stress, sleep deprivation, lack of exercise, air pollution and a host of other factors also play a role. But processed food is the elephant in the room. We're so caught up in diet wars, we've missed the essential point: eliminate processed food and our health will automatically improve — regardless of whether we choose to go keto, paleo, vegan, vegetarian or Mediterranean.

The problem is not that we don't have the answer to what constitutes a healthy diet. The problem is that the food industry doesn't like the answer. And what does big business do when they don't like an answer? They shroud it in complexity. They pretend there isn't enough information. They incite bickering over details. They instigate paralysis by analysis.

Recall the fight put up by the tobacco industry when cigarettes were found to cause cancer, emphysema and heart disease. The food industry is putting up the same fight and employing the same underhand tactics. It's déjà vu. There is no confusion about the toxic effects of processed foods. The food industry is *creating* confusion. And if we're honest with ourselves, we — the consumer — are quietly complicit because we don't like the answer any more than they do. We enjoy the easy pleasure of processed foods and we fear that our lives will be lacking without them. The opposite is true. We'll flourish without processed foods.

---

[7] Mayonnaise is not inherently unhealthy. Industrially produced mayonnaise is a problem because it contains sugar, vegetable oils and other additives. Try making your own mayonnaise using eggs, olive oil, vinegar, lemon juice and salt. Ask chef Google for mayonnaise recipes that use olive oil. It's not only healthier but much tastier than store-bought mayonnaise.

Nothing tastes as good as healthy feels. And quite frankly, when we've retrained our palate, nothing tastes as good as real, whole, unadulterated food.

Can you see why Lao Tzu's three treasures are the keys to healthy eating?

- The exciting **simplicity** of rediscovering real food.
- **Patience** while making incremental changes.
- Self-**compassion** when it feels like an overwhelming effort.

CHAPTER 39

The Noxious List

It is not because things are difficult that we do not dare; it is because we do not dare that things are difficult.

SENECA (4 BCE – 65 CE)

I t's time to act.

How do we break free from our reliance on processed foods when they're so deeply embedded in our culture and our day-to-day lives?

One simple step at a time.

Start by memorising the ingredients that mess with our brain and body. Knowledge is the first rung on the ladder of empowerment. Write down the following checklist — **The Noxious List**[8]— and take it with you whenever you go shopping. These are the ingredients to remove from our diet. I mentioned them in the previous chapter but here is a more detailed look.[9]

1. **trans fats** — to date, these are the worst culprits. Several European and South American countries have banned their use. Other governments prefer to allow their citizens to develop heart disease rather than upset food manufacturers.
2. **hydrogenated, partially hydrogenated** or **inter-esterified fats and oils**
3. **vegetable oils** — which are in fact industrially processed seed oils

---

[8] You can download The Noxious List from outwittingalzheimers.com/resources

[9] Fats, oils and margarine will be discussed in Chapters 44–46, 'What the fat is going on?', 'The fat is in the fire' and 'The fat hits the fan'.

4. **margarine** and **shortening** — shortening = fats used to make baked goods that are crisp and crumbly, e.g. pastries, pie crusts and biscuits.

5. **sugar** — see Chapter 41 'Fifty shades of sugar' for the more than 50 different names the food industry uses for sugar. This is a deliberate ploy to conceal the presence of sugar. I invite you to play a game of hide-and-seek. Food companies try to camouflage the sugar by using obscure terminology on the back of the product. Armed with your list, you will now be able to outwit manufacturers and identify all the hidden sugars.

6. **emulsifiers** — these substances are used to hold mixtures together and to make the texture of foods more appealing. Certain emulsifiers, e.g. carboxymethyl cellulose (designated E566) and polysorbate-80 (E433) cause gut bacteria to produce a protein called flagellin, which triggers inflammation. The more we study emulsifiers, the more we discover they mess with our gut.

7. **thickeners** and **bulking agents**

8. **anti-foaming** and **anti-caking agents**

9. **foaming, gelling, glazing** and **carbonating agents**

10. **artificial flavourings** and **flavour enhancers**

11. **colourings**

12. **compound chocolate** — the main ingredients in compound chocolate are sugar and vegetable oils. If you want to eat chocolate, make sure cacao or cocoa is the first ingredient and cocoa butter is the second ingredient. Dark chocolate is better than milk chocolate because it has a higher concentration of cacao and lower concentration of sugar. See Chapter 53 'The charms of chocolate'.

13. **white chocolate** is a misnomer as it doesn't contain any cocoa solids. It is made of cocoa butter, sugar, milk and flavourings. White chocolate is simply an ultra-processed sugar bomb.

14. **white, bleached** or **refined wheat flour** — see Chapter 42 'Carb correction'.

15. ingredients identified by **numbers**

16. ingredients you would not be able to cook with yourself.

In an ideal world, we would avoid everything on the foregoing list. In the real world, do the best you can. **The more you avoid**

these ingredients, the more you avoid injury to your brain. The simplest solution is to buy as few packaged foods and as much fresh produce as possible. Reading nutrition panels can be laborious to begin with, but once you've laid the groundwork and established which products are free of toxins, you'll know what to buy. You don't have to overhaul every aspect of your diet at once. Work at your own pace. Every step you take will boost your confidence and increase your sense of self-mastery. Any early struggles will be more than compensated by your subsequent surge in energy, vitality and joie de vivre. The human body is remarkably resilient and we can bounce back even after years of noxious insults.

EVERYTHING offered at fast-food outlets is LOADED with ingredients from **The Noxious List**. Almost all food outlets — including fish shops, cafés and restaurants — employ cheap industrial seed oils for frying. And refrying. **Fast food is a fast route to Alzheimer's.** Ditch the deep-fried options and choose steamed, poached, grilled, baked, barbecued, stewed, sautéd or roasted instead (in that order). Most restaurants use vegetable oils for all cooking that requires oil but at least the non-fried options deliver a smaller dose. Ask the café or restaurant which oils they use and request olive oil, butter or coconut oil as an alternative. The more that diners ask for healthy options, the more rapidly we will change our food environment. It will take time, but with persistence, anything is possible.

In 2019, a study at the University of New Hampshire showed that 40–60 minutes **after a single fast-food meal** consisting of a Big Mac hamburger and medium French fries, **the coronary arteries in healthy young people became stiffer.** This means their arteries were not able to supply the heart with as much oxygenated blood as prior to the meal. Arterial stiffness is a response to large amounts of sugar, refined starches, salt and additives. When heart muscles don't receive enough oxygenated blood, we are at increased risk of a heart attack and compromised oxygen delivery to the brain. **Repeated shortfalls in brain oxygen set the stage for Alzheimer's and other neurodegenerative diseases.**

Salt is essential for life but remember Goldilocks: not too much and not too little. Nutritional experts are still debating how much salt (sodium) we need for optimal health. Most heart associations (including the Australian Heart Foundation) recommend an upper limit of 2 grams of sodium per day for adults. This is equivalent to 5 grams of salt — roughly one teaspoon per day. Other researchers suggest we are safe — even better off — to consume twice as much as this. Here is another example of individual differences. People require varying amounts of salt depending on a range of factors including genes, hormones, kidney function, blood pressure, exercise levels, physical environment and diet composition. If you eat a low carbohydrate diet, you will need to eat more salt. If you eat a salty meal that contains carbohydrates, drink more water. It isn't the absolute amount of salt that matters most; it's the concentration of salt in our blood. Therefore, before you consume a meal that is high in salt, drink a large glass of water to dilute it. If you're still unsure how much salt to consume, aim for one teaspoon a day and visit your doctor at least once a year to check your blood pressure and overall health. If you only eat real food, you are unlikely to be eating too much salt. The problem is not the salt we use in home cooking or add to food at the dinner table. The problem is the massive amounts of hidden salt in processed foods. Any time we eat a packaged or fast-food meal, we are more than likely exceeding our daily salt requirement.

If you're faced with nothing but fast-food outlets and you're ravenously hungry, what are the best options?

- Grilled meats with steamed vegetables
- Salads with dressing on the side so you can judge whether you really need the dressing. Better still, can you request a mixture of olive oil and vinegar? It's unlikely a fast-food outlet will have olive oil but there's no harm in asking. Toss out the croutons and dried fruit that are often sprinkled on top.
- Sandwiches can range from nutritious to little more than junk food. It depends on the quality of the bread, spread and fillings. Unfortunately, most store-bought breads contain many ingredients on **The Noxious List,** especially sugar, vegetable oils and refined grains. Wholegrain sourdough is likely to be your best option.

- Find a sushi store and choose sashimi (but not if you're pregnant) with salad and pickles. Your next best option is sushi made with wholegrain rice (brown, red or black) and topped with raw fish, prawns, avocado, raw or pickled vegetables and seaweed. Regrettably, sushi is often a sugar bomb. Fast-food outlets add three to four teaspoons of sugar to every cup of cooked rice. Fillings made with cooked tuna usually include mayonnaise and extra sugar. Avoid battered vegetables (tempura) and creamy dipping sauces. A sachet of soy sauce and wasabi (Japanese horse radish) are acceptable. Try eating only half the rice that comes with each sushi roll.

Before your next visit to the grocery store, do an audit of every box, tin, jar, bottle, packet and packaged food in your pantry, fridge and freezer. Read the ingredients itemised on the back. They are listed in order of highest to lowest amount. If the first item is sugar, this is the main ingredient in the product.

Do the same with all the beverages in your house.

Are you shocked to find how many breakfast cereals, soups, pasta sauces, salad dressings, savoury snacks, breads and frozen meals contain substantial amounts of sugar and vegetable oils? Are you shocked that most of the products in your kitchen contain at least one item on **The Noxious List?**

Not all processed foods are harmful to heath; it depends on the ingredients. The items below can go either way. If nothing from **The Noxious List** has been added, feel free to use them.

- Frozen raw vegetables
- Frozen berries
- Tinned vegetables — these sometimes contain acidity regulators, food acids (e.g. citric acid) and firming agents (e.g. calcium chloride, calcium sulphate and magnesium sulphate). I rarely use tinned vegetables so the few times I do, I am not concerned about these particular additives.
- Tinned fish — this is where many people get caught out — pun intended. Fish in spring water or brine is fine. Fish in any of the vegetable oils is not. Food companies often state 'tuna in olive

oil blend' on the front of the packaging to make you think you're buying tuna in olive oil. NEVER trust the front. Read the back and you'll find that 'olive oil blend' means 1% olive oil mixed with 99% soy bean oil. No thank you.

- Yoghurt — the only ingredients in healthy yoghurt are milk and bacterial cultures. The minute you find emulsifiers, thickeners, sugar, honey, fruit juice or flavourings (even if it states 'natural flavours'), give it a miss.
- Non-dairy milks — the only ingredients in healthy non-dairy milks are water, soybeans, almonds, macadamia nuts, coconut or hazelnuts. Unfortunately, many non-dairy milks include vegetable oils and sugar. Give these brands a miss.
- Nut butters — the only ingredients in healthy nut butters are nuts. This makes them more expensive hence manufacturers often add vegetable oils, sugar and other nasties. Stick to nut-only nut butters.

This is not an exhaustive list but you now have enough information to determine for yourself what is healthy and what is not.

Having identified the processed foods that are eroding our health, how do we go about eliminating them from our diet? Replace them with delicious real foods that you prepare at home. It doesn't have to be complicated or time-consuming. More than anything, it involves a shift in mindset. As soon as you commit to making healthy eating a top priority, you will find ways to plan, shop and organise your household to make it happen.

Our food preferences are learned, not fixed. It won't take long to recalibrate your tastebuds to appreciate the more deeply satisfying flavours of real, whole, unadulterated food.

Here are some **simple swaps** to get you started:

- Replace soft drinks with plain mineral water, still bottled water or tap water. All carbonated drinks erode tooth enamel, even if they have no added sugar.
- Replace all snack foods and roasted nuts with raw unsalted nuts — commercially roasted nuts are usually drenched in vegetable oil and salt.

- Replace commercial salad dressings with a home-made mixture of extra virgin olive oil and lemon juice or vinegar (balsamic or apple cider vinegar provide a lovely flavour).
- Replace margarine with butter or avocado.
- Replace vegetable oils with olive oil, coconut oil, avocado oil, macadamia nut oil, ghee or lard.
- Replace breakfast cereals with home-made porridge using chia seeds, quinoa or steel-cut oats. Or switch to eggs your way with spinach, mushrooms, avocado and tomato.
- Replace pasta with spiralised zucchini, spaghetti squash, soybean spaghetti or konjac/shirataki noodles.

This is not a quick fix or annual detox. **It's an exciting, empowering, lifelong project in building a sharper brain and stronger body.**

Unfortunately, many people fear that healthy eating is bland and boring or expensive and time-consuming. These beliefs are the result of billion-dollar marketing campaigns by clever food companies. Their profits rely on convincing us that real food is dull while fake food is fun; that real food is arduous while fake food is time- and money-saving. This is a big fat myth. Fake food costs a lot more in terms of brain fog, medical bills, time spent visiting doctors and hospitals, days off work, loss of productivity, reduced quality of life, shorter life-span and the need to buy larger amounts of food because it doesn't keep us satisfied. When we eat real food, we don't need snacks because our meals are far more satiating.

Nutritious and delicious go hand in hand.

To remind you of the relationship between food and brain health, I've swapped some of the words in Tina Turner's song *What's Love Got to Do With It?* to create the song *What's Food Got To Do With It?* Here is the first verse. For the complete song, see the Song section at the back of this book.

What's **Food** Got to Do With it?

*You must understand, though the **taste** of your **snack***
*Makes **your brain** react*
*That it's only the thrill **of a quick sugar hit***
And our brain's been hacked
It's physical
Only logical
We** must try to ignore **all the slick tempting ads

*Oh-oh, what's **food** got to do, got to do with it?*
*What's **food** but **the fuel for all our brain power***
*What's **food** got to do, got to do with it?*
*Who needs **to eat junk** when **junk causes brain fog?***

*It may seem to you that I'm **being too strict***
Saying no soft drinks
Having water instead clears our skin and our head
Research shows the links
There's a name for it:
Being smart and fit
*But whatever the reason, **fresh food helps us think***

*Oh-oh, what's **food** got to do, got to do with it?*
*What's **food** but **the fuel for all our brain power?***
*What's **food** got to do, got to do with it?*
*Who needs **fast food** when **fast food slows** our **brain down?***

CHAPTER 40

Sweet talk

Even a mistake may turn out to be the one thing necessary to a worthwhile achievement.

Henry Ford (1863–1947)

The bad news: sugar damages brain cells and impairs brain function.

The good news: the poison lies not in a single grain of sugar but in the dose and type of sugar.

The mindset we need to overcome: that something as longstanding, ubiquitous and delicious as sugar can cause devastating effects on our brain and body.

The questions that trip us up:

- Haven't humans been eating sugar for centuries?

Answer: Yes, but in much smaller quantities than today. For example, in 1909, Americans consumed an average of 40 kg (88 pounds) of sugar per person per year. This equates to nine and a half teaspoons per day. Less than 90 years later, in 1997, sugar consumption had almost doubled to 70 kg (154 pounds) per person per year or 16 and a half teaspoons per day. Today the figure has doubled again to over 30 teaspoons per day. Much of the sugar we consume is hidden in processed foods that we perceive to be healthy and don't even suspect contain sugar. Stay tuned.

- Isn't sugar found naturally in fruit and vegetables?

Answer: Yes, but eating sugar in the form of whole fruits and vegetables is not the problem. Extracting sugar from cane, beets, rice, corn, coconut, dates or any number of other crops, and adding it to 80% of food products found in our grocery stores, is the problem. The sugar consumption reported in the previous answer only refers to sugar that has been added to processed food and drinks or used in home baking, not the relatively small amounts of sugar we consume by eating whole fruits and vegetables.

- Isn't the anti-sugar bandwagon just another fad?

Answer: No. Eliminating added sugar from our food supply is supported by extensive and unequivocal scientific evidence. The only groups arguing against the harms of sugar are those with a financial interest in our ongoing consumption of sugar, such as the processed food industry and its affiliates.

- If sugar is really so damaging, why have its harms only recently come to light?

Answer: The fattening and tooth-eroding impacts of sugar have been known since the days of corpulent kings and queens with their terrible dental caries (because, in the past, only the wealthy were able to afford sugar). The advent of fluoride allowed us to transiently mask sugar's assault on our teeth. However, tooth decay and excess body fat are only the tip of sugar's toxic iceberg. The introduction of blood tests and organ imaging techniques have given modern medicine a much bigger window into sugar's destructive trail throughout our body.

The mystery: how did we come to be eating so much sugar?

The explanation: our governments told us to! Huh? When US President Dwight Eisenhower suffered a heart attack in 1955, his doctor gave a press conference instructing Americans to stop smoking (good advice) and to cut down on dietary fats (bad advice). Based on flawed research and biased opinions, this advice was incorporated into the first US government dietary guidelines of 1980 and soon adopted by governments worldwide. The key message was to eat less saturated fat and to eat more carbohydrates. In good faith, food companies reformulated their products to remove the fats and replace them with sugars and seed oils. It was an error of colossal proportions and it set off worldwide epidemics of obesity and chronic diseases.

The numbers speak for themselves.
- In 1950, fewer than one in eight Americans were obese (12% of the population).
- In 1980 — 30 years later — just over one in seven Americans were obese (15% of the population).
- In 2000 — 20 years later — more than one in three Americans were obese (35% of the population). Similar trends were seen in Australia and the UK. The rest of the world has now followed suit.

Human history is littered with myths, mistakes and misconceptions. In ancient times, python bile was applied to female genital ulcers. Arsenic was used to treat fevers and syphilis. Trepanning (drilling a hole in the skull) was employed to relieve headaches; and bloodletting was a remedy for just about everything from high blood pressure and smallpox to gonorrhoea and pneumonia. We used to believe the earth was flat, the sun revolved around the earth and that sugar was harmless. Why are we still following outdated dietary advice from more than half a century ago? Because there are too many financial interests and egos at stake. Profit before people. Wealth before health. The food industry is big business and governments are too gutless and shortsighted to stand up to them. The food industry has convinced us that we can't live without their convenient and tasty products. Sweet lies. Millions of people have made the switch to home cooking with real, whole, unadulterated foods — and so can you. Thinking that it can't be done is our biggest hurdle.

The goal: to empower ourselves and our fellow humans to:
1. understand what 'sugar' actually means
2. recognise which foods contain added (and hence harmful) sugars
3. remove added sugars from our diet or at least cut back to less damaging levels.

The starting point: what is sugar?

Understanding the term 'sugar' is critical to making brain-healthy food choices.

Sugar is a type of carbohydrate. Think of sugar as a brick and carbohydrate as a wall. All carbohydrates are made by joining different sugars in various combinations. The type and number of sugars (bricks) that make up a carbohydrate (wall) determine how the carbohydrate is digested, absorbed and metabolised by our body. Digestion, absorption and metabolism of carbohydrates involves enzymes, hormones and gut bacteria.

Carbohydrates — referred to as saccharides in biochemistry — are molecules composed of carbon, hydrogen and oxygen, hence the name *carbo-hydrates.* All plants make carbohydrates from carbon dioxide and water using energy from sunlight. The process is called photosynthesis.

Carbohydrates are divided into four groups, based on how many chains of carbon atoms they contain. The first two groups are referred to as simple sugars or just sugars. These are the potential villains in our diet. When we consume them in whole fruit, they are not a problem. When we consume them in juices, sweets and processed foods, they cause havoc to our health. The second two groups are designated complex carbohydrates. They are found in grains, legumes and starchy vegetables. These carbohydrates cause health problems when refined and consumed in excess.

The official names for the two groups of simple sugars are monosaccharides and disaccharides. The official names for the two groups of complex carbohydrates are oligosaccharides and polysaccharides.

1. **Monosaccharides** consist of a single chain of carbon atoms. Hence the designation *mono* indicating one chain. Examples are **glucose, fructose and galactose.** They are the final breakdown products of all other carbohydrates. These three sugars occur naturally in all fruits and vegetables but eating whole plant foods is not where most of the sugars in our diet are coming from. By far our biggest source of sugars is soft drinks, baked goods and processed foods. When we have a blood sugar test, we are measuring the amount of glucose in our blood.

2. **Disaccharides** are composed of two chains of carbon atoms. Hence the designation *di* indicating two chains. Disaccharides

are made up of two monosaccharides joined together. Examples are **sucrose, lactose and maltose.**

    (a) sucrose = glucose + fructose = table sugar, the white stuff you're trying to avoid

    (b) lactose = glucose + galactose = the sugar found in milk and dairy products = a problem for people with lactose intolerance

    (c) maltose = glucose + glucose = the sugar produced by sprouting seeds and used in brewing beer.

People with lactose intolerance are deficient in the enzyme lactase, which is required to break down lactose into its constituent monosaccharides, glucose and galactose. If a lactose-intolerant person consumes lactose, they experience a variety of symptoms such as gas, bloating, abdominal pain, diarrhoea or, more rarely, constipation, fatigue and headaches. Some people with lactose intolerance need to avoid lactose altogether while others can tolerate small amounts. Lactose intolerance can be diagnosed by a blood test or hydrogen breath test. People who have no problems digesting lactose need not avoid it.

Because of their different chemical structures, the six simple sugars listed above (glucose, fructose, galactose, sucrose, lactose and maltose) all have different effects on our brain and body.

3. **Oligosaccharides** consist of three to nine chains of carbon atoms and are found in foods such as chicory root, Jerusalem (f)artichoke, onions, garlic, leeks, legumes, wheat and asparagus. *Oligo* means 'few' and refers to the few (three to nine) linked chains of monosaccharides. The human digestive tract has a hard time breaking down many of these carbohydrates and most of them remain undigested until they reach the colon. Here they serve as prebiotics, i.e. food for our gut bacteria. When the bacteria ferment the oligosaccharides, they produce gaseous byproducts that can cause bloating and flatulence. For some people, this is too much of a good thing.

4. **Polysaccharides** are made up of 10 or more monosaccharides joined together. Hence the designation *poly* meaning 'many'. Polysaccharides have two main roles:

(a) to form part of the physical structure of plants, e.g. **cellulose**. This is what constitutes dietary fibre.

(b) to store energy in the form of **starch** (in plants) and **glycogen** (in animals). Starch and glycogen are both composed of multiple chains of glucose. Sources of dietary starch include grains (wheat, rice, oats, cornmeal, rye, millet and barley) and vegetables such as corn, potatoes, peas, parsnip, taro, yams, beetroot and butternut squash.

Classification of carbohydrates

	Simple sugars		Complex carbohydrates	
Official name	monosaccharides	disaccharides	oligosaccharides	polysaccharides
Number of carbon chains	1	2	3–9	10 or more
Examples	glucose (glc) fructose (fru) galactose (gal)	sucrose = glucose + fructose (table sugar) lactose = glucose + galactose (milk sugar) maltose = glucose + glucose (malt sugar)	maltotriulose = glc + glc + fru raffinose = gal + glc + fru kestose = glc + fru + fru	cellulose (dietary fibre) starch glycogen The three polysaccharides above are all made by linking glucose molecules in different ways.

To recap: monosaccharides are the building blocks of all carbohydrates. The different combinations of monosaccharides and the way they are joined together are what give different carbohydrates their individual properties. Hence carbs refers to a wide variety of foods with vastly different effects on our body.

The most damaging carbohydrate is the simple sugar fructose, followed closely by sucrose (because it contains fructose), then glucose and maltose. When we are told to reduce our sugar intake, these are the four sugars that health authorities are referring to. Why are these sugars a problem and where do they lurk in our diet?

All plant foods eventually get broken down into glucose, fructose or galactose. However, if we only ate sugars in the form of real, whole, unadulterated foods — i.e. unrefined carbohydrates such as vegetables, nuts, seeds, legumes and fruit — we would be unlikely to overdose on sugar, whether in the form of fructose, sucrose, glucose or maltose. This is because nature packages sugar with generous amounts of fibre, water, vitamins, minerals and polyphenols. Fibre, water, vitamins (especially vitamin C), minerals and polyphenols slow down the absorption and metabolism of sugar and put the brakes on over-consumption. Your body will tell you if you've eaten too much fruit. Many years ago, I was picking cherries on a beautiful fruit farm in Tasmania. The owners allowed us to eat as many cherries as we wanted while we were picking. I love cherries and there were so many explosively flavourful varieties to taste. By the early afternoon, I felt very bloated and suffered an upset stomach. I've learnt my lesson.

On the other hand, if we extract fructose, sucrose, glucose or maltose from cane, beets, rice, corn, coconut or dates, and refine them to produce crystalline powders or sticky syrups, they are extremely easy to overeat. Removing nature's control mechanisms (fibre and water) sets the stage for dangerously high levels of sugar consumption. It doesn't matter whether it's called raw, organic, natural, granulated or any of the 50+ names for sugar found on food packaging; extracted sugar, regardless of the source, provides a rapidly absorbed hit of empty calories and the equivalent of machine gunfire on our liver and brain. Empty calories are calories that provide no vitamins, minerals or other essential nutrients. Since sucrose (table sugar) is a combination of fructose and glucose, whenever we consume table sugar we are consuming both fructose and glucose. The same goes for high fructose corn syrup (HFCS), a man-made mixture of fructose and glucose used in soft drinks and processed foods produced in the USA.

The all-important point is that nature never intended carbohydrates to enter our bodies without their chaperones: fibre, water, vitamins, minerals and polyphenols. These chaperones stop sugar from misbehaving and inflicting damage. The minute humans started separating sugars from their chaperones and adding them to every food product imaginable, sugar started running amok in our bodies. Adding back some token fibre or vitamins (which breakfast cereal boxes often brag about) does not compensate for having isolated the sugars from their natural sources in the first place. Sugar has been set free to run riot.

The fate of fructose

When we eat a piece of fruit, the fructose it contains is absorbed from our gut into our bloodstream and taken to the liver where it is metabolised with no ill effects. However, when we consume fructose in large amounts — such as that contained in a can of soft drink (375 mL in Australia or 12 ounces in the USA) — the liver converts (metabolises) the fructose into fat (triglycerides). This activates a chain of reactions leading to:

- fatty liver
- insulin resistance (our organs become less responsive to the hormone insulin)
- hyper-insulin-aemia[10] (elevated blood insulin levels)
- elevated blood glucose levels
- eventually, type 2 diabetes.[11]

I will explain all these conditions shortly. You'll soon become familiar with the terms 'insulin resistance' and 'hyperinsulinaemia' because they're the basis for most of the chronic diseases of our modern world: heart disease, stroke, type 2 diabetes, obesity and Alzheimer's. All the diseases induced by insulin resistance are referred to as metabolic diseases or metabolic disorders. The good news is that they're all reversible through dietary and lifestyle measures.

---

[10] I've written hyper-insulin-aemia using hyphens to make it easier to see how the word is constructed. Hyper means 'too much' and aemia denotes that a substance is present in blood. Whatever is inserted between hyper and aemia means there is too much of it in our blood.

[11] Type 2 diabetes and type 1 diabetes are opposite conditions. Type 1 diabetes is a disease of too *little* insulin while type 2 diabetes is a disease of too *much* insulin. In type 1 diabetes there is autoimmune destruction of the insulin-producing cells of the pancreas. It is NOT caused by excess refined carbohydrate consumption, and the only treatment to date is a low carbohydrate diet and lifelong daily insulin injections. In type 2 diabetes, excess refined carbohydrate consumption leads to insulin resistance, which leads to excessive insulin production, which leads to the pancreas giving out. Everything I discuss in this book relates to type 2 diabetes.

If these were the only afflictions associated with fructose, it would be bad enough. But it's just the beginning. Fructose metabolism depletes liver cells of energy and generates the waste product uric acid. Elevated uric acid levels contribute to high blood pressure, gout, kidney stones and a host of other diseases. In addition, fructose can erode our intestinal lining and give rise to a leaky gut, chronic inflammation and food intolerances. If these processes continue unchecked, fructose-induced fatty liver can progress to cirrhosis, cancer and liver failure.

One in four Australian adults have fatty liver disease due to excessive sugar consumption. Many people don't know they have it because there are no obvious symptoms. One clue is the presence of dark brown patches of skin in the folds of the neck, armpits, groin, navel, knuckles, elbows or knees. This is known as acanthosis nigricans. Fatty liver is sometimes picked up by routine liver function tests (blood tests) but a definitive diagnosis requires a liver scan. The condition was originally called non-alcoholic fatty liver disease (NAFLD) to differentiate it from alcohol-induced liver disease. It is now called metabolic-associated fatty liver disease (MAFLD) because it foreshadows type 2 diabetes, heart disease and ultimately Alzheimer's. Fortunately, MAFLD and its corollaries can be rectified by restricting sugar intake. The damage that fructose inflicts on our liver is an indirect means by which fructose contributes to the development of Alzheimer's.

Fructose can also directly interfere with brain function. Fructose can make its way into the brain where it alters hundreds of genes and proteins that regulate learning, memory, metabolism and hunger. Consuming fructose does not lead to satiety and thereby drives overeating and a self-perpetuating destructive spiral. Fructose causes mitochondrial damage, impairs signalling between neurons and creates toxic byproducts. Rats fed high amounts of fructose showed a drop in their ability to learn and remember new information, accompanied by a shrinkage of their hippocampus (the brain's major memory centre), after just one week. In another study, mice fed sugar for several months exhibited features of ADHD, sugar addiction and significant impairment of memory and learning.

Research on fructose and human brain function corroborates these findings. In 2011, a study of 737 Puerto Ricans aged 45 to 75 found that greater intakes of sugar-sweetened beverages and added sugars (not sugars occurring naturally in fruits and vegetables) was linked to lower cognitive function and diminished ability to learn lists of words.

A 2016 New York study of 800 men and women aged 23 to 98 found that the higher their intake of sugar-sweetened soft drinks, the worse their performance in tests of memory, concentration, decision-making and problem-solving. The sugar in the soft drinks was either sucrose or high fructose corn syrup, both of which are combinations of fructose and glucose.

A 2019 study of 1200 Malaysian men and women aged 60 and over found that higher intake of food and drinks containing fructose, sucrose, glucose and maltose was linked to lower MMSE (Mini-Mental State Examination)[12] scores and poorer overall memory and cognition. In contrast, the more real, whole, unadulterated foods and home-cooked meals they ate, the better their brain function.

Need I go on? Many more studies support the same conclusion: **excessive consumption of fructose and sucrose is a major risk factor for Alzheimer's.** Fructose not only directly injures brain cells, it contributes to other risk factors for Alzheimer's, such as high blood pressure, cardiovascular disease, insulin resistance and type 2 diabetes.

What about glucose? As mentioned earlier, sucrose (table sugar) is made up of 50% fructose and 50% glucose. Is glucose just an innocent bystander or can glucose cause problems in its own right?

The fate of glucose

Consuming too much glucose is also a health hazard, but for different reasons to fructose. Sucrose is one source of glucose; carbohydrates such as grains, rice, pasta, bread and potatoes (starches) are also broken down into glucose. Eating glucose stimulates the release of insulin — a hormone produced by the pancreas. One of insulin's

---

[12] For a review of the MMSE, see Chapter 8 'In search of memory' and Appendix 1 .

many roles is to enable glucose to enter our cells where it is either converted to energy or stored as glycogen. When blood glucose levels are higher than what can be stored as glycogen (primarily in the muscles and liver), the excess glucose is turned into triglycerides and accumulates as body fat. Once glucose is converted to fat, insulin locks the fat inside fat cells. In other words, insulin allows glucose to enter cells but it does not allow fat to exit cells. **To shed excess body fat, we have to dial down our insulin production.** This is achieved by reducing glucose intake in the form of both sucrose and starches. You'll recall that fructose also raises blood insulin levels, albeit indirectly, so fructose intake also needs to come down. This trifecta — lowering fructose, glucose and starch consumption — is the key to reducing body fat and preventing and curing type 2 diabetes. It's also the key to keeping our brain in optimal working order.

Keeping blood glucose within a safe range is critical. This is why the pancreas pumps out insulin at the first hint of glucose — to get glucose out of our blood and into our cells. If insulin fails to achieve this, sustained high blood glucose levels (chronic hyperglycaemia) damage the cells that line the inner surface of blood vessels (endothelium). This has downstream effects on almost every organ of the body. The most devastating impacts are seen in the eyes (retinopathy), kidneys (nephropathy), nerves (neuropathy) and penis (erectile dysfunction), which can ultimately lead to blindness, kidney failure and limb amputations (don't worry, the penis is spared). These are the endpoints of type 2 diabetes if it is not treated appropriately. As mentioned earlier, type 2 diabetes is curable and its complications are avoidable.

The bottom line is that the more sugar and refined starches we eat, the more glucose enters our bloodstream and the more insulin we need to siphon the glucose into our organs (especially the liver) to be stored as fat. Sugar and refined starches are collectively known as refined carbohydrates. Refined starches are starches that have had their protective chaperones (notably fibre) removed. Examples are white flour, white rice, white pasta, noodles, peeled potatoes and instant oats.

What happens when we eat too many refined carbohydrates over many years?

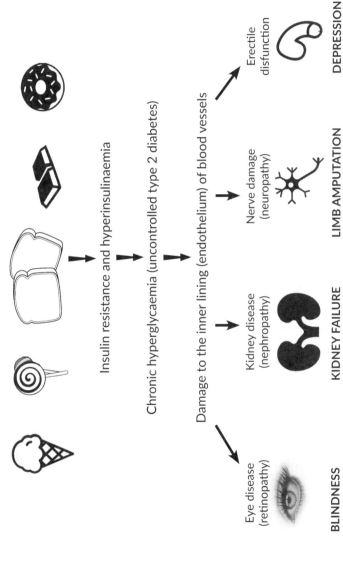

Insulin resistance and hyperinsulinaemia

Chronic hyperglycaemia (uncontrolled type 2 diabetes)

Damage to the inner lining (endothelium) of blood vessels

Eye disease (retinopathy)

BLINDNESS

Kidney disease (nephropathy)

KIDNEY FAILURE

Nerve damage (neuropathy)

LIMB AMPUTATION

Erectile disfunction

DEPRESSION

Eventually the liver becomes so full of fat that it simply can't accept any more glucose and it starts to resist the action of insulin. This is known as liver insulin resistance. In response, the pancreas churns out even more insulin to force more glucose into the liver. This gives rise to elevated blood insulin levels — hyperinsulinaemia. For a time (sometimes for many years) hyperinsulinaemia keeps blood glucose levels in check but at the expense of multiple organ damage and ongoing body fat accumulation. The liver fights back because the increasing fat is deranging the liver's ability to carry out its functions. As the liver increases its resistance, the pancreas increases its output of insulin. Other organs can also become insulin resistant and start to malfunction, including the pancreas itself. Blood glucose levels now start to creep up and the condition is referred to as pre-diabetes. In pre-diabetes, blood glucose levels aren't high enough to be classified as type 2 diabetes, but blood vessel and organ damage has already begun. If refined carbs are not eliminated from the diet, blood glucose will continue to rise until it hits the threshold for type 2 diabetes.

In some cases, the pancreas gets so worn out that it stops making insulin altogether. This prompts doctors to prescribe glucose-lowering medications and insulin injections but these measures are simply bandaids on a gushing wound. At this stage, it is not enough to remove only refined carbs from the diet. All carbs need to be curtailed until insulin sensitivity is restored.

Cutting out carbs gives the pancreas a rest from producing insulin and allows fat to exit our overstuffed liver. The released fat (which is also coming from other organs and body fat stores) can now be used as energy. This reduces hunger and facilitates weight loss. After a period of weeks, months or years (depending on the individual and how long they've had type 2 diabetes), insulin sensitivity returns and our pancreas kickstarts back into action.

Another way to boost insulin sensitivity is to increase our muscle mass through strength training. Larger muscles means they are able to take in more glucose and remove some of the strain on the liver. Other factors such as sleep deprivation, stress and smoking also contribute to insulin resistance — see the Seven S's listed in

Chapter 16 'What's happening to the brain?' Avoiding the Seven S's (sugar, starches, seed oils, sedentary living, sleep deprivation, chronic stress and smoking) almost guarantees we will avoid becoming insulin resistant and diabetic.[13] In our current world, this is easier said than done but it doesn't require perfection. Just keep moving in the direction of fewer S's and you'll be amazed at the positive difference that small daily changes can make.

What does all this glucose dysregulation have to do with the brain and Alzheimer's? Our brain gets caught in the crossfire.

You'll recall from my discussion with Jasmin in Chapter 16 'What's happening to the brain?' that one of the first things that happens in Alzheimer's is a reduction in the brain's capacity to use glucose for fuel — a condition known as cerebral glucose hypo-metabolism. Just as the liver and muscles can become insulin resistant, so can the brain. This means that brain cells are not able to take in glucose and use it for energy. This causes brain cells to starve, malfunction and die off.

Insulin resistance goes hand-in-hand with increased amounts of insulin floating around. Insulin eventually has to be cleared away and one of the enzymes that performs this function is called (not surprisingly) insulin degrading enzyme (IDE). It turns out that IDE is also required for the breakdown of amyloid beta (Aβ)! Therefore, if IDE is preoccupied with removing insulin, Aβ is left to accumulate and form plaques. Insulin also has structural and regulatory roles in the brain, which are likewise compromised when the brain becomes insulin resistant. Hence insulin resistance is a multi-pronged assault on the brain:

---

13 In addition to type 1 and type 2 diabetes, a rare form of diabetes called monogenic diabetes or MODY (which stands for Mature-Onset Diabetes of the Young) is caused by a change in a single gene inherited from one or (extremely rarely) both parents. The gene disrupts the ability of the pancreas to make and release sufficient insulin. Therefore, a person with MODY can make some, but not enough, insulin. It is usually diagnosed in adolescence or early adulthood and is not necessarily associated with excess body fat. Depending on the specific gene mutation, a person with MODY may or may not need insulin injections or oral glucose-lowering medication. In many instances, a person with MODY can remain medication-free by eating a low carbohydrate diet and engaging in regular strength training and endurance exercise. The diagnosis of MODY is confirmed by genetic testing.

- Insulin resistance impairs the brain's ability to use glucose for fuel.
- Insulin resistance hinders the clearance of Aβ, leading to destructive plaque formation.
- Insulin resistance promotes the build-up of tau tangles, and tau tangles accelerate insulin resistance, thereby creating a vicious cycle of ongoing brain damage.

Insulin resistance is a fundamental cause of Alzheimer's. Insulin resistance is a domino that sets off a cascade of events that culminate in diminished brain function. This is not to say that everyone with insulin resistance will go on to develop Alzheimer's. Everyone who smokes does not develop lung cancer. However, insulin resistance is a warning that the brain's energy supply is under threat. A Finnish study of 980 people aged 69 to 78 (349 men and 631 women) found that hyperinsulinaemia (which inevitably accompanies insulin resistance) is associated with a higher risk of Alzheimer's than carrying an APOE4 gene.

The dietary measures that dramatically reduce our risk of Alzheimer's are screaming at us: **we need to eat in a way that prevents insulin resistance and reduces inflammation.** The following 10 steps will enable us to achieve this (in order of priority).

1. **Quit soft drinks** and all sugary beverages including sports drinks, energy drinks, fruit juices, fruit smoothies, cordials, flavoured mineral waters, milk shakes, flavoured milks and flavoured yoghurt drinks. They are all sugar bombs. Obviously, some drinks have more sugar than others but, as a general rule, consuming any of these beverages is akin to throwing a hand grenade into our brain: destruction and devastation. Read the nutrition panel on the product. You'll be shocked at the amount of sugar in one small drink. Replace them with water.

2. **Quit added sugars** — or at least reduce your daily intake to comply with World Health Organisation (WHO) guidelines. See Chapter 42 'Carb correction'.

3. **Quit refined carbohydrates** (refined starches). These include biscuits, pastries, cakes, donuts, muffins, scones, white bread, bagels, croissants, white rice, white pasta, pizza dough, crackers,

noodles, French fries, potato chips, corn chips, instant mashed potato, instant oatmeal, muesli, granola and breakfast cereals.

4. **Quit vegetable oils** (industrially processed seed oils). Throughout this book I use the terms 'vegetable oils' and 'seed oils' interchangeably. These include sunflower oil, safflower oil, soybean oil, corn oil, cottonseed oil, rice bran oil, grape seed oil, canola (rapeseed) oil and margarines. Despite being promoted as heart-healthy, vegetable oils are nothing of the sort. This will be discussed in Chapters 44–46, 'What the fat is going on?', 'The fat is in the fire' and 'The fat hits the fan'.

5. Having implemented the above, you can now **ADD generous amounts of healthy fats** to your diet. These include olive oil, coconut oil, avocado oil, macadamia nut oil, butter, lard, ghee and duck fat. Use them as desired in cooking, making sauces and splashing over salads, vegetables and meats. **Dietary fat is NOT fattening** *unless it is combined with sugar or refined starches.* You do not need to trim the fat off meat or take the skin off chicken. And by all means enjoy your pork crackling and full fat cheeses! If you think I've suddenly gone mad, jump ahead to Chapter 44 'What the fat is going on?'

6. **Quit processed foods** (aka fake foods) that contain any of the ingredients on **The Noxious List**. If you've accomplished steps one to five, you've probably already quit most processed foods. Good on you!

7. **If you have been diagnosed with type 2 diabetes,** pre-diabetes or fatty liver (NAFLD or MAFLD), you may also need to cut down on starchy vegetables (e.g. corn and potatoes), legumes (e.g. beans and chickpeas) and grains — even whole grains. These foods are NOT inherently harmful, however when a person has developed insulin resistance, they need to minimise all sources of carbohydrates in order to regain insulin sensitivity. Note that gluten-free does not mean carb-free. Gluten-free products often contain even *more* added sugar than their regular counterparts.

8. **Eat as much real, whole, unadulterated food** as you need to feel satiated. All real food is on the menu if you enjoy it and it

agrees with you (other than starches, legumes and grains if you have diabetes or insulin resistance). Meat, eggs and dairy often come under fire but there is no evidence they are detrimental to our health UNLESS they've been fried in vegetable oils or laced with ingredients from **The Noxious List**.

9. Include as many **BRAIN FOODS** and **SMASH** seafoods as you can. See Chapter 35 'Does what we eat really matter?' for a refresher on the acronyms.

10. Take note of how you respond to each dietary change you make. Do you have more energy? Are you thinking more clearly? Are you sleeping better? Has your mood improved? How do you feel physically and mentally? View nutrition as a way to discover your best self — because it is. **Every meal is truly an opportunity to heal.** This is not just empty rhetoric. Eating is something we do several times every day — how can it not have enormous impacts on every aspect of our health? People on medication for diabetes, high blood pressure and a range of other conditions are often able to come off their pills after revamping their diet. PLEASE only reduce your medication dose in consultation with your doctor. Educating ourselves about food and how it affects us is incredibly empowering and exhilarating. It's the most important lifelong adventure you'll ever embark on.

CHAPTER 41

Fifty shades of sugar

People only see what they are prepared to see.

RALPH WALDO EMERSON (1803–1882)

If you're looking for another party trick (the first one I offered was to stand on one leg with your eyes closed doing complex mental arithmetic — see Chapter 30 'Tip the balance') this one is sure to impress: rattle off the following 50-plus aliases for sugar. I provide this list to enable you to identify added sugars in products that you might not have suspected contained sugar. They all end up as either fructose or glucose and lead to the associated harms. The list is also a great cure for insomnia. Forget counting sheep — count sugar instead.

But why *fifty* shades of sugar?
- Because of the many different *lights* in which sugar is portrayed in science, the media and food marketing.
- Because of sugar's *shady* reputation in relation to our health.
- Because there are more than 50 different names for sugar sprinkled liberally throughout our food supply. (You'll notice there are in fact more than 70 different names for sugar but 'Fifty shades' has a more provocative ring to it …)

If you come across an alias I haven't mentioned, please visit the contact page on outwittingalzheimers.com and inform me of my omission. I'd be delighted to hear from you.

SUGARS THAT CONTAIN FRUCTOSE		
Sugars that are at least honest enough to include sugar in their name	**Sugars that go by the name of syrup**	**Sugars that are particularly well camouflaged by exotic names**
1. Barbados sugar	26. buttered syrup	46. agave nectar
2. beet sugar	27. carob syrup	47. attar or qattar
3. brown sugar	28. flavoured syrup	48. blackstrap molasses
4. cane sugar	29. fruit syrup	49. caramel
5. caster sugar	30. golden syrup	50. chashni
6. coconut sugar	31. high fructose corn syrup (HFCS)	51. date honey
7. confectioners' sugar	32. honey syrup	52. demerara
8. dark brown sugar	33. invert syrup	53. dried fruit
9. date sugar	34. maple syrup	54. Florida crystals
10. golden sugar	35. palm syrup	55. honey
11. granulated sugar	36. refiners' syrup	56. kuromitsu
12. grape sugar	37. rose syrup	57. molasses
13. icing sugar	38. sorghum syrup	58. muscovado
14. invert sugar	**Sugars that go by the name of juice**	59. panela
15. organic sugar		60. rapadura •
16. palm sugar	39. cane juice crystals	61. treacle
17. powdered sugar	40. evaporated cane juice	
18. raw sugar	41. fruit juice	
19. raw organic sugar	42. fruit juice concentrate	
20. sanding sugar	**Sugars that go by their chemical name**	
21. superfine sugar		
22. table sugar	43. crystalline fructose	
23. turbinado sugar	44. saccarose	
24. unrefined sugar	45. sucrose	
25. yellow sugar		

SUGARS THAT CONTAIN MOSTLY GLUCOSE		
Syrups	Malts	Chemical names
62. barley malt syrup	70. malt sugar	73. dextrose
63. corn sweetener	71. maltose	74. glucose solids
64. corn syrup	72. maltobiose	
65. corn syrup solids		
66. high maltose corn syrup (HMCS)		
67. malt syrup		
68. rice malt syrup		
69. rice syrup		

CHAPTER 42

Carb correction

If someone is able to show me that what I think or do is not right, I will happily change, for I seek the truth, by which no one was ever truly harmed. It is the person who continues in his self-deception and ignorance who is harmed.

MARCUS AURELIUS (121–180 CE)

While I passionately advocate for everyone to follow the 10 steps outlined in Chapter 40 'Sweet talk', different people can tolerate different amounts of sugar, refined starches and grains before they run into trouble. These differences are influenced by our genes, microbiota (gut bacteria), life circumstances, muscularity, level of physical activity, chronic stress and other components of our diet.

Many Asian cultures have been consuming copious amounts of white rice for centuries without suffering epidemics of obesity and type 2 diabetes. How so? Their diets were devoid of sugar and fake foods, while simultaneously rich in fermented vegetables and real foods. They also had active outdoor lives, better quality sleep and supportive social networks. It's the totality of our lives that ultimately makes the difference. Now that we've screwed up so many aspects of our lives, we have little to buffer a high carb diet.

How does a person know if they're consuming too many carbs? In other words, how do you know if you are insulin resistant and at heightened risk of Alzheimer's? **There are 10 Telltale Signs** — all of which are referred to as metabolic disorders or metabolic diseases — that indicate you are eating more sugar, refined starches and grains than your body can handle. Any one of these is a sign of hyperinsulinaemia and insulin resistance and calls for cutting back on carbs:

1. pre-diabetes or type 2 diabetes
2. fatty liver disease (NAFLD or MAFLD)
3. high blood pressure (hypertension) — consistently above 130/80
4. acanthosis nigricans — see Chapter 40 'Sweet talk'
5. gout
6. polycystic ovarian syndrome (PCOS)
7. erectile dysfunction
8. abdominal obesity, i.e. a waist circumference greater than 80 cm for women or 94 cm for men, or a waist-to-hip ratio of >0.85 (women) or >0.9 (men)
9. constant hunger and difficulty feeling satiated
10. any one of the following blood tests reveals higher than normal levels:
    (a) fasting glucose
    (b) fasting insulin
    (c) fasting triglycerides
    (d) OGTT = oral glucose tolerance test
    (e) HbA1C
    (f) uric acid
    (g) C-peptide.

The following signs *hint* at insulin resistance but they can also occur for other reasons:

11. you have irregular periods
12. you don't feel as sharp or energetic as you'd like to feel
13. you have tried calorie-restriction or low-fat diets and they don't work for you
14. you have rheumatoid arthritis or other inflammatory conditions.

As soon as you reduce the insulin-spiking foods in your diet (sugar, refined starches and grains) all these metabolic disorders will start to improve. Some people feel immediate benefits after taking only the first two steps in Chapter 40 'Sweet talk'. Great for you! Other people will need to take things further. The brilliant news is that all the above conditions are curable through the recommendations in this book — thereby significantly lowering your risk of Alzheimer's. I'll repeat that in case you thought it was a typo: despite what anyone tells you (including your doctor), **all 14 conditions can be cured through dietary and lifestyle interventions.** However, NEVER stop taking a prescribed medication without medical supervision, and consult your doctor to monitor your progress upon changing your diet.

What if you have no telltale signs but are nonetheless concerned you might be eating too much sugar? Is there a 'safe' level of sugar consumption just as there is a 'safe' level of alcohol consumption? (The latter is debatable — see Chapter 49 'Drink to me only with thine eyes'.)

The World Health Organisation (WHO) recommends the following upper limits for daily added sugar intake. 'Added sugar' refers to the sugar in processed foods and beverages, not the sugar in whole fruits and vegetables. The latter do not count towards our daily limits.
- Children under the age of two years — NIL
- Children under the age of 12 years — four teaspoons (16 grams)
- Women — six teaspoons (24 grams)
- Men — nine teaspoons (36 grams)

Personally, I think these amounts are overly generous and I aim for as little sugar as possible. You don't have to go cold turkey. Just keep moving in the direction of eating less and less sugar. One teaspoon is equivalent to 4.2 grams but to make the maths easy, divide the number of grams by four to convert to teaspoons. On the other hand, some people find it easier to eat zero sugar than small amounts of sugar. Use the approach that works best for you. Eating sugar is a learned habit and has the potential to become an addiction. **The less sugar we eat, the less sugar we crave.** Quitting sugar is not as difficult as we expect it to be. The biggest hurdle is pushback from family and friends. (Give them this book.) There are many great low carb organisations, websites, podcasts and online communities that provide support, recipes and practical advice. Excellent resources can be found at:

dietdoctor.com
lowcarbdownunder.com.au
defeatdiabetes.com.au
adaptyourlifeacademy.com

If you struggle with emotional eating, I recommend reading my book *NeuroSlimming — Let your brain change your body*.

Before concluding the subject of sugar, it's necessary to expose **The Great Pretenders:** foods that deceive people because they carry a self-righteous health halo.

The Great Pretenders include fruit juice, fruit smoothies, dried fruit, breakfast cereals, granola, muesli bars, honey, maple syrup and a subset of wholegrain products. These foods are heavily marketed as 'healthy choices' but are wolves in sheep's clothing. Front-of-pack labelling such as 'low fat', 'no added sugar', 'all natural ingredients' or 'fortified with vitamins and minerals' are red flags for being high carb and highly processed so the vitamins and minerals had to be added back. The term 'all natural' is meaningless because it is open to vast interpretation. How often have you heard sugar described as 'natural' because it comes from sugar cane? Just because something originated in nature doesn't mean it retains its natural properties when it ends up in a box. Meanwhile, 'no added sugar' frequently means the product contains so much dried fruit or artificial sweeteners that the manufacturer didn't need to add any more sugar. Alternatively, 'no added sugar' can be a case of semantics in which the manufacturer does not acknowledge that honey or maple syrup qualify as sugar. They most definitely do — just ask your liver. Occasionally, 'no added sugar' really does mean no added sugar. You'll have to read the nutrition panel on the back to find out. Look through the list of ingredients and see if they include one (or frequently more) of the 70+ names for sugar you memorised from the previous chapter. Then note how many grams of sugar are documented in the contents table.

While **honey and maple syrup** contain antioxidants and trace amounts of minerals (especially zinc and manganese in the case of maple syrup), these constituents do NOT offset their high sugar content. One tablespoon of either honey or maple syrup contains about 16 grams (4 teaspoons) of sugar. Vegetables are incomparably richer and healthier sources of both antioxidants and minerals. Honey can serve as a cough suppressant so reserve it as a medicine when coughing interferes with a restful night. Honey applied to the skin can aid in healing burns, wounds and diabetic foot ulcers.

If you implement the suggestions in this book, you won't ever have to deal with a diabetic foot ulcer.

The worst way to consume sugar is to drink it. Sugary beverages are much more likely to cause obesity and metabolic derangements than are sugary foods. We tend to drink more quickly than we eat and this results in high amounts of sugar arriving at the liver in a short space of time. A 12-ounce can (355 mL) of soft drink contains 10 teaspoons of sugar. This onslaught of fructose on the liver and brain triggers the chain of reactions leading to mitochondrial stress, uric acid production and insulin resistance. Soft drink companies know this. A deceptive way to design studies on sugary beverages is to tell participants to sip their juice or soda over a period of several hours. The slow trickle of fructose and glucose entering the bloodstream gives the liver time to metabolise the sugars with no ill effect in the short term. Liar liar, liver on fire. Who takes three hours to finish drinking a small can of soft drink?

What about **fruit juice** that is made from 100% fruit with nothing added? What about fruit that you juice yourself at home? There are more than 20 grams or 5 teaspoons of sugar in one cup (250 mL) of orange juice. When we juice fruit, we ingest a much larger quantity of fruit than when we eat it. Juicing removes the fibre and speeds up absorption so we're left with a big dose of liquid sugar. Blood levels of fructose, glucose and insulin spike rapidly and our liver is left to clean up the mess. I shudder when I hear someone going on a juice cleanse. Whether it is cold pressed or freshly squeezed, juice is a tidal wave of sugar causing destruction in its wake. There is no need to drink fruit. We can obtain all our vitamins and minerals from eating whole foods.

What about **fruit smoothies** that retain the fibre? Most smoothies involve pulverising the fibre so it loses its functionality. This means there are no brakes on the speed at which the sugar enters our bloodstream. In addition, smoothies pack in a LOT of fruit — much more than we would ever eat in a single sitting. Fruit smoothies are still a sugar bomb unless you keep the fruit to a minimum (such as half a cup of berries) and use ingredients such as spinach, kale and avocado instead.

Dried fruit presents another vehicle for rapid ingestion of large amounts of sugar. Removing water removes bulk and leaves us with highly concentrated sugar. Try eating the same number of grapes as there are sultanas in the tiniest available packet. You'll finish the sultanas in a matter of seconds but you're likely to get a stomach ache before you get through the grapes. Eat fruit as nature provided it, including all edible peels.

Breakfast cereals = refined carbs + sugar + very savvy marketing. Even cereals labelled wholegrain often contain large amounts of dried fruit, added sugars and vegetable oils.

Granola and muesli bars = various combinations of refined carbs, dried fruit, nuts and seeds. Depending on the brand, they can also include added sugars, vegetable oils and flavourings. They are yet another synonym for sugar bomb.

The subject of **grains** is highly divisive. I've seen nutrition experts shouting at each other defending their polarised positions. Let's tackle the topic at the grassroots level (pun intended) so you can determine for yourself whether or not to include grains in your diet.

Grains are the seeds of grassy plants called cereals. Common grains include wheat, rice, corn (maize), rye, triticale (a hybrid of wheat and rye), barley, oats, sorghum, millet, farro and teff. Pseudo grains are the seeds of pseudo cereals (non-grasses) but they are used in a similar way to grains. Examples of pseudo grains are quinoa, chia, amaranth and buckwheat. Unless otherwise stated, when I use the term 'grains', I'm referring to both true grains and pseudo grains.

Grains have three parts:
- a hard outer shell called the bran (also known as the seed coat or pericarp)
- a middle layer called the endosperm
- an inner layer called the germ or embryo.

Bran = undigestible carbs + small amounts of protein = a source of dietary fibre (prebiotics).

Endosperm = starch (glucose) + small amounts of protein = empty carb calories.

Germ = oils + significant amounts of protein + minerals = a source of healthy fats, proteins and minerals.

Here is the same information in a table:

Part of the grain	What it contains	Is it good for health?
bran (outer layer)	indigestible fibre (prebiotics) + small amounts of protein	yes
endosperm (middle layer)	starch (glucose) + small amounts of protein	yes — if eaten as part of the whole grain no — if it is removed from the bran and germ and eaten as a refined grain
germ (inner layer)	fat + protein + minerals	yes

The exact proportion of carbs, proteins and oils varies between different types of grains. Chia seeds have the highest amounts of fibre, oils and protein. They stimulate the smallest insulin response of all grains.

When a grain is refined, the outer shell and inner germ (nature's chaperones) are both removed. All that remains in a refined grain is the carb-rich, insulin-spiking endosperm devoid of nutritional value. It's akin to eating sugar.

In contrast, wholegrain products retain all three parts. However, whole grains are nonetheless frequently processed by cracking, crushing, rolling or pulverising them. The more a grain is smashed to smithereens (e.g. made into very fine flour), the more we lose the protective effect of its chaperones (particularly fibre) and the more our blood glucose and insulin will spike. For instance, steel cut oats are healthier than rolled oats are healthier than quick oats are healthier than instant oats.

Another example is eating cooked whole wheat berries (the name given to whole grains of wheat) versus grinding wheat berries into flour and eating them as bread. Even though the bread is made from whole grains, the grains have been changed in a way that produces more rapid increases in blood glucose levels than when eating the intact wheat berries mixed through a salad. The degree to which a grain is processed matters. The more a food has been altered from its original form, the less healthful it is likely to be. The faster it cooks, the faster we digest it and the faster our blood glucose shoots up. Thus, eating grains — even wholegrain products — can contribute to insulin resistance.

Another problem with many wholegrain products such as bread and crackers is that they often have added sugar, vegetable oils, colourings and flavourings. The bottom line: if a person is insulin resistant — and especially if they have type 2 diabetes — they have become carbohydrate intolerant. Their body is no longer able to metabolise carbs without causing harm. They can continue to eat non-starchy vegetables (essentially all vegetables that grow above the ground) but they need to abstain from starchy vegetables (potatoes, parsnip, butternut squash) and grains (other than chia seeds). This dramatically curtails insulin production and enables a person to burn fat for fuel. Many type 2 diabetics are able to stop their insulin injections within a few days of cutting out carbs. This makes perfect sense. If you don't eat carbs you don't need insulin. Although proteins also stimulate insulin production, they do so to a far lesser degree than carbs. Many ex-diabetics find that after a period of months or years (depending on how long they had diabetes and how much damage their pancreas sustained) they can slowly reintroduce a range of carb-containing whole foods.

The take home message is that all grains — whole or otherwise — are a rich source of carbs. Even though whole grains provide fibre and minerals, there is nothing in grains that we can't obtain from other food sources such as meat and vegetables. Grains are not an essential component of the human diet. However, if you are insulin sensitive and enjoy a handful of grains as part of a salad or side dish, choose 100% whole grains with nothing added.

An excellent rice replacement is cauliflower pulsed through a food processor for 10 seconds. A bonus is that it cooks in much less time than rice. Google 'cauliflower rice' for recipes. As for bread, there are hundreds of delicious low carb bread, cracker and pizza base recipes all over the internet. It's worth the minimal effort and great satisfaction of home baking. Another bread alternative is to use cabbage, cos or iceberg lettuce leaves to wrap around sandwich fillings and home-made burgers.

As mentioned earlier, all potatoes (white, brown, orange, red and purple) get broken down into glucose and are too high in carbs for someone with insulin resistance. Swap mashed potato for mashed cauliflower.

A simple way to reduce blood glucose and insulin levels resulting from foods such as potatoes, rice and pasta is to cool them down after cooking and either eat them cold (e.g. potato salad and sushi) or reheat them the following day. The effect of cooling is to convert a large percentage of the cooked starch into crystals that are resistant to digestive enzymes. If we are not able to break down starch, we are not able to absorb glucose. The process is called starch retrogradation and the crystals are designated resistant starch. Resistant starch behaves like insoluble fibre and is fermented by colonic bacteria to produce gut-friendly compounds known as short chain fatty acids (SCFA) — a win for both us and our gut bacteria. Reheating does not convert resistant starch back into insulin-spiking starch.

This chapter is not intended to engender a fear of carbs but rather a healthy respect for them. Traditional cultures that subsisted on grains and starchy vegetables have demonstrated that as long as we avoid fake food and don't overdose on sugar and refined starches, we can maintain lifelong insulin sensitivity and enjoy carbohydrates in the form of vegetables, fruits, legumes and whole grains.

Now that we've sorted out the carbs, we can add back all the fabulous fats we've been denying ourselves! Fats do not raise insulin levels. Contrary to the perception that eliminating sugar and refined carbs is a restrictive way of eating, it creates space for a whole smorgasbord of delectable healing foods.

CHAPTER 43

Insulin overhaul

When everything seems to be going against you, remember that the airplane takes off against the wind, not with it.

HENRY FORD (1863–1947)

By now it should be evident that hyperinsulinaemia and insulin resistance are core drivers of many metabolic diseases including Alzheimer's. It should also be evident that too much sugar and refined starches are major causes of insulin dysregulation but they are not the only causes. Various other factors play a role in determining whether our organs respond to insulin.

The following table summarises the most common contributors to insulin resistance and hence to Alzheimer's. I've tried to list them in order of impact, but the relative importance for each individual person is highly variable. I first touched on these in my conversation with Jasmin in Chapter 16 'What's happening to the brain?' where I referred to them as **The Seven S's**. Here I've expanded the seven to **17 S's**. (By now it should also be evident that I'm partial to alliteration.)

Factors that contribute to insulin resistance	How to reverse insulin resistance
1. Soft drinks and sports drinks	Quit all soft drinks, sports drinks, fruit juices, fruit smoothies, cordials, flavoured milks and other sugary beverages like iced tea.
2. Sugar	See Chapter 40 'Sweet talk'.
3. Starches (refined)	See Chapter 42 'Carb correction'.
4. Seed oils (contribute to inflammation)	See Chapter 44 'What the fat is going on?'
5. Synthetic food (fake food)	See Chapter 39 'The Noxious List'.
6. Sarcopenia (muscle loss)	Engage in strength training at least two times per week. See Chapters 27 and 28 'Resistance is not futile' and 'Get a grip'.
7. Sedentary living = lack of physical exercise and sitting for prolonged periods	Move in a way that you enjoy for at least 150 minutes per week. See Chapter 25 'No pain, more gain'. Stand up for 2 minutes every 20 to 30 minutes. See Chapter 26 'Jack-in-the-box'.
8. Size = having a waist circumference of >80 cm for women and >94 cm for men. This is because visceral (abdominal) fat contributes to chronic inflammation.	There is a two-way relationship between visceral obesity and insulin resistance, i.e. insulin resistance leads to visceral obesity and visceral obesity leads to insulin resistance. The above steps all promote visceral fat reduction. See Chapter 42 'Carb correction'.
9. Sleep deprivation and sleep apnoea	Aim for 7–9 hours of good quality sleep per night. See Chapters 17 and 19 'Snore no more' and 'Let sleep be your medicine'.
10. Shift work	Try to have regular shifts rather than a continually changing roster so that you can establish a routine. Get as close as possible to 7–9 hours of sleep per 24-hour period. See Chapter 51 'Good timing'.
11. Stress (severe and chronic)	Give yourself permission to take time out and do nothing. Learn to manage stress through breath work, meditation, music, yoga, CBT and doing things just for fun.
12. Smoking and air pollution	See Chapters 57 and 75 'Smoke alarm' and 'Something's in the air'.

Factors that contribute to insulin resistance	How to reverse insulin resistance
13. Sepsis (infections), e.g. gingivitis or inflammatory conditions, e.g. rheumatoid arthritis, Crohn's disease	Prolonged infections can lead to insulin resistance because they are accompanied by prolonged inflammation. See Chapter 72 'Mental floss'.
14. Sex hormones scaling down, e.g. menopause in women (low oestrogen) and andropause in men (low testosterone)	Severe hot flushes and night sweats have been associated with greater insulin resistance in women who are going through menopause. Discuss the possibility of Menopausal Hormone Therapy (MHT) with your doctor.
15. Shortfall in thyroid hormones — symptoms include fatigue, increased cold sensitivity, dry skin, constipation, expanding waistline, puffy face, thinning hair, muscle weakness, painful swollen joints, slowed heart rate, depressed mood and impaired memory. The thyroid gland may or may not be enlarged.	If you have an underactive thyroid gland (known as hypothyroidism) you may need Thyroid Replacement Therapy (TRT).
16. Side effects of certain medications, e.g. steroids, statins and antipsychotics	Not all antipsychotics and statins contribute to insulin resistance. Speak to your doctor about whether insulin resistance is a potential side effect of any medications you are taking.
17. Sweeteners, e.g. saccharin, sucralose and sugar alcohols	See Chapter 71 'You can't fool your brain'.

CHAPTER 44

What the fat is going on?

*No diet will remove all the fat from your body because the brain
is mostly fat. Without a brain, you might look good,
but all you could do is run for public office.*

GEORGE BERNARD SHAW (1856–1950)

Puppy fat, belly fat, subcutaneous fat, visceral fat.

Saturated, unsaturated, monounsaturated, polyunsaturated.
Omega-3, omega-6, trans and hydrogenated.
Virgin, extra virgin, cold pressed, hot pressed.

What the fat is going on?

What constitutes healthy and unhealthy fat in our bodies and on our
plates? When orthodox nutrition experts talk about 'bad fats' they're
usually referring to saturated fats — butter, coconut oil and fatty
meat. When health-conscious consumers talk about 'bad fats' they're
referring to polyunsaturated vegetable oils and margarines. Who's
right? Who's confused? Who's bamboozled about butter? There's
an ever-widening chasm between various schools of thought and
the general public is caught in the crossfire. How do we dissect fat
from fiction? Moreover, what does fat have to do with Alzheimer's?

To answer these questions we need to examine not only the science
of fat but also the economics and politics of fat. Science and politics
have been on a long collision course that has blown up into a health
crisis of massive proportions (pun intended).

Body fat, technically known as adipose tissue (AT), is fascinating stuff.

Of all the constituents of the human body, it's the one that varies the most between individuals. For adult men, a healthy amount of body fat is 10–22% of total body weight and, for women, 16–30%. This difference is largely due to oestrogen hormones, which reduce a woman's capacity to burn energy after eating. This allows her to convert more calories into body fat. The extra fat stores prepare her to nourish a developing foetus during pregnancy and breastfeed without jeopardising her own energy requirements. When we're born, we have a higher percentage of body fat than any other species on the planet. The purpose of all this baby fat is to help fuel our rapidly developing energy-demanding brains.

Fat tissue is composed mainly of fat cells (called adipocytes) but it also contains immune cells. The various cells within body fat produce over 80 different chemicals that influence many of our bodily functions and susceptibility to disease.

When it comes to body fat, what matters is location, location, location. **Subcutaneous fat (SAT)** is the layer of fat under our skin. Sub means 'under' and cutaneous refers to skin. Colloquially it is known as 'the inch you can pinch'. Subcutaneous fat is found all over our body: hips, thighs, arms, back, belly, palms and soles of our feet. Subcutaneous fat serves as an energy reserve and insulates us from the cold. Carrying large amounts of subcutaneous fat is not a health hazard unless it gets to a level that impedes our ability to move or breathe.

The fat that surrounds and infiltrates the organs inside our abdomen is another story. This is known as **visceral fat (VAT)** from the word 'viscera' meaning 'internal organ'. Colloquially it is known as belly fat or beer belly. Small amounts of VAT line the inner surface of our abdomen and are of no concern. However, if we develop insulin resistance, increasing amounts of VAT are deposited throughout our abdomen and internal organs: liver, pancreas, kidneys and heart. This is bad news because VAT produces hormones and inflammatory compounds that drive up heart disease, type 2 diabetes, cancer (especially breast, uterus, colon and kidney), Alzheimer's and vascular dementia. Thus belly fat is not just another place we store excess calories. Belly fat behaves differently from the fat on our hips and thighs. VAT *mis*behaves by spitting out harmful chemicals that wreak havoc throughout our body. One way of keeping VAT in check is daily physical exercise. Why? It's not about burning calories. It's because **the hormonal and metabolic effects of physical exercise are the exact opposite of the hormonal and metabolic effects of excess VAT.**

VAT is not visible to the naked eye but, for most people, waist circumference is a close and useful approximation. As a rough guide, **men with a waist greater than 94 cm and women greater than 80 cm begin to increase their risk of chronic diseases including Alzheimer's.** Waist circumference is a much more accurate predictor of future health problems than is body weight or body mass index (BMI).[14] Swap the bathroom scales for a tape measure.

Therefore, the all-important question is: what drives visceral fat production? Is it simply a matter of eating too much and exercising too little? Far from it. *What* and *when* we eat is just as important as *how much* we eat. **Insulin resistance is both a cause and consequence of VAT.** Thus sugar and refined starches are a major stimulus for VAT accumulation. If you don't recall why (and I don't blame you as it's a complex topic), reread Chapters 40 and 42 'Sweet talk' and 'Carb correction'. In contrast, eating fat does NOT make us fat — unless the fat comes from industrially processed vegetable oils (seed oils). Why?

The following chapter explains why fats in real food keep us healthy and fats in processed food make us sick. It's a heavy chapter with respect to the science because I don't want you to take my word for it that vegetable oils are toxic. I want you to see it for yourself by understanding their chemical properties. Read on to discover a seedy affair …

---

[14] BMI = weight (in kilograms) divided by the square of your height (in metres). For example, a person weighing 100 kg who is two metres tall would have a BMI of $100/4 = 25$. A healthy BMI is deemed to range from 20 to 25 but this does not apply to someone who is very muscular. Don't worry about BMI. Measure your waist circumference instead.

CHAPTER 45

The fat is in the fire

*The only real mistake is the one from which
we learn nothing.*

HENRY FORD (1863–1947)

The previous chapter was about the fat in our body. This chapter is about the fat on our plates — and what happens to it when it is assimilated into our body.

Fats are of different types and found in varying amounts in a range of foods. Fats are also extracted from foods like milk, olives and seeds to make butter, olive oil and sunflower oil respectively. Oils are simply fats that are liquid at room temperature. Fats/oils in their natural state are healthy. Fats/oils extracted from foods may be healthy or unhealthy depending on how they are extracted, processed and heated.

Fats do much more than provide us with energy; they are components of all our cell membranes. This means they influence the transport of substances into and out of cells, and they're vital to a vast number of cellular processes.

All fats have the same number of calories — nine Calories per gram. **All fats in real whole unadulterated foods play a role in keeping us healthy.** Fats also help us absorb vitamins A, D, E and K because these vitamins dissolve in fat. Hence the recommendation to drizzle extra virgin olive oil over your salads, mushrooms and steamed vegetables. Or add a dob of butter if you prefer. It was only when humans started extracting oils from seeds (such as sunflower seeds, safflower seeds, cotton seeds, rapeseeds, corn, rice bran, soybeans etc.), using heat, pressure, solvents, bleaches and deodorisers, that we started to mess up our metabolism.

Fats are made up of fatty acids (FAs) just as carbohydrates are made up of sugars. Fatty acids are designated as saturated, monounsaturated or polyunsaturated depending on the number of double bonds in their chemical structure. Mono- and polyunsaturated FAs are collectively referred to as unsaturated.

A double bond means the fatty acid has a free hand (carbon atom) to grab onto passing oxygen atoms. This chemical reaction is known as **oxidation,** and it leads to **rancidity.** Rancid oils have a bitter taste and unpleasant odour. More importantly, they are damaging to our health. The more double bonds, the less stable the FA and the more it needs to be protected from oxygen, heat and light to prevent it from going rancid.

1. **Saturated** fatty acids (SFAs) have NO double bonds. This makes them solid at room temperature, e.g. butter, lard and coconut oil.

2. **Monounsaturated** fatty acids (MUFAs) have ONE double bond. This makes them liquid at room temperature but they will solidify in the fridge, e.g. olive oil.

3. **Polyunsaturated** fatty acids (PUFAs) have TWO or more double bonds. This enables them to remain liquid even when placed in the freezer, e.g. fish oil, sunflower oil, soybean oil, rice bran oil.

Unsaturated FAs need to be kept in dark airtight bottles or metal containers and stored in a dark cool place. Don't leave them out on your kitchen benchtop or near your stove. Unsaturated fatty acids are classified according to where their double bonds are located.

If the first double bond occurs between the third and fourth carbon atoms from what is known as the omega end of the molecule, it is called an **omega-3** fatty acid and is written as n-3 or ω-3. Examples of omega-3 fatty acids are alpha-linolenic acid (ALA), eicosa-pentaenoic acid (EPA) and docosa-hexaenoic acid (DHA). ALA is found mainly in plant foods such as flaxseeds (linseeds), hemp seeds, chia seeds, walnuts, soybeans, edamame (young soy beans harvested before they have ripened or hardened), tofu, tempeh and dark leafy greens.

EPA and DHA are found in seaweed, fatty fish (e.g. salmon, trout, herring, sardines, anchovies and mackerel), oysters, mussels, shrimp and prawns. **There is no debate about the health benefits and anti-inflammatory properties of omega-3 fatty acids. Everyone gives them a big tick, especially in relation to brain and heart health.**

If the first double bond occurs between the sixth and seventh carbon atoms from the omega end, it is called an **omega-6** fatty acid and is written as n-6 or ω-6. The predominant omega-6 fatty acid in the human diet is linoleic acid (LA). It is found in most nuts and seeds (including those that also contain n-3), peanuts (which are legumes, not nuts), soybeans, margarine and vegetable (seed) oils. **Omega-6 fatty acids sit at the heart of a raging debate.** More about this later.

If the first double bond occurs between the ninth and tenth carbon atoms, it is called an **omega-9** fatty acid and is written as n-9 or ω-9. The most common omega-9 fatty acid in our diet is oleic acid. It is found in olives, macadamia nuts, avocados, almonds, hazelnuts, pecans, peanuts, cashews, pistachios, eggs, cheese, tallow (beef fat) and lard (pig fat). **As with omega-3 fatty acids, everyone agrees that oleic acid is anti-inflammatory and improves brain and heart health. Eat it to your heart's content — literally.**

Omega-3 (ALA, EPA and DHA) and omega-6 (LA) are the predominant PUFAs in the human diet. Omega-9 (oleic acid) is the predominant MUFA in the human diet.

Classification of unsaturated fatty acids

Monounsaturated	Polyunsaturated	
omega-9	omega-3	omega-6
oleic acid	ALA, EPA, DHA	LA

One more distinguishing feature of unsaturated fatty acids is whether they are straight (trans) or bent (cis). Unsaturated FAs in nature are bent (cis) and liquid at room temperature. A significant proportion of industrially produced FAs used in processed foods are straight (trans), which makes them solid at room temperature. All scientists, health professionals and even governments agree that trans fats are toxic. See Chapter 46 'The fat hits the fan' for a discussion of trans fats.

Why does all this matter? The chemical structure of a fatty acid determines how it behaves in our body. In other words, the functions of different fatty acids depend on:

- the length of the carbon chain
- the number of double bonds (saturated, monounsaturated or polyunsaturated)
- the location of the double bonds (omega-3, omega-6 or omega-9)
- the orientation of the hydrogen atoms (cis or trans).

For a deep dive into fat biochemistry, refer to Appendix 5. The present chapter includes just enough detail to clarify why SFAs, MUFAs and natural PUFAs (both omega-3 and omega-6) are healthy (unless heated past their smoke point) and why industrially produced omega-6 PUFAs are toxic.

All fats in our diet contain a mixture of SFAs, MUFAs and PUFAs. Thus, although olive oil is composed mainly of MUFAs, it also contains SFAs and PUFAs. Dietary fats are labelled saturated, monounsaturated or polyunsaturated based on which fatty acids predominate. The following table lists common sources of dietary fats and their fatty acid composition as a percentage of their total fatty acid content. All percentages are approximations and can vary between different brands.

Dietary fat or oil	Saturated (SFA) %	Mono-unsaturated (MUFA) %	Poly-unsaturated (PUFA) %
Fats that are labelled as **saturated**			
coconut oil***	92	6	2
palm kernel oil from the seed of the plant	82	15	3
butter	68	28	4
ghee (clarified butter)	65	32	3
palm oil (palmolein) from the flesh of the fruit	52	38	10
Fats that are labelled as **monounsaturated**			
hazelnut oil	7	82	11
high oleic sunflower oil**	10	81	9
macadamia nut oil	15	80	5
olive oil***	14	75	11
avocado oil***	12	74	14
almond oil	9	73	18
canola (rapeseed) oil*	8	64	28
duck fat	35	50	15
peanut oil	18	48	34
margarine — frequently marketed as polyunsaturated because it contains more PUFAs than butter	20	47	33
lard — frequently demonised as saturated but it contains similar amounts of SFAs and MUFAs	41	47	12
rice bran oil*	21	42	37
Fats that are labelled as **polyunsaturated**			
safflower oil*	7	15	78
flaxseed oil	9	17	74
grapeseed oil*	10	17	73
sunflower oil*	11	20	69
walnut oil	10	24	66
soybean oil*	16	24	60
corn oil*	14	29	57
cottonseed oil*	27	19	54
pumpkin seed oil	21	31	48
sesame oil	15	41	44

*These **seed oils** are marketed as vegetable oils. They are the products of large-scale industrial processing and are referred to as refined, bleached, deodorised (RBD) oils because it describes the way they are manufactured. Oils are extracted from seeds by the following series of steps:

- removing the hulls
- grinding the seeds into a powder
- heating and mechanically pressing the powder to obtain oil
- treating the residual powder with chemical solvents (usually hexane) to extract even more oil
- boiling the oil to evaporate the solvent
- heating the oil AGAIN and mixing with alkaline additives to decolourise it and get rid of the otherwise bitter taste
- degumming the oil to prevent fermentation of the oil
- bleaching the oil
- deodorising the oil by subjecting it to extremely high temperatures that transform some of the cis double bonds into trans double bonds. The significance of this alteration is discussed in Chapter 46 'The fat hits the fan'.

Surely food was never meant to be this complicated!

**High oleic sunflower oil is made from sunflower seeds that have been genetically modified to contain substantially higher amounts of oleic acid. The purpose of the modification is to enable sunflower oil to withstand higher cooking temperatures and to extend its shelf life. It is therefore marketed as healthier (less prone to cause inflammation) than regular sunflower oil. While this is true from the perspective of its FA profile, high oleic sunflower oil still undergoes the same processing as regular sunflower oil.

***Coconuts, olives and avocados are botanically classified as fruits. A fruit comes from the ovary of a plant and the ovary is in the flower. Oil is obtained from fruits by pressing the flesh of the fruit. Fruit oils do not need to undergo the processing that is required for vegetable (seed) oils. Always choose **unrefined** fruit oils because this indicates that no heat or chemicals have been used to produce them. Exceedingly few vegetable oils are available as unrefined. One example is virgin unrefined canola oil. This is very different (and healthier) than canola oil available in grocery stores. You will need to hunt long and hard and pay a much higher price for unrefined canola oil. The name 'canola' comes from splicing the words '**Can**ada', '**o**il' and '**l**ow **a**cid'. Canola oil is made from an edible version of the rapeseed plant developed by Canadian scientists. Rapeseeds belong to the mustard family and contain the toxic compounds erucic acid and glucosinolates. When these compounds were crossbred out of the plant, the product was designated low (erucic) acid and deemed safe for human consumption.

Most vegetable oils cannot be produced without extensive refining as described above. If they happen to be unrefined, the producers will make a big deal about it on the packaging. If the bottle does not specify whether a vegetable oil is refined or unrefined, you can be certain the oil is refined.

Nut and seed oils in the preceding table that are not marked with an asterisk can either be refined (industrially processed) or unrefined (pressed or crushed without using heat or chemicals). Always choose oils in dark bottles and labelled raw, virgin, cold pressed or unrefined. The more refined an oil, the more it is stripped of its nutritional value and the more harmful chemicals it is likely to contain.

What are the differential effects of dietary saturated, monounsaturated and polyunsaturated fats in our bodies?

The fate of dietary saturated fatty acids

SFAs are found predominantly in coconut oil, butter, meat, cheese and full-cream dairy products. Because they have no double bonds, they are the most chemically stable. Chemically stable means two things:
1. They melt at a higher temperature compared to MUFAs and PUFAs and therefore tend to be solid at room temperature.
2. They do not react with oxygen because they have no free bonds to grab onto oxygen atoms.

What role do dietary SFAs play in our body?
* They provide us with energy.
* They are important components of cell membranes.

- They regulate much of the traffic going into and out of our cells, thus affecting many cellular functions.

They do NOT clog our arteries and they do us NO harm.

Why then, have we been told that saturated fats cause heart disease and we should avoid eating them? **Doctors made a big fat mistake.** It began with a flawed 1950s hypothesis that saturated fats cause heart disease. This hypothesis engendered a series of poorly designed studies, biased interpretations and food companies bribing scientists to blame saturated fat for our health problems. Why would the food industry do this? To ramp up sales of their vegetable oil and sugar-laden products. The only time that saturated fat-containing products are harmful is when they're combined with unhealthy additives to create processed foods. Natural sources of SFAs — coconut oil, butter, meat and cheese — pose no threat to our health.

In the last decade, rigorous worldwide research involving hundreds of thousands of people has exonerated saturated fats from causing heart disease or any of the other diseases for which it was condemned.

In 2010, an analysis of 11 American and European studies involving 344 696 participants showed that **replacing saturated fats with carbohydrates was associated with an INCREASE, rather than a decrease, in heart disease.**

In 2014, a group of British scientists reviewed 76 studies with a total of 659 298 participants and found NO association between saturated fat consumption and heart disease. In 2017, another five randomised controlled trials (RCTs) with 12 000 people demonstrated NO cardiovascular benefits in replacing saturated fats with vegetable oils.

Unfortunately, **it takes several decades for information to flow down from academia to medical practice.** It takes even longer for people in power to admit they were wrong. And too many big companies have too many financial reasons for making sure we keep consuming vegetable oils. Hence many doctors still advocate shunning saturated fats. Look around you. Read the medical headlines. Despite dutifully cutting back on saturated fats, have we reduced our rates of obesity, heart disease and Alzheimer's? Definitely not.

You can find all the studies I've mentioned at <u>outwittingalzheimers.com/references</u>. I also highly recommend the following books and documentaries:

1. *Big Fat Surprise* by Nina Teicholz
2. *Toxic Oil* by David Gillespie
3. *Eating Ourselves Sick* by Louise Stephen
4. *Good Calories Bad Calories* by Gary Taubes
5. *Metabolical* by Dr Robert Lustig MD, MSL
6. *The Magic Pill* — a documentary by Colin Gara and Rob Tate
7. *Fat Fiction* — a documentary by Jennifer Isenhart.

The fate of dietary monounsaturated fatty acids

As mentioned earlier, this is one group of fatty acids that everyone agrees about: MUFAs are heart-healthy, brain-healthy and anti-inflammatory. Case closed. Foods that are high in MUFAs are listed in the earlier discussion of omega-9 fatty acids. MUFAs are less stable than SFAs because they contain a double bond. This has two implications:

1. MUFAs melt at a lower temperature than SFAs. Hence when MUFAs are extracted from their sources (olives, avocados and nuts), they tend to be liquid at room temperature.
2. MUFAs must be kept away from heat, light and oxygen to stop them going rancid. Rancidity occurs when an oxygen atom reacts with a double bond to form what is known as a radical or reactive oxygen species (ROS). A radical is highly reactive and wants to react with something else. This sets off a chain of reactions that continue to degrade the quality of the oil. Never cook with or consume rancid oils because ingesting radicals can damage our DNA and increase our risk of cancer, heart disease and cognitive impairment.

The fate of dietary polyunsaturated fatty acids

Omega-3 and omega-6 FAs are often lumped into one group despite their opposing functions because they are the only true essential fatty acids (EFAs). Essential means we need to obtain them from food because they are essential for human health but our body is not able to make them. How much do we need? Scientists have not come to a definitive conclusion but the general recommendation is

1.5 grams of each of omega-3 and omega-6 FAs per day. This is easy to achieve if you eat one or two servings of oily fish or seafood per week — see the tables that follow. Other fats (SFAs and MUFAs) required by our body can be made by our liver, brain and fat cells hence they are not labelled as essential. Yes, we need them, but we can synthesise them if we don't consume them in our diet.

Because of their multiple double bonds, PUFAs are even less stable than MUFAs and are highly prone to oxidation and rancidity when exposed to air, light and heat. **Do NOT cook with polyunsaturated oils.**

Omega-3 FAs are critical to the development and preservation of a healthy brain. Our brain is 60% fat and the most abundant FA in our grey and white matter is DHA. DHA deficiency in babies causes problems with vision, balance, coordination and cognition. Omega-3 FAs are important structural components of cell membranes and they play a role in regulating:
- brain cell survival
- neurogenesis (the growth of new brain cells)
- synaptic function (communication between brain cells)
- brain inflammation
- mood and cognition
- blood flow throughout the body.

Changes in the ratio of omega-3 to omega-6 FAs in the brain (i.e. too little n-3 and too much n 6) have been implicated in depression, schizophrenia, multiple sclerosis, ADHD and Alzheimer's. Although observational studies suggest that diets high in omega-3 FAs are associated with a lower risk of all these conditions, there is no compelling evidence that taking omega-3 supplements is protective or improves brain function in people who have already been diagnosed with Alzheimer's. The benefits appear to come from eating real whole food throughout life rather than popping pills when health problems start to surface. It is highly likely that foods rich in omega-3 FAs also contain other micronutrients we have not yet identified as vital to brain health. Nonetheless, omega-3 supplements are a multibillion-dollar industry and the focus of ongoing brain and heart research. See Chapter 47 'Something's fishy' for a closer look at supplements.

The following table lists common foods that contain omega-3 FAs. Aim for at least 1.5 grams per day from a mixture of marine (DHA and EPA) and plant (ALA) sources. Tinned fish is fine as long as it is in spring water, brine or olive oil and not in a sauce or any type of vegetable oil. Omega-3 content of foods can vary widely depending on where a plant is grown and what an animal is eating. The purpose of this table is not to get obsessed with adding up grams of FAs in everything we eat. It's to demonstrate how easy it is to obtain adequate omega-3 FAs in our diet. There are many other foods not listed that contain trace amounts of omega-3 FAs.

Foods that contain ALA	How much ALA is in 100 grams of food? (approx.)
flaxseeds (also known as linseeds)	22 grams
hemp seeds	21 grams
chia seeds	17 grams
walnuts	8 grams
mustard powder	4.6 grams
edamame (green soy beans)	0.4 grams
tofu	0.4 grams
kale	0.2 grams
spinach	0.1 grams
Foods that contain DHA and EPA	How much DHA or EPA is in 100 grams of food? (approx.)
caviar	6.5 grams
mackerel	2.3 grams
herring	2.0 grams
anchovies — canned	2.0 grams
salmon — canned	1.7 grams
salmon — wild	1.4 grams
salmon — farmed	highly variable
sardines — canned	1.4 grams
rainbow trout — wild	1.0 grams
oysters	0.6 grams
mussels	0.5 grams
shrimp	0.4 grams
prawns	0.4 grams
tuna — canned	0.3 grams
ling	0.2 grams

Omega-6 FAs

Omega-6 FAs (linoleic acid) have roles complementary to omega-3s and we need to consume them in similar amounts — about 1.5 grams per day. **The correct dietary ratio of omega-3 to omega-6 FAs is critical to staying physically and mentally healthy. The optimal ratio is likely to be 1:1** but we can probably get away with eating three times as much omega-6 as omega-3. Unfortunately, in the last hundred years, omega-6 FAs from industrially produced vegetable (seed) oils have flooded our food system. These oils did not exist until the 20th century and their PUFAs are almost exclusively omega-6s that have been subjected to extremes of heat and pressure. Not only are seed oils erroneously promoted as heart-healthy spreads and cooking oils (which they are absolutely NOT), they are used in almost ALL processed foods. Look at the list of ingredients in biscuits, chocolates, breads, pastries, cakes, donuts, sauces, dips, pestos, salad dressings, instant noodles and frozen meals. They all contain vegetable oils of one type or another. All fast-food chains and most cafés and restaurants use vegetable oils for frying and even grilling. Furthermore, in many regions of the world, livestock feed has shifted from omega-3-rich grasses to omega-6-rich grains. As a result, eggs and meat from grain-fed animals contain mostly omega-6 FAs while eggs and meat from pasture-fed animals contain significantly more omega-3 FAs. Meat from wild animals has the most DHA of all — even free-range organically reared animals don't come close to having the DHA content of venison and buffalo. We are drowning in omega-6 FAs.

Humans evolved to eat roughly equal amounts of omega-3 and omega-6 FAs but most people in industrialised nations now consume 10–20 times more omega-6s than omega-3s! This massive imbalance is making us very sick — physically and mentally. How?

While omega-3s stimulate production of anti-clotting (anti-thrombotic) and anti-inflammatory compounds, omega-6s are precursors to pro-clotting (pro-thrombotic) and pro-inflammatory molecules. We need them both. We don't want to bleed to death after a penetrating injury and we don't want a blood clot to cause a stroke or deep vein thrombosis (DVT). Similarly, pro-inflammatory compounds are essential components of the body's response to infection and injury — they are part of the healing process. Goldilocks was a guru: not too much (clotting) and not too little; not too hot (inflammation) and not too cold (inability to fight infections).

Excessive consumption of omega-6 FAs leads to excessive inflammation, which starts to damage healthy tissues. Chronic (prolonged) inflammation contributes to insulin resistance, type 2 diabetes, abdominal obesity, allergies and mental health problems as well as heart disease, cancer, autoimmune diseases and Alzheimer's. In an experiment involving college students, those whose blood tests revealed a high ratio of n-6 to n-3, produced more inflammatory proteins when they had to take a stressful exam. Too much n-6 weakens our resilience to stress.

Inflammation is just one of the health hazards associated with over-consuming omega-6 FAs. When we change the PUFA balance in our diet we also change the PUFA balance in our cell membranes. Replacing DHA (n-3) with linoleic acid (n-6) makes cell membranes less flexible and leads to malfunctioning cells, especially in the brain and retina. Hence excess linoleic acid is associated with an increased risk of macular degeneration. Oxford University emeritus professor of neuroscience, John Stein, fears that omega-6s are forcing omega-3s out of our brain cells and this is contributing to the worldwide explosion of mental health problems and neurodegenerative diseases such as Alzheimer's. Similarly, omega-6s are replacing saturated fatty acids in the cells lining our blood vessel walls. In this location, omega-6s promote both inflammation and oxidation (the latter because of their double bonds) which drives up cardiovascular disease.

If that wasn't bad enough, cooking with PUFAs releases high concentrations of toxic chemicals called lipid oxidation products (LOPs), which cause cancer, atherosclerosis, heart muscle damage, type 2 diabetes, birth defects, rheumatoid arthritis, digestive issues, gastric ulcers and dementia. The higher the temperature, the longer the oil is heated and the more times the oil is reused, the more LOPs are generated. These LOPs have been designated as carcinogenic (cancer-causing), teratogenic (toxic to the developing foetus), genotoxic (toxic to DNA) and cytotoxic (toxic to cells).

A review of the diets of 3000 men found that a higher consumption of deep-fried foods using vegetable oils — especially French fries, fried chicken, fried fish and donuts — was linked to a higher likelihood of developing aggressive prostate cancer. A similar study in women found that consuming foods fried in vegetable oils was associated with a greater risk of breast, endometrial and ovarian cancers. In both sexes, frying with vegetable oils has been linked to higher rates of laryngeal and colorectal cancers. Even just inhaling fumes from heated vegetable oils is harmful. A study in 2013 found that non-smoking Chinese women who regularly wok-fried food in vegetable oils had an elevated incidence of lung cancer.

One of the scientists leading the research on heated vegetable oils, Professor Martin Grootveld of De Montfort University in Leicester (UK), was shocked to discover that a single serving of fish and chips fried in vegetable oil contained up to 200 times more toxic aldehydes (a type of LOP) than the safe daily limit set by the World Health Organisation (WHO). When the same foods were fried in coconut oil, butter or lard, much lower levels of aldehydes were detected. The oil that produced the lowest amounts of harmful chemicals when heated was coconut oil — possibly because coconuts grow in tropical climates and are designed to resist heat.

Scientists are urgently calling for governments and health authorities to warn the public about the dangers of consuming foods cooked in vegetable oils, but their pleas are being ignored. Why? Because the information would put processed food companies, fast-food outlets and makers of frozen meals out of business overnight — unless they changed their cooking oils. This would be a huge blow to vegetable oil producers and create a lot of unhappy stakeholders. Profit tramples over people yet again.

The good news is that it's an easy fix: quit vegetable (seed) oils, including canola oil. This equates to home cooking with SFAs and MUFAs. Most SFAs and MUFAs can be used for oven-roasting and pan or wok-frying. If you *must* deep fry, the best options are avocado oil, ghee, lard, tallow or fat drippings. Eating out is guaranteed to be a feast of vegetable oils unless you ask the café or restaurant to use butter or olive oil to prepare your meal. Restaurants and eateries have adapted to provide gluten-free and vegan options so why not also vegetable oil-free options? **Consumers can and do drive change.**

The following table lists common foods that contain omega-6 FAs. It is obviously not an exhaustive list. You'll notice that several nuts and seeds contain both omega-3 and omega-6 FAs. Real whole foods that are high in omega-6 FAs also tend to be rich in nutrients that mitigate their inflammatory potential. For example, sesame seeds, tahini and sesame oil contain potent anti-inflammatory and antioxidant compounds called sesamin, sesamol and sesamolin. These three substances are being studied for possible neuroprotective effects. As discussed, most of the omega-6 FAs in our diet do not come from real foods. Instead, they come from processed and fast foods that are full of industrially made vegetable oils that have been stripped of their protective elements and corrupted by pressure, heat and toxic chemicals. This table should reassure you that quitting vegetable oils will not leave you with a deficit of omega-6 FAs in your diet.

Foods that contain LA (linoleic acid)	How much LA per 100 grams of food? (approx.)
walnuts	43.3 grams
sunflower seeds	34.5 grams
Brazil nuts	29.0 grams
tahini (ground sesame seeds)	27.9 grams
sesame seeds	21.4 grams
peanuts	15.0 grams
almonds	12.8 grams
olive oil	7.6 grams
mustard powder	7.3 grams
pork chops	5.9 grams
avocado	2.8 grams
mutton	1.6 grams
corn	1.3 grams
eggs	1.1 grams
lamb	1.1 grams

Conclusions about fat

1. Belly fat, NOT body weight, is associated with an increased risk of Alzheimer's.
2. Eating fat does NOT make us fat. Fat has important structural and biochemical functions in our body. Sugar and refined starches are the primary causes of obesity, heart disease and type 2 diabetes.
3. Saturated fats (found in coconut oil and animal foods) are NOT associated with an increased risk of heart disease or Alzheimer's. The advice to limit saturated fats is outdated and was based on an untested hypothesis. There is no need to restrict our intake of saturated fats if our diet is low in carbohydrates and founded on real whole unadulterated foods.
4. Monounsaturated and omega-3 fatty acids unequivocally contribute to a healthy heart and optimally functioning brain. Eat a variety of foods that are rich in MUFAs and omega-3 PUFAs.
5. Omega-6 fatty acids are also an essential component of our diet HOWEVER if we over-consume them in the form of vegetable (seed) oils and especially if we use them in cooking, they contribute to widespread chronic inflammation, cell damage, insulin resistance, type 2 diabetes, obesity, cardiovascular disease, cancer and Alzheimer's. It is just as important to avoid vegetable oils as it is to avoid sugar and refined starches.

CHAPTER 46

The fat hits the fan

All truth passes through three stages. First, it is ridiculed.
Second, it is violently opposed. Third, it is accepted
as being self-evident.

ARTHUR SCHOPENHAUER (1788–1860)

There's one more big problem with vegetable (seed) oils —
trans fats.

Trans fats are created when vegetable oils are blasted with hydrogen
under extreme heat. During this process, hydrogen atoms grab
onto double bonds to create partially unsaturated (i.e. partially
hydrogenated) fatty acids. This straightens out the FA chains so they
can be more tightly packed together and thereby become semi-solid
(like margarine and shortening[15]) at room temperature.

Hydrogenation was a huge windfall for the food industry because
hydrogenated vegetable oils were cheap to produce, had a longer
shelf life than existing fats and improved the texture of products
that contained them. One of the first trans fat-containing products
was Crisco — erroneously marketed as a healthy alternative to
butter. It is mind-boggling that no one ever tested the consequences
of consuming a chemical substance that had only just been created.
Nor did anyone question the manufacturer's claims that it was
healthier than the fats we'd been consuming for millennia.

By the mid 1900s, hydrogenated vegetable oils were used in almost
all industrially made baked goods such as cakes, biscuits, pies,

---

[15] Shortening is named for the 'short' or crumbly texture it imparts to baked products such
as puff pastry, pie crusts and shortbread biscuits.

pastries and pizza dough, as well as in margarines and shortenings sold for home use. These newfangled Franken-fats[16] also became the first choice for fast-food outlets, restaurants and potato chip makers because the oil could be re-used for deep frying more often than other fats. Every time the oil is re-used, more trans fatty acids are produced.

Finally, in the 1990s, the fat hit the fan. **Trans fats were discovered to cause heart attack, stroke and type 2 diabetes**. The more trans fats a person ate, the more damaged their blood vessels became, the worse their cholesterol profile and the more likely they were to develop diabetes. The 14-year Nurses' Health Study followed more than 80 000 women aged 34 to 59 years and found that every 2% increase in trans fat consumption almost doubled the risk of heart disease. Meanwhile, animal studies revealed that trans fats displaced DHA in the brain. Study after study showed that trans fats were nothing short of toxic to our brain and body. It was the food industry's worst nightmare.

In response, governments around the world started legislating against the use of trans fats in foods. In 2003, Denmark was the first country to ban foods containing more than 2% trans fats. Prior to this, foods could contain unlimited amounts of the stuff. In June 2018, the American Food and Drug Administration (FDA) likewise banned the use of partially hydrogenated oils in processed foods. Products made prior to this date were given until January 2020 to be removed from distribution.

However, manufacturers in the USA are still permitted to label a product 'free from trans fats' if there are fewer than 0.5 grams per serving. This allows for exploitation of a loophole: what constitutes one serving? Given that serving size is an arbitrary measure, food producers can simply nominate a serving size that contains less than 0.5 grams of trans fats and voila! They don't have to disclose the trans fat content.

Shamefully, Australia has no bans on the use of trans fats. Manufacturers don't even have to list the presence of trans fats

---

[16] Franken is a reference to Frankenstein and denotes a modified version of something that is grotesque and unnatural.

on the nutrition information panel. This is despite overwhelming evidence that such measures would save thousands of lives lost to heart attacks and complications of type 2 diabetes.

How then, can we avoid consuming trans fats?

The simplest way — surprise, surprise — is to avoid all processed and fast foods. Even though food companies have genuinely reduced the trans fat content of their products, small amounts can quickly add up to a significant toxic load. *Reduced* does not mean eliminated. ALL vegetable oils contain at least trace amounts of trans fats because they are generated during the deodorisation stage of their production. If you are consuming vegetable oils you are also consuming trans fats, even if they are not mentioned on the nutrition panel.

Fried fast foods such as French fries, battered fish, fried chicken, fried noodles, hamburgers and donuts are all perfect examples of trans fats sneaking into foods via multiple routes.
Route 1 = the foods are fried in vegetable oils that contain trans fats.
Route 2 = frying at high temperatures creates more trans fats.
Route 3 = each time the oil is reused, the trans fat content increases.
Conclusion = it is impossible to avoid trans fats if one consumes fried fast foods.
Fried fast foods = Franken-fat bombs.

As for processed foods in supermarkets, carefully read the nutrition panel on every food product you plan to buy (which you're no doubt in the habit of doing by now). If anything in the list of ingredients is hydrogenated or partially hydrogenated, it is code for hiding trans fats. Even if there is nothing suspicious on the label, foods likely to contain furtive trans fats include margarines, shortening, copha (hydrogenated coconut oil), flaky and puff pastry products, sweet and savoury pies, sausage rolls, biscuits, muffins, frozen pizzas, microwave popcorn,[17] non-dairy coffee creamers or coffee whiteners, ready-made cake icing / frosting and potato chips or corn chips that

---

[17] Popcorn is not inherently unhealthy. Just buy a bag of natural (NOTHING added) kernels for popping on a stovetop. The problem with microwave popping corn (and the popcorn sold at movie theatres) is that it contains vegetable oils. In addition, some brands of microwave popping corn contain a chemical called diacetyl to give the product a buttery flavour and aroma. Diacetyl is linked to lung damage (bronchiolitis obliterans) when inhaled in large amounts.

do not specify which oils they use for frying. Just as well you gave up eating processed foods before getting to this chapter.

Trans fatty acids (TFAs) are also produced when bacteria digest grass in the stomach of ruminant animals such as cows, sheep and goats. TFAs are therefore present in small amounts in meat fat (3–9% of the fat in meat) and dairy fat (2–6% of the fat in dairy products such as milk, cheese and butter). These naturally occurring TFAs are called vaccenic acid and rumenic acid or conjugated linolenic acid (CLA). They are NOT the same as the artificial TFAs created from vegetable oils and they pose no threat to our health. I merely mention them for completeness.

PART FIVE

Slow ageing despite fast living

One of the illusions of life is that the present hour is not the critical decisive hour. Write it on your heart that every day is the best day of the year.

RALPH WALDO EMERSON (1803–1882)

CHAPTER 47

Something's fishy

When the music changes, so must the dance.

AFRICAN PROVERB

In November 2014, research published in the journal *Cerebral Cortex* made omega-3 supplement makers very happy. The paper was titled 'Long-chain omega-3 fatty acids (i.e. DHA and EPA) improve brain function and structure in older adults'.

Sixty-five healthy men and women aged 50 to 75 years took either fish oil supplements (2.2 grams per day consisting of 1320 mg EPA plus 880 mg DHA) or a placebo for six months. Before and after the trial, participants were given a battery of blood tests, brain scans and cognitive assessments. At the end of the study, those who had been taking omega-3 supplements showed an increase in brain grey matter, structural improvements in white matter, higher levels of brain-derived neurotrophic factor (BDNF), improved blood glucose regulation and lower levels of inflammatory markers. They also performed better in tests of thinking, memory and processing speed. What's not to get excited about?

The headlines promoting the benefits of fish oil (omega-3) supplements don't stop at brain health. Heart disease, diabetes, arthritis, multiple sclerosis, depression, ADHD, exercise-induced asthma, breast cancer, macular degeneration and fertility have all had positive press when it comes to consuming fish oil. Here are two of my favourite reports:

1. Men taking fish oil supplements for more than 60 days in a three-month period had bigger testicles and produced 40 million more sperm (an eighth of a teaspoon) per sample than the average man.

2. Young offenders at a maximum security institution who were given omega-3 supplements for nine months had a 37% reduction in violent offences compared with those given a placebo.

So why aren't we all dosing up on omega-3 capsules? Because the situation is far more nuanced than sensational headlines will have us believe. For every study that demonstrates brain, heart or mood benefits with omega-3 supplements, there is an equally convincing study that shows no improvements at all. How can we reconcile these discrepancies?

As with all things food and medicine, different supplements affect each of us differently depending on our age, genetics, body composition (muscle-to-fat ratio), gut bacteria, pre-existing health conditions, geographical location, diet, exercise habits, workload, stress levels, sleep patterns and other lifestyle factors.

If that wasn't enough to confound the results, omega-3 supplements in different studies comprise a range of types (EPA, DHA, ALA or mixtures), sources (fish vs krill vs algae), doses, formulations, ratios, brands and duration of use (months vs years vs decades). DHA, EPA and ALA have distinct roles in different organs and tissues of our body. **DHA is the most important and abundant omega-3 in the brain and retina** and contributes to the formation of neuronal synapses. **EPA prevents brain and blood vessel inflammation** and serves as a signalling molecule. A purified, concentrated EPA supplement called Vascepa has been approved in the USA as a prescription medicine for lowering blood triglyceride (TAG) levels because high TAGs are associated with an increased risk of heart disease. However, in March 2021, a study of over 70 000 UK citizens found that only people who carry a specific variant of a gene called GJB2 (AG) experience a reduction in TAGs when taking fish oil supplements. Those with a different variant (AA) may actually see an increase in their TAGs! This highlights the **need for personalised dietary and supplement recommendations based on an individual's unique genetic composition**. As for ALA, its role in human health is still being unravelled.

Although it is possible to convert dietary ALA to EPA and DHA in the body, the conversion process is very inefficient and only about 5% of ALA is converted to EPA while less than 0.5% of ALA is made into DHA. In people consuming a diet rich in omega-6 fatty acids, the conversion is further reduced by 40–50%. This puts vegans and vegetarians who do not eat seafood at risk of DHA and EPA deficiency since the latter are only found in seafood and animal products. Research suggests that non-fish eaters who eat high amounts of ALA from plant sources develop the capacity to convert a larger percentage of ALA into EPA and DHA but the amount is still suboptimal. Vegans and vegetarians are therefore advised to take an algal-based DHA and EPA supplement of 1 to 1.5 grams per day.

Women are slightly better at converting ALA to EPA and DHA, possibly due to their higher oestrogen levels. This contributes to having sufficient DHA in pregnancy to enable normal foetal brain development. Human studies have shown that **babies fed breast milk that is deficient in DHA have poorer academic outcomes and visual impairment**.

Even when trying to control for all the above variables, no consistent results from omega-3 supplementation have emerged. Some scientists argue that because EPA is best for the heart and DHA is best for the brain, the two supplements should not be administered together because they might counteract each other. This does not make sense from a dietary perspective because EPA and DHA occur together in many foods. However, when removed from their natural sources, it's conceivable they might behave differently.

The 2019 REDUCE-IT trial of 8179 heart disease patients serves as an example of ongoing controversies. Half of the participants were given purified EPA and half were given a mineral oil placebo. After five years, those taking EPA had significantly fewer heart problems than those taking the placebo. However, critics argue that the mineral oil *increased* heart disease rather than EPA *decreased* it. We will not know if this is the case until the study is repeated with a different placebo.

Many studies also show that high dose omega-3 supplementation can elevate the risk of an abnormal heart rhythm known as **atrial fibrillation (AF).** The higher the dose, the more likely a person will develop AF. At a dose of 4 grams per day there was almost a doubling of AF cases compared with the placebo, while a dose of 840 mg per day was deemed safe. Atrial fibrillation can cause palpitations, lightheadedness, fainting, breathlessness or chest pain. It raises a person's risk of stroke, heart failure, Alzheimer's and vascular dementia — the very conditions that omega-3 supplements are supposed to prevent. If you are taking high dose omega-3 supplements, periodically check your pulse for fast irregular beats and inform your doctor if you have any of the aforementioned symptoms.

Omega-3 fatty acids also interact with blood-thinning medications such as warfarin and aspirin by increasing the likelihood of excessive bleeding or gastric ulcer irritation. Healthy people who are not on blood-thinning medications need not be concerned about bleeding problems in response to taking a daily 1–2 gram omega-3 supplement.

Most people experience no adverse side effects but a few may notice a fishy taste or odour in their mouth, burping, nausea, vomiting, diarrhoea or constipation. Lowering the dose or taking the supplement with food may reduce or eliminate these issues.

There is no denying that DHA and EPA are essential for normal brain development and cognition from the time we're in the womb to the day we die. As outlined in the previous chapter, omega-3 fatty acids cannot be made by our body and must therefore be consumed in our diet. Omega-3 deficiency is associated with lower intelligence, depression, anxiety disorders, heart disease, arthritis, cancer and Alzheimer's. Mice that are not fed DHA during the first few months of life have smaller brains and poorer brain function than those receiving DHA. However, this does not mean that consuming more than the required 1.5 to 2 grams per day will turn us into Einstein or eliminate heart attacks. Always remember Goldilocks: not too little, not too much.

This is also not to say that specific health conditions or circumstances (such as pregnancy and vegetarianism) don't warrant supplementation. Several studies provide compelling evidence that 4 grams of daily **DHA supplements can help protect the brain from injury** caused by head knocks or concussions in sports such as boxing, football, rugby, ice hockey and soccer. It is postulated that DHA provides a scaffolding function that makes it harder for the brain to be shaken around in the skull after impact.

APOE4 carriers appear to have a unique response to omega-3 consumption. PET scans have demonstrated that under the age of 50, APOE4 carriers have a greater uptake of DHA in the brain than non-carriers. This is good news for APOE4 carriers because a diet rich in fish and dark leafy greens has been shown to lower the risk of developing Alzheimer's in both APOE4 carriers and non-carriers. However, after a certain age (and we don't yet know what that age happens to be), the brain of an APOE4 carrier is *less* able to absorb omega-3 fatty acids (FAs). Therefore, the advice to APOE4 carriers is to eat lots of fish and plant sources of omega-3s while you're young to provide a buffer against Alzheimer's as you age. As long as an APOE4 carrier does not develop Alzheimer's, they are likely to benefit from a high omega-3 diet. Non-APOE4 carriers, on the other hand, appear to maintain the ability to take up omega-3s into their brain even after showing signs of cognitive impairment. As such, non-carriers *may* benefit from supplementation even after receiving a diagnosis of Alzheimer's.

To clarify these observations, a two-year trial led by Hussein Yassine called PREVENT-E4 is currently underway at the University of Southern California. The purpose of the trial is to answer the following questions:

- Does DHA enter the brain in sufficient amounts when taking supplements?
- Does being an APOE4 carrier make a difference to how much DHA is taken up by the brain?
- Does DHA supplementation result in changes in brain structure and function as assessed by MRI scans?
- Does DHA supplementation improve cognition?

The study is estimated to finish in May 2024 with the results published by May 2025.

In the meantime, where does that leave you and me in terms of whether or not to take omega-3 supplements to prevent Alzheimer's or heart disease? The more I delve into the research on DHA, EPA and

ALA, the more seemingly discordant results I find. I say 'seemingly' because future studies may uncover subsets of people who clearly benefit and those who don't. Reputable scientists currently sit on both sides of the supplement fence: many vehemently recommend that everyone should take a good quality DHA and EPA supplement, while others maintain there is simply not enough evidence to support their use, other than in specific situations of overt deficiency or when treating head injuries.

The one thing everyone agrees on is that we need to eat foods that contain DHA, EPA and ALA at a level that provides an average of 1.5 grams per day or 10.5 grams per week. At least 75% (8 grams per week) needs to come from marine sources. See the table in Chapter 45 'The fat is in the fire' for a list of foods that are rich in omega-3 FAs. Avoiding deficiency is more important than taking extra, and eating food sources is better than swallowing supplements.

How does a person know if they are deficient in DHA and EPA? Many cardiologists recommend a test called the **Omega-3 Index** which measures the percentage of DHA and EPA in our red blood cell (RBC) membranes. Numerous (but not all) studies have found that the lower the concentration of EPA and DHA in RBC membranes, the higher the risk of having a heart attack. Conversely, increasing our Omega-3 Index may be an easy way to reduce heart disease. Only one drop of blood is required and it can be done at home and mailed to a company called OmegaQuant. You will receive your result within four weeks. Visit omegaquant.com to order your collection kit. Founded in the USA by Dr William Harris and Professor Clemens Von Schacky, OmegaQuant has partnered with laboratories in Scotland and Australia to offer the Omega-3 Index test to people living in the USA, European Union (EU), Australia and Asia-Pacific region (APAC).

What do the results mean?

An Omega-3 Index of less than 4% is associated with a high risk of having heart disease. A score of 4–8% is associated with moderate risk and a score of over 8% is linked to low risk. Australians and Americans tend to have scores in the 4–5% range while the Japanese score between 8–10%. This reflects their significantly higher seafood consumption. The only way to increase your score is to eat more marine sources of DHA and EPA or take a DHA plus EPA supplement. The omegaquant.com website is unsurprisingly in the pro-supplement camp but this does not negate the value of the test.

Personally, I live by a food-first approach. Dad, Felix and I ate at least three servings of fish per week — a combination of New Zealand or Alaskan salmon, tinned sardines, mackerel or anchovies and my home-made marinara (containing prawns, mussels, scallops and squid) with spinach and spiralised zucchini. Raw oysters are a treat if we eat out. This maintains our Omega-3 Index above 8% and until I learn of evidence to the contrary, I'm satisfied with that.

If you choose to take supplements, ensure that you find a reputable brand from a marine source and store the airtight bottle in the fridge or freezer to prevent oxidation.

Marine omega-3 supplements come in three forms:
1. fish oil — as ethyl esters or re-esterified triglycerides
2. krill oil — as phospholipids
3. algal oil — as triglycerides.

What difference does this make?

Krill oil comes from tiny crustaceans called Antarctic krill, which are a food source for whales, seals and penguins. The FAs in krill oil have a different structure to those in fish oil and micro algae, which some studies have found make them easier to absorb. Proponents of krill oil suggest that we need only two-thirds as much krill oil as fish oil to achieve the same blood levels. More research is needed to substantiate this claim. Krill oil also contains an antioxidant called astaxanthin (which gives it a reddish colour) that is not found in most fish oils. Astaxanthin *may* make krill oil more resistant to going rancid but this too needs verification. A notable disadvantage of krill oil is that it is less readily available and substantially more expensive than fish oil due to its harvesting and processing methods.

Algal oil is made from specific species of marine micro algae that contain DHA, EPA and omega-9 FAs. Micro algae produce omega-3 FAs from exposure to UV light, oxygen, sodium and glucose. They are the mother of all DHA and EPA because they provide omega-3

FAs for the fish we eat, both wild and farmed. The advantages of algal oil are that it appears to have equivalent effects as fish oil but is more environmentally sustainable because it doesn't contribute to overfishing. It is also free from toxic metals (that might be present in fish oil) and has been associated with fewer digestive side effects. Algal oils are an excellent plant-based source of DHA and EPA for vegans, vegetarians and people who do not tolerate seafood.

CHAPTER 48

Vitamins for vitality

Not how long, but how well you have lived is the main thing.

Seneca (4 BCE – 65 CE)

What do the following six groups have in common?

1. strict vegans
2. heavy alcohol drinkers
3. bariatric surgery patients (e.g. for obesity or type 2 diabetes)
4. people who regularly take antacids to treat stomach ulcers, hiatus hernia or indigestion
5. people who have an underactive thyroid (hypothyroidism)
6. 50-plus year-olds

They all put a person at risk of vitamin B12 deficiency. Why? And what does this have to do with Alzheimer's?

Vitamin B12 (also known as *cobalamin* because it contains the element cobalt) is involved in many biochemical processes that affect the health of our brain, nerves and red blood cells. B12 deficiency causes a specific type of anaemia called *pernicious* or *megaloblastic macrocytic anaemia* that leads to weakness, fatigue and breathlessness. Low levels of B12 are also associated with headaches, depression, memory problems and numbness or tingling in the hands and feet.

When cells don't have enough B12, they are not able to break down an amino acid called homocysteine, which is toxic to neurons. **High blood levels of homocysteine are linked to brain shrinkage, cognitive decline and increased risk of Alzheimer's.** Therefore, making sure we do not develop B12 deficiency is an important piece of the Alzheimer's puzzle.

Vitamin B12 is found only in animal foods including fish (especially shellfish), crab, caviar, dairy, liver, meat and poultry. Animals store B12 in their liver and muscles and pass varying amounts into their eggs and milk. Duck eggs provide 10 times more B12 than chicken eggs. Goose eggs provide 20 times more B12 than chicken eggs (just in case you were wondering). Faeces is also a rich source of B12 hence rabbits, dogs and cats sometimes eat faeces. But let's not go there.

Sources of B12 for vegetarians include milk, cheese, yoghurt, eggs, some yeast extracts and fortified products like tofu, soy and breakfast cereals. If buying fortified foods, read labels to avoid added sugar, vegetable oils, emulsifiers and other nasties. Most breakfast cereals qualify as junk food and are not recommended. Cheeses contain varying amounts of B12, with Swiss, mozzarella and feta being good options (in that order). Vegans obviously need synthetic B12 in fortified foods or supplements.

B12 is unique among the B vitamins in that it can be stored in the liver for two or more years. Consequently, deficiency develops insidiously over several years and early symptoms are often vague and falsely attributed to stress or ageing. With prolonged deficiency, neurological complications gradually progress from tingling and numbness to impaired co-ordination, visual disturbances, memory loss, disorientation and eventually dementia.

B12 absorption requires adequate amounts of two agents that tend to decline with age: stomach acid and a carrier protein called intrinsic factor (IF). Thirty per cent of people over the age of 50 have reduced absorption of B12. Excessive alcohol consumption leads to inflammation and disruption of the stomach lining impairing our ability to absorb B12. Similarly, gastric surgery that decreases stomach volume will also reduce stomach acid and IF.

The recommended daily dose of B12 is 2.4 micrograms (μg) per day. One serving of fish provides adequate daily needs. If you eat a diet that includes a selection of the aforementioned B12-containing foods, you will be consuming sufficient amounts.

You will need more than 2.4 µg/day if you are pregnant or breastfeeding (2.6 µg/day), belong to one of the six risk groups or have a medical condition such as Crohn's or coeliac disease that make it difficult to absorb B12 from food. In many of these instances, regular supplementation with synthetic B12 is required. Synthetic B12 does not require stomach acid for absorption. B12 can also be given as an intramuscular injection.

How do you know if you are low in B12? The following blood tests are used to assess a person's vitamin B12 status and whether or not they need supplementation:
1. Vitamin B12 (cobalamin)
2. Vitamin B9 (folate)
3. Vitamin B6 (pyridoxine)
4. Homocysteine
5. Methylmalonic acid (MMA).

Why so many tests?

The reason for measuring the three B vitamins is that they work together in lowering homocysteine levels. It's important to know your homocysteine concentration because it can start to rise and cause brain shrinkage before blood levels of the B vitamins begin to drop. Some studies also point to high homocysteine levels contributing to heart disease and stroke, further increasing the risk of dementia. Likewise, high MMA levels can also be a sign of B12 deficiency.

A ground-breaking two-year Oxford University study (called VITACOG) of 70-plus year-old adults with high homocysteine levels and mild cognitive impairment (MCI), found that supplementation with high doses of vitamin B12 (0.5 mg/day), B9 (0.8 mg/day) and B6 (20 mg/day) slowed brain shrinkage and cognitive decline. Thus the VITACOG study highlights two important principles:

1. **If vitamin deficiencies are corrected soon enough, brain decline can be slowed, if not stopped.**
2. To stay healthy, our brain requires sufficient levels of all vitamins (A, B, C, D, E, K), minerals (sodium, potassium, calcium, phosphorus, chloride, magnesium, iron, zinc, iodine, sulphur, cobalt, copper, fluoride, manganese and selenium) and essential

nutrients (such as proteins, PUFAs and choline). Focusing on a select few 'brain-boosting supplements' is not the answer to averting Alzheimer's. **The totality of our diet and lifestyle is what determines the destiny of our brain.**

Another B vitamin that deserves particular attention is B1 (thiamine) because it is critical to brain glucose metabolism. In laboratory animals, B1 deficiency exacerbates Aβ plaque formation, promotes phosphorylation of tau and impairs memory. When the animals are given a synthetic B1 supplement called benfotiamine (which is better absorbed than giving straight B1) the symptoms of Alzheimer's are reversed. Benfotiamine is used to treat nerve damage (peripheral neuropathy) in people with diabetes; however, trials of benfotiamine in Alzheimer's patients have been minimally effective. Scientists are working on understanding why this is the case. People who drink more than two standard alcoholic drinks a day are at risk of B1 deficiency. See Chapter 49 'Drink to me only with thine eyes' for more details.

Thus, mega-dosing on multivitamins and minerals is not the answer. The key is avoiding deficiencies. Some vitamins and minerals can be toxic in excess, particularly vitamins A and E and minerals iron, copper and fluoride. Always remember Goldilocks: not too much and not too little. In an ideal world, we would obtain sufficient vitamins, minerals and nutrients from food. When this is not possible, supplements can be helpful. If you have concerns about your nutritional status, ask your doctor to do the relevant tests. When you have the results, discuss whether adjusting your diet or supplementation is the best solution.

CHAPTER 49

Drink to me only with thine eyes

I used to think drinking was bad for me …
so I stopped thinking.

Research on alcohol has yielded a barrage of conflicting results. One week, alcohol is a leading cause of premature death and the next week it is hailed as heart healthy. Different countries have different government guidelines for safe levels of alcohol consumption and many countries have no safe drinking guidelines at all. Some nations such as the USA, Canada and New Zealand have separate drinking recommendations for men and women, with safe levels for women in the US being half that for men. Meanwhile in the UK, Australia, Grenada, Portugal and South Africa, alcohol advice for men and women is the same.

Many factors influence the rate at which a person metabolises alcohol, including age, sex, body weight, muscle mass, concurrent food and water consumption and habitual alcohol use.

Bearing all the above in mind, **which of the following statements about alcohol are true and which are false?**

1. Alcohol has been linked to more than 60 acute and chronic diseases.

2. Heavy alcohol consumption over the course of a lifetime can lead to dementia.

3. Alcohol is a carcinogen (capable of causing cancer).

4. Alcohol can exacerbate or cause mental illness, in particular depression, anxiety and self-harm.

5. Alcohol accelerates ageing by shortening our telomeres (the protective caps on the ends of our chromosomes).

6. Alcohol consumption produces changes in our gut bacteria.

7. Binge drinking during adolescence can cause gene alterations in the brain leading to long-term reduced cognitive functioning.

8. People for whom drinking only small amounts of alcohol causes facial flushing are 10 times more likely to develop oesophageal cancer if they are regular drinkers than people who do not get red in the face.

9. One night of binge drinking reduces the ability to perform complex memory tasks for as long as four days later.

10. There are genetic differences in the way people respond to alcohol.

11. Red wine and dark-coloured spirits such as brandy, whisky and rum induce more severe hangovers than white wine or vodka because red and brown drinks contain aromatic fermentation products called congeners.

12. When you drink on an empty stomach you feel the effects of alcohol more quickly.

13. Carbonated alcoholic drinks cause a faster rise in blood alcohol level (BAL) than non-carbonated drinks, which means you'll feel intoxicated more quickly drinking champagne than wine.

14. Alcohol within three hours of bedtime causes fragmented sleep (frequent waking throughout the night even if you don't remember waking).

15. Alcohol within three hours of bedtime reduces the time a person spends dreaming.

16. Alcohol within three hours of bedtime increases the number of times a person will need to visit the bathroom. This is not

only because you're consuming a liquid but because alcohol interferes with a hormone called vasopressin that inhibits nighttime urination.

17. If a person consumes more than 30 grams of alcohol per day (about 300 mL of wine) they need to take a vitamin B1 (thiamine) supplement.

18. Thiamine deficiency puts a person at risk for a specific type of dementia called Wernicke-Korsakoff Syndrome (WKS). See Appendix 1: 'Types of dementia'.

19. We tend to be more sensitive to the effects of alcohol in our 40s than in our 20s, i.e. we get intoxicated more quickly as we age.

20. Balance problems in an older person are sometimes misdiagnosed as an inner ear infection (labyrinthitis) when the cause is actually alcohol consumption.

21. Forgetfulness and confusion in an older person are sometimes misdiagnosed as Alzheimer's when the cause is actually alcohol consumption.

22. For the same amount of alcohol, women tend to have a higher BAL than men. This means women get drunk more quickly than men.

23. There is no safe level of alcohol consumption for a woman who is pregnant or breastfeeding because the brain of a foetus and newborn is highly vulnerable to the damaging effects of alcohol.

24. Alcohol concentration in breast milk is the same as in blood.

25. It takes twice as long for alcohol to be cleared from breast milk as from the blood.

26. Alcohol reduces male fertility and sperm quality and contributes to miscarriages and negative health outcomes in their offspring.

27. Medications such as cough syrups and laxatives can contain as much as 10% alcohol and amplify the effects of drinking.

28. Drinking alcohol while taking certain painkillers, antidepressants and anti-anxiety medications can be fatal.

29. Aspirin combined with alcohol increases the risk of bleeding from the stomach or intestines.

30. Antihistamines (anti-allergy medications) taken with alcohol can make a person feel sleepy.

31. Even some herbal remedies can be dangerous when consumed with alcohol.

32. The amount of alcohol in one standard drink in the USA is different from a standard drink in Australia, the UK and Europe. In fact, individual countries vary widely in what is regarded as one drink.

33. Many countries recommend abstaining from alcohol for one to three days per week, depending on the country.

34. It is worse for our brain and body to have seven drinks in one sitting (binge drinking) than to have one drink per night for seven days.

35. The more you drink, the more you shrink (your brain).

All 35 statements are true.

According to the World Health Organisation (WHO) as at May 2022, **harmful use of alcohol results in three million deaths worldwide every year.** That's more than 8000 deaths due to alcohol every day. But what constitutes harmful use? Is there a safe level or is zero alcohol the best choice for optimal brain health and longevity? Does advice need to be tailored to each individual or to change as we age?

Despite the alarming number of alcohol-related deaths, the WHO has not determined what constitutes a safe level of alcohol consumption. This is why every country has its own arbitrary set of guidelines — if they have any guidelines at all. To make matters even more confusing, different countries have different definitions for what constitutes a standard drink. The following table illustrates how one standard drink in Austria is equivalent to two and a half standard drinks in the UK.

How much alcohol is in a standard drink?

Country	Amount of alcohol in a standard drink
World Health Organisation (WHO)	10 grams (12.5 mL of pure alcohol)[1]
United Kingdom (UK) and Iceland	8 grams
Australia, New Zealand, China, Singapore, Vietnam, France, Germany and India	10 grams
Switzerland	10–12 grams
Denmark	12 grams
Luxembourg	12.8 grams
Bulgaria	13 grams
Canada	13.6 grams
USA, Mexico, Chile, Grenada and The Philippines	14 grams
Austria	20 grams

These variations are one of the reasons that research on alcohol has yielded discordant results. If researchers talk about standard drinks do they mean a standard drink as defined by the WHO, UK or USA? Inconsistent guidelines across the globe erode public confidence that we know anything conclusive about the health effects of alcohol. Inaccuracies are also due to poor methods of research. Many studies on alcohol have relied on asking people how much they drink. This is fraught with problems because people frequently under-estimate or don't remember how much they consume. They also admit to *hoping* that a few drinks are good for them.

On closer examination, studies that support a protective effect of low to moderate alcohol consumption failed to take into account what is known as the **healthy user bias.** In other words, people who drank a glass or two of wine several times a week were of a higher socio-economic status, better educated, more likely to exercise and eating a healthier diet than teetotallers who could not afford quality food, alcohol or gym membership. Obviously, there are exceptions in both groups but this pattern was seen often enough to obliterate the purported health benefits of mild to moderate drinking. Thus the observation that drinkers had fewer heart attacks than teetotallers was

---

[1] Ten grams or 12.5 mL of pure alcohol is approximately 100 mL (3.38 ounces) of wine, 30 mL of spirits or 285 mL (0.6 pints) of full-strength beer.

due to lifestyle factors other than alcohol. Scientists are increasingly concluding that **the safest level of drinking is none.**

Notwithstanding the shortcomings of alcohol research, **10 common cancers have been definitively linked to alcohol:** mouth, pharynx, larynx, oesophagus, breast, liver, stomach, bowel, kidney and pancreas. The evidence for other tumours is inconclusive but melanomas and cancers of the lung, gallbladder and prostate are also likely to be increased. The three cancers most commonly associated with alcohol are oesophagus, liver and breast. In Australia, one in five breast cancers are attributable to alcohol consumption and one in 20 people who exceed 14 (Australian standard) drinks per week (e.g. 1.5 litres of wine) are predicted to develop cancer. Each additional drink adds to the risk for cancer.

How does alcohol give rise to cancer? The liver breaks down alcohol into a toxic compound called acetaldehyde, which damages DNA and drives uncontrolled cell proliferation leading to cancer. Acetaldehyde is subsequently metabolised to acetate by an enzyme called aldehyde dehydrogenase 2 (ALDH2). More than a third of East Asians (Chinese, Japanese, Koreans and Taiwanese) have a deficiency of ALDH2, which means it takes them longer to rid their body of acetaldehyde. In addition to being a carcinogen, acetaldehyde causes facial flushing, nausea and tachycardia (an abnormally rapid heart rate). This is why people who experience what is termed alcohol flushing syndrome are at much higher risk of oesophageal cancer if they are regular drinkers: the prolonged accumulation of acetaldehyde results in more DNA damage.

We also know that **alcohol causes brain shrinkage.** After ruling out the effects of sex, height, weight, genetics, head size, smoking and socioeconomic status, MRI scans of 36 678 men and women aged 40 to 70 years showed that by the age of 50, two standard UK drinks per day (= 16 grams of alcohol or 160 mL of wine = just over one and a half standard Australian drinks or just over one US drink) accelerated brain ageing by two years. Thus, the brain of a 50-year-old light drinker looked like the brain of a 52-year-old teetotaller. This may not seem like much of a difference, but for every added drink per day, brain ageing increased exponentially.

Brain ageing means structural damage, loss of connectivity and less grey and white matter.

The following table summarises the findings.

Number of daily UK standard drinks (one drink = 8 g of alcohol or 80 mL of wine)	How much does alcohol age your brain?
<2 drinks per day (<160 mL wine or 48 mL spirits or 456 mL beer)	No difference seen on MRI scan
2 drinks	2 years
4 drinks (320 mL wine or 96 mL spirits or 900 mL beer)	10 years

Unfortunately, just because brain changes are not detectable on MRI scans doesn't mean that brain deterioration is not occurring. Studies of identical twins found that consuming more than **40 grams of alcohol** *per week* (four standard drinks in Australia and three standard drinks in the USA) **tripled the risk of dementia** compared with consuming less than 40 grams per week. This is a small amount of alcohol by most people's reckoning — roughly 400 mL of wine per week (not per day). For some drinkers, it equates to just two home-poured glasses.

Thus, up to one Australian standard drink every second day *may* be safe but any more than this starts to compromise brain function. This means our government guidelines — which focus on reducing cancer rather than dementia — are not stringent enough when it comes to protecting our brain. The fine print commentary explains that 'zero alcohol confers the greatest health benefits but we need to be realistic about making the guidelines achievable'. Sadly, dangerous drinking is considered normal social behaviour throughout most of the world, and weekend binge drinking is par for the course with university students. It's up to you to decide how much cognition you are willing to risk for the transient pleasure of alcohol. Personally, I'd rather you drink to me only with thine eyes.

Why is a given amount of alcohol more damaging for a woman than a man? Alcohol is broken down by an enzyme found in the stomach and liver called alcohol dehydrogenase (ADH). The more ADH in our stomach, the less alcohol we absorb into our blood and body. Men have more ADH in their stomach than women so they take up less alcohol in the first place. Secondly, for the same height and weight, men have a higher percentage of body water due to their greater musculature than women. Since alcohol dissolves in water, it is more concentrated in a woman's body than a man's. The higher the concentration of alcohol, the greater the damage it exerts. This may be another reason why Alzheimer's is more common in women: drinking the same amount results in higher levels of alcohol reaching their brain. The recommendations for safe levels of alcohol should therefore be much lower for women than for men. Regrettably this is not the case in Australia.

The **Australian Alcohol Guidelines** are summarised here:

Guideline 1: Healthy men and women should drink no more than 10 standard drinks a week and no more than 4 standard drinks on any one day. The less you drink, the lower your risk of harm from alcohol.

Guideline 2: Young people should not start drinking before the age of 18 years. The longer they abstain, the better their brain performance in the short and long term. (In the United States, the minimum legal drinking age is 21.)

Guideline 3: There is no safe level of alcohol consumption from the moment of conception to the end of pregnancy. Women who are trying to fall pregnant are therefore advised not to drink any alcohol in order to avoid physical, mental and emotional harm to their child.

Guideline 4: There is no safe level of alcohol consumption during breast feeding because the alcohol concentration in breast milk is the same as in blood.

CHAPTER 50

Fast to last

Fasting is the greatest remedy — the physician within.

PHILIPPUS PARACELSUS (1493–1541)

What is the fast-food industry's greatest nightmare?

Fasting!

We are bombarded with advertising urging us to eat at every opportunity. Yet human beings evolved to wake up and hunt for food — akin to exercising on an empty stomach. Likewise, snacking between meals is not a natural human imperative — it's an invention of snack food companies.

Fasting to cleanse the body and sharpen the mind is practised in one form or another by all major religions and has been used for medicinal purposes by healers throughout history. The first books on therapeutic fasting were published in the early 1900s but it took scientists another 100 years to work out the mechanisms by which fasting confers health benefits. Unfortunately, the media has turned fasting into 'just another fad diet' but fasting is not a diet and not a fad.

Fasting is a way of living that incorporates periodically abstaining from food for long enough to cause our body to switch from using sugar (glucose) to using fat (from fat cells) for fuel. This takes a minimum of 12 hours and is referred to as **metabolic switching**. I say 'a way of living' because **if we want an optimally functioning brain and body, fasting is something we need to engage in at regular intervals** for the duration of our lives.

Thousands of studies in animals and humans have shown that **intermittent fasting (IF) can help protect us from obesity, type 2 diabetes, heart disease, fatty liver, cancer, Alzheimer's and a host of other chronic diseases**. Intermittent fasting can even help cure a person already afflicted with a chronic disease.

How can **not eating** have such a powerful positive effect on our biology? And what exactly does intermittent fasting entail? First and foremost, intermittent fasting does NOT mean starving ourselves of calories and nutrients so that we lose excessive amounts of weight, weaken our immune system and potentially develop an eating disorder. Intermittent fasting means different things to different people and includes the following subcategories.

Overnight fasting = the period of time between our last bite of food at night and our first bite of food the next day. To qualify as *therapeutic* fasting, this needs to be a minimum of 12 hours because that's how long it takes for the liver to run out of glucose. Overnight fasting is recommended as a lifelong habit for everyone over the age of five years.

Time restricted feeding (TRF) or **time restricted eating (TRE)** = extending the overnight fast beyond 12 hours. In fasting vernacular, this is referred to as 13/11, 14/10, 15/9 or 16/8, where the first number indicates how many hours without food and the second number is the hours within which food is consumed. Thus 16/8 means a person only eats during an eight-hour window, e.g. from 11 am to 7 pm every day.

To date, there have been few head-to-head comparisons between different TRF regimes but they all confer health benefits. 16/8 appears to lead to greater reductions in visceral fat, type 2 diabetes and inflammation than 13/11, but if you don't need to shed excess body fat or reverse an inflammatory condition, choose whichever pattern best suits your family and lifestyle. You can also practise 13/11 on some days and go longer without food on others. TRF is recommended as a lifelong habit for everyone over the age of 17 years.

5:2 fasting = eating without any restrictions for five days a week and eating only 500–600 Calories for two non-consecutive days of the week. A good way to ease into or out of a 5:2 fast is the 6:1 fast, i.e. eating 500–600 Calories one day a week. The 500–600 Calories are usually consumed as one protein-rich meal at your chosen time of day. If you prefer, you can split it into two small 250–300 Calorie meals. This was conceived by prominent fasting researcher and neuroscientist Dr Mark Mattson and popularised by British TV journalist Dr Michael Mosley. The 5:2 fast (together with TRF, not instead of) is an effective adjunct in treating people with obesity, type 2 diabetes, fatty liver or any other condition linked to insulin resistance. When you have achieved your health goal, go back to only TRF. The 5:2 fast is not necessary for people who are lean and fit.

Prolonged fasting = going without any food at all for 24 to 72 hours, a few times a year. This can be a further boost for people with obesity or who simply want to amplify the benefits discussed below. Please consult your doctor before embarking on a fast that is longer than 24 hours.

Because **fasting lowers blood pressure, blood sugar and insulin levels**, if you are taking medications for hypertension, pre-diabetes or diabetes, speak with your doctor about checking your blood pressure and blood glucose levels several times a day, and potentially lowering your drug dose in response to the effects of fasting. If you take any other medications or supplements, check whether fasting impacts their absorption or effectiveness.

TRF is the most natural, simple and sustainable way to reduce our risk of all chronic diseases including Alzheimer's. Eating the same number of calories and the same foods in an eight-to-11-hour window is healthier and leads to less body fat than consuming the exact same foods during a 12-plus hour window. Why?

Constant eating does not leave the brain and body time to repair, detoxify and remove damaged or dysfunctional cells. This leads to the accumulation of molecular garbage and defective cells, which can eventually cause organs to malfunction and cancers to develop. Fasting also allows our bowels to get into a better rhythm because they aren't continually dealing with food. Many of our beneficial gut bacteria subsist on the mucous that lines our intestines, but in the presence of perpetual food, they don't get their fair share of mucous. This upsets the balance of bacteria in our gut and can lead to leaky gut syndrome and increased risk of allergies and autoimmune diseases. Furthermore, intermittent fasting turns down inflammation, improves blood sugar regulation, lowers blood pressure and switches on genes that slow ageing. All these factors enhance brain function and protect against dementia. In fact, **intermittent fasting directly reverses many of the degenerative processes occurring in the brain of a person with Alzheimer's**.

When rats are only fed on alternate days, their brain cells become resistant to developing Alzheimer's and Parkinson's. They also experience improvements in heart health, insulin sensitivity and physical endurance. No one is suggesting that a human should only eat every other day. The same benefits can be achieved through daily TRF of at least 13/11. If you need to shed excess body fat or reverse type 2 diabetes, add a 5:2 fast for a few months. Although these regimes may sound daunting, it takes the brain and body only four weeks (in some cases even shorter) to adjust to intermittent fasting, and you'll find that you no longer feel hungry or cranky during times of not eating. In addition, you'll be sharper, more productive and have more energy.

When you first start TRF, take small steps and adjust your eating incrementally by having breakfast half an hour later than usual and cutting out after-dinner snacking. When this becomes comfortable, push breakfast back another half hour or eat dinner half an hour earlier. Continue extending the time between dinner and breakfast until you reach your desired time frame. My personal daily routine is TRF 15/9. I eat one hearty meal at 11.30 am and another at 6.30 pm so that I finish by 7.30 pm. Only after our last bite of food can our brain and body begin to wind down and prepare for the nightly work of detoxification. This is why it's important to leave at least three hours between finishing dinner and going to bed. This also allows enough time to digest most of our food and prevent acid reflux. Eating late at night disrupts our sleep and goes against our circadian rhythm (our body's 24-hour internal clock). More about living in alignment with our circadian rhythm in Chapter 51 'Good timing'. Many people (like myself) find that TRF simplifies life because it means only two meals a day are needed. Less time preparing food means more time having fun. I enjoy cooking but twice a day is enough. If a special event interferes with your fasting, no matter. The aim is to enhance our quality of life, not to become obsessive about sticking to a rigid plan, 365 days a year. Most of the time is good enough. Return to your fasting routine after the festivities are over.

During the fasting period, water, black coffee and black tea are permitted. The minute you add milk, sugar or an artificial sweetener to your beverage, the pancreas starts producing insulin, gut muscles start contracting and the fast is broken. Some medications (especially cough syrup) contain sugar or artificial sweeteners so taking them would also break your fast. During your eating window, there is no need to restrict calories — eat to satiety. However, TRF and 5:2 are NOT licence to eat rubbish during our eating windows.

Humans evolved to function optimally when we were in a fasted state so that we could outsmart our prey and forage for edible plants. Intermittent fasting is the natural way of living; having food available 24 hours a day is not. Intermittent fasting only seems abnormal because our current lifestyles are far removed from the natural order of things.

When we eat, energy obtained from food is used to fuel our everyday activities. Any calories not immediately needed are stored as glycogen (chains of glucose molecules) in the liver. The liver can stockpile up to 500 Calories of glucose and when this limit is reached, glucose is converted to fat and stored in fat cells distributed throughout our body. When we are not eating, it takes at least 12 hours to use up the glucose in our liver. Only after this time, do we begin to release fat from our fat cells and switch on what is colloquially termed 'fat-burning'. The fat is carried to our liver where it is broken down into water-soluble molecules called **ketone bodies.** This process is known as **ketogenesis.** Ketone bodies (also referred to as endogenous ketones or simply ketones) are then released from the liver into blood and transported to our muscles, heart, brain and other organs to be used as energy. Thus ketone bodies are an important fuel source when glucose is not available. This is particularly relevant in Alzheimer's because one of the characteristic features of the disease is that the brain is struggling to obtain energy from glucose.

There are two main reasons for this:
1. Delivery of glucose from the blood to the brain becomes compromised because of damage to the blood-brain barrier (BBB).
2. Brain cells develop insulin resistance so that even if glucose can reach them, glucose is not able to enter the cells.

This results in an energy crisis whereby neurons are starved of fuel, are unable to perform their functions and begin to die off. As more and more brain cells start dying, more and more symptoms of Alzheimer's emerge. However, if the brain is supplied with ketones (as it is during fasting), it can use ketones for energy in place of glucose. Alzheimer's is averted.

The switch to using ketones for fuel is accompanied by other health-promoting changes throughout our brain and body. These changes include an enhanced ability of cells and organs to prevent and repair damage, resist stress, and clear out garbage through a process known as **autophagy.** All these factors further protect our brain from Alzheimer's. Fasting and ketones also promote the production of BDNF (brain-derived neurotrophic factor), which, you will recall, stimulates the formation of new brain cells and enhances neuroplasticity.

All the beneficial effects of intermittent fasting are further enhanced by exercising during the fasting period. Fasting, together with exercise, supercharges our brain and body so that we perform at our peak and stay healthy for life. Exercising on an empty stomach speeds up depletion of glucose from the liver and accelerates ketone production. Hence, I exercise in the morning before my first meal of the day.

Is there anyone for whom fasting is not recommended? Fasting overnight for up to 14 hours is unlikely to cause problems for anyone. Longer periods without food or 5:2 fasting is not recommended for the following groups unless supervised by a health professional and undertaken for a specific therapeutic purpose:
• anyone who is underweight
• anyone with a history of an eating disorder such as anorexia nervosa, bulimia nervosa or binge eating disorder

- anyone taking medications for hypertension (high blood pressure) or diabetes[2]
- women who are pregnant or breastfeeding
- prepubescent children
- someone with dementia who is struggling to eat enough calories in the first place.

Women sometimes find it more difficult to practise 5:2 fasting or TRF longer than 14/10 during the week before their period. If this is your experience, listen to your body, choose real whole foods and eat when you're hungry (which we should all be doing anyway).

Obese teenagers can benefit from TRF but special care is needed to ensure they don't develop an unhealthy relationship with food and they have adequate intake of vitamins, minerals, protein and fat. Nutritional deficiencies in children can affect bone growth and delay the onset of menstruation. It is best if TRF is adopted by the whole family so that it becomes a normal way of life (which it is).

For more practical advice about fasting, I highly recommend Ben Tanner's website fastingwell.com. He offers a free *Intermittent Fasting Checklist* and fortnightly fasting tips. Ben Tanner PA-C is a physician assistant (similar to a doctor but with a narrower scope of practice) with a wealth of scientific knowledge and hands-on experience in various types of intermittent fasting.

My overriding message is to **make whatever tweaks you can to reduce the amount of time you spend eating.** Many people avoid making a start because they don't believe they will ever get their eating to a narrow enough window. There is no need to go as far as 16/8 if it doesn't suit your lifestyle. Any move in the right direction will bring benefits. Recall the Chinese proverb: 'The person who moves mountains begins by carrying away small stones.'

---

2 Fasting is very effective in reducing the need for medication in people with hypertension and type 2 diabetes. Hence the importance of involving your doctor.

CHAPTER 51

Good timing

*Of all the liars in the world, sometimes the worst
are your own fears.*

RUDYARD KIPLING (1865–1936)

Not only is timing important in relation to eating, timing of all our daily activities is an overlooked factor that contributes to health or disease. Almost every cell in our body has an internal clock that tells the cell when to carry out its specific functions. Biological processes do not happen at random times. Our alertness, energy levels, hormone production, body temperature, immune system, hunger and digestive activities increase and decrease at predetermined times of the day to optimise our overall functioning and wellbeing. For example, in the early hours of the morning our body goes through a series of changes that prepare us to wake up and seize the day. We shut down production of the sleep hormone melatonin and increase production of the stress hormone cortisol. Our breathing and heart rate speed up and our blood pressure and body temperature rise. All this occurs without our conscious awareness, in the service of getting us out of bed. The reverse happens at the end of the day.

The cyclical changes that take place in our body on a daily basis are referred to as our **circadian rhythms**. The term 'circadian' comes from the Latin *circa* meaning 'approximately' and *diem* meaning 'day'. In the same way that sunrise and sunset do not occur precisely every 24 hours, neither do our circadian rhythms. The study of circadian rhythms is called **chronobiology**.

In addition to every organ having its own clock governing the timing of particular tasks, there is a master clock in the brain that keeps all the other clocks in sync. This master clock is called the suprachiasmatic nucleus (SCN) and is located in a region of the brain called the hypothalamus. A distinct protein in our eyes called melanopsin detects the presence of light (even in people who are blind) and immediately conveys this information to our SCN, which in turn tells the other clocks in our body to stop our nightly repair work and shift into gear for our day jobs. Changing the times at which we're exposed to light (for instance, when we travel to a different time zone) resets our circadian rhythms but it can take a few days for everything to get in sync again. The discomfort associated with this transition is known as jet lag. You'll recall from Chapter 31 'Mind over muscle' that jet lag is also influenced by our beliefs about jet lag. Believing that we will seamlessly adjust to a new time zone helps to reset our SCN more quickly.

Unfortunately, we don't need to travel vast distances to disrupt our circadian rhythms. Bright lights at night time can turn off melatonin production and delay our ability to fall asleep. Blue wavelength light activates melanopsin more powerfully than red light and is therefore more likely to forestall sleep. Conversely, blue light is desirable during daylight hours because it improves alertness, mood, learning and productivity. To operate at our best, we need to maximise our exposure to natural outdoor light during the day and minimise bright light (especially blue) during the evening. Hence the emergence of blue-blocking glasses and apps that filter out blue wavelength light from devices after sundown. Do not wear blue-blocking glasses during the day. See Chapter 19 'Let sleep be your medicine' for a caveat regarding blue-blocking apps on devices.

Research from Northwestern University's Feinberg School of Medicine in Chicago has shown that even low levels of light *while* we sleep raise our heart rate, blood glucose and insulin, thus increasing our risk of heart disease, type 2 diabetes, obesity and Alzheimer's.

What constitutes low levels of light? A bedside lamp, keeping the TV on, or street lights shining through thin curtains. Participants in the study spent two nights in a sleep laboratory. On the first night they all slept in a dark room. On the second night, half of them slept in a room with a low level of light (<100 lux). On both mornings, everyone had their blood sugar and insulin measured. Those who'd slept in the light room saw a rise in their glucose and insulin, while those who'd spent both nights in a dark room saw no change. Even though participants did not report any noticeable difference in the quality of their sleep, their brain was nonetheless affected.

Despite our eyes being closed, our SCN registers ambient light. This activates our fright, flight, fight response and puts our body in a mild state of stress. As a result, our breathing becomes irregular and shallow and we spend less time in slow wave and REM (dream) sleep, thus also exacerbating obstructive sleep apnoea.

A sleep study in Japan that ran from 2010 to 2014 found that even minimal light exposure — above 5 lux or 60 cm (2 feet) away from a candle — while a person sleeps increases the likelihood of developing depression, even when other predisposing factors are ruled out.

Thus **we need to block out all light while we sleep**. Invest in opaque curtains and an eye mask, and if you use a digital clock or phone as an alarm, turn them upside down or cover them with a dark cloth so you're not exposed to light from the clock numbers or incoming messages. This is an easy fix that can make a big difference to our physical and mental health.

Light is the most potent factor affecting the SCN in our brain, but food has the biggest regulatory role when it comes to timing the activities of our liver. When mice were fed during their sleep time instead of their usual feeding times, almost every function in their liver was reset to match food intake rather than light exposure. Likewise, all the organs involved in digestion (pancreas, gut, gall bladder and intestinal bacteria) need to adjust the timing of their tasks to coordinate with incoming food. This has a knock-on effect on our muscles, kidneys and fat tissues due to the unexpected presence of insulin and glucose in our blood. Because our body and gut bacteria are not designed to deal with food during the night, digestion is slower, less efficient and often incomplete. Hence night-eating substantially contributes to heartburn, obesity and type 2 diabetes. In the morning when light signals our SCN to wake up our organs, if they've been processing food during the night, they are instead ready to shut down. Even if we don't eat during the day, the mismatch between light and food compromises all our circadian rhythms and we are more prone to gut problems and feeling under par. This highlights the importance of overnight fasting and TRF.

Eating at erratic times throughout the day also causes circadian confusion. Stick to eating meals at the same time where possible and **avoid snacking**. Every time we eat, we stimulate insulin release from the pancreas. This further disrupts the biological clocks in our pancreas, liver and entire digestive tract and we increase our risk of insulin resistance, obesity and gut disorders. Chapter 42 'Carb correction' explains why keeping insulin in check is so important for every aspect of our health. If you get hungry between meals, it means that one of several things may be going on:

- You are not eating enough food at mealtimes.
- You are not eating enough protein at each meal. You are eating non-satiating, high-carb (high-GI) foods at mealtimes.
- Your hunger is emotional, not physical.
- You have created a snacking habit that is driven by brain circuits signalling a desire to eat in response to specific triggers or times of day.

To get on top of recalcitrant snacking, read my book *NeuroSlimming — Let your brain change your body* (<u>winningatslimming.com</u>).

What about timing of physical exercise? Researchers are still investigating whether there is an optimal time to exercise. The good news is that exercising either in the morning or late afternoon bolsters all our circadian rhythms. Outdoor exercise in bright morning light is a great way to enhance mood and brain function, and mitigate jet lag or sleep deprivation. You'll discover this is the best way to increase your productivity. If you go to the gym in the morning, try to find an area near a glass window that allows exposure to natural light. Exercising before our first meal of the day is also the best option for fat burning and enhancing all the benefits of TRF discussed in the previous chapter.

On the other hand, exercising between 3 pm and dinner may result in better performance because this is the time when our muscle tone, strength and coordination are at their peak.

If your work or commitment to caring for someone do not enable you to exercise until after dinner, this is still better than not exercising at all. Although exercise spikes alertness, it lowers post-meal blood glucose levels and has a beneficial effect on all our organs. Exercising in any capacity for just 10 minutes after each meal — either a brisk walk or pumping a few weights is fine — lowers potential glucose spikes and reduces the risk of type 2 diabetes.

A 12-week study in 2022 involving 27 women and 20 men aged 25 to 55 found that exercising at different times of day had differential effects in men and women. All participants followed the same healthy meal plan and were trained by coaches for one hour four days a week. On the days that participants engaged in strength training and HIIT, they ate a small amount of food (250–300 Calories) one hour prior to exercising. On the days they did endurance training or stretching, the morning group did not have their first meal until after their workout, and the evening group did not eat for at least four hours prior to training.

The only difference was that some people exercised in the morning between 6 and 8 am and others in the evening between 6.30 and 8.30 pm. At the end of three months everyone had reduced their body fat and blood pressure, and improved their strength, fitness, flexibility, mood and food satiety. However, in men the improvements were greater in those who exercised in the evening. In women, different parameters saw bigger improvements at different times of day. Morning exercise produced greater reductions in visceral (belly) fat and blood pressure, while evening exercise resulted in greater strength, endurance, satiety and mood enhancement.

Note that this was only a small study and participants were active and healthy prior to the trial. We do not know if older or younger populations, people with obese levels of body fat or exercising later in the morning or earlier in the afternoon would change the results.

The bottom line is to exercise when you most enjoy exercising. After that, be guided by what you are trying to achieve and when you can fit it in.

Chronically living in opposition to our circadian rhythms increases the risk of developing a wide range of diseases because our bodily processes aren't occurring at their designated times. This means that jobs aren't being done as well as they should be. Imagine a production plant (analogous to our body) in which goods (proteins, hormones, neurotransmitters) are manufactured through a series of orderly steps. If something is mistimed or machines (organs) are not serviced and the factory is not cleaned after hours, glitches start to arise. Over time this results in faulty products (diseases) or a slower, less efficient system (indigestion, fatigue and low mood).

Shift workers are a prime example of living in contravention of our circadian rhythms and having greater susceptibility to obesity, heart disease, type 2 diabetes and cancer as a consequence. For non-shift workers, the three biggest circadian rhythm disruptors are:

1. working late into the night (be that school work, studying, spillover from our day job or scrolling through social media) while exposed to blue wavelength light
2. eating beyond a 12-hour window
3. sitting for prolonged periods and not getting any exercise.

Conversely, trying to live as closely aligned with our circadian rhythms as possible will improve our mood, increase our sense of wellbeing, elevate our energy, strengthen our immune system, lower our risk of chronic diseases and boost our brain. If you are a shift worker, this obviously entails more than the steps outlined below and I recommend you read Dr Satchin Panda's book *The Circadian Code*. For the rest of us, restoring our circadian rhythms means incorporating as many of the following strategies as you can.

1. Expose yourself to natural outdoor light as soon as possible after waking. Open the curtains, throw on some joggers and go for a brisk morning walk without sunglasses — as little as five minutes will make a positive difference. If you work from home, eat your first meal of the day outside in the sun. Even on an overcast day, outdoor light is many times brighter than indoor light.
2. Expose yourself to natural outdoor light as much as possible throughout the day. If your work necessitates that you stay

indoors for eight or more hours, make certain you have bright lighting and take outdoor breaks whenever you can.

3. Leave a minimum of 12 hours between your last and first meal of the day — in other words, practise TRF.

4. Get out of the habit of snacking. Eat two to three satisfying meals at roughly the same times every day.

5. Do not eat for at least three hours before bed.

6. Try not to eat for as long as possible after waking. I know this goes against the notion that 'breakfast is the most important meal of the day'. There is absolutely no science to support the idea that we should eat shortly after waking. The opposite is true.

7. Dim all the lights two hours before bedtime. Invest in faint red lights for your night lighting. This is also the time to turn off phones and screens. Avoid doing anything rousing or stimulating two hours before bedtime.

8. Sleep in a completely darkened cool room — below 19 degrees Celsius (67 Fahrenheit) is ideal.

9. Get seven to nine hours of sleep every night — determined by your personal sleep requirement.

10. Go to bed and wake up at the same time every day including weekends. We need variety in how we spend our days but consistency in how long and when we sleep. If circumstances have put you in a sleep-deprived state and you have the opportunity to go to bed earlier or to sleep in, please do so before re-establishing your regular sleep routine.

In the latter stages of Alzheimer's, the SCN can start to degenerate and cause disruption to a person's sleep-wake cycle, bowel habits, appetite regulation and sense of time. This makes it even more critical to follow as regular a routine for sleeping, eating and exercising as possible.

CHAPTER 52

Cholesterol controversies

Until we have begun to go without them, we fail to realise how unnecessary many things are. We've been using them not because we needed them but because we had them.

SENECA (4 BCE – 65 CE)

'Why is nothing in medicine straightforward?' Jasmin opened our conversation. 'Having high cholesterol in midlife is listed as a risk factor for Alzheimer's. But then I read that the most common medicines used to treat high cholesterol — called statins — can *impair* memory and brain function! So what does one do? My grandmother has been taking a statin called atorvastatin (Lipitor) for over 10 years. Has this done more harm than good?'

'Doctors all around the globe are asking the same question,' I replied. 'Cholesterol is a very complex subject and the cause of a lot of controversy. The first thing to understand is that **there is nothing inherently bad about cholesterol** — in fact, cholesterol is essential for life. It's a critical component of all our cell membranes and a precursor for making oestrogen, testosterone, adrenal hormones, vitamin D and bile acids.'

'Doesn't the brain contain about a quarter of all the cholesterol in our body?' she asked

'Yes. **The brain contains more cholesterol than any other organ.** Without it, brain cells would not be able to communicate with each other. Cholesterol is an indispensable part of the myelin sheath that surrounds the axons (long tails) of brain and nerve cells. This sheath acts like insulation and allows for efficient transmission of electrical impulses along the length of the cell. Cholesterol is also important for mitochondrial function.'

'Damage to myelin results in multiple sclerosis, doesn't it?' Jasmin interjected.

'Yes. However, myelin is only one of cholesterol's many roles within the brain. Scientists are even investigating how cholesterol metabolism might influence amyloid β (Aβ) plaque formation.'

'If cholesterol is so important for our brain, why is high cholesterol a problem? Shouldn't *low* cholesterol be the worry?'

'Always remember Goldilocks. The brain needs to have the *right* amount of cholesterol for optimal functioning — too little interferes with brain cell signalling and too much could lead to Aβ accumulation. Hence brain cholesterol levels are strictly regulated, and the amount of cholesterol in our blood does not reflect the amount of cholesterol in our brain. They're two separate systems. The brain makes its own cholesterol from readily available raw materials. The brain is not going to leave it to our fickle food preferences to provide it with one of its most vital molecules. A very tight barrier exists between the contents of our blood and the contents of our brain. It's called the blood-brain barrier or BBB and is formed by walls of closely knit cells and proteins that only allow certain substances to cross the border. This is to protect the brain from toxins, bacteria and viruses that might be circulating in our blood. It also makes it difficult for many drugs to enter the brain. In most cases that's a good thing; in the case of developing medications to treat Alzheimer's, it adds to the challenge.'

'Can statins cross the blood-brain barrier?'

'In certain circumstances, some of them can. There are multiple factors at play.'

'That's your favourite answer,' Jasmin accused teasingly.

'That's the way it is,' I affirmed cheerfully. 'There are currently seven different statins on the market, all of which block an enzyme called HMG-CoA reductase in our liver and other organs. This enzyme is necessary for the production of cholesterol. Because statins reduce cholesterol production in the liver, it takes up more LDL-cholesterol from the blood, thus lowering blood cholesterol levels. Statins can also reduce inflammation, and each of the seven statins has its own distinct properties and side effects. Some statins can dissolve in fat while others can't. Researchers originally thought that if a statin was fat-soluble (referred to as lipophilic or hydrophobic), it was better at crossing the BBB and exerting an undesirable effect on the brain, but the situation has turned out to be far more nuanced. Statins probably interact with the BBB in several different ways. If someone has an illness that punches holes in the BBB, statins of all types could slip through and interfere with brain cholesterol production. In most people this would be a bad thing. In some people, if the statin decreased brain inflammation and prevented micro haemorrhages it might be a good thing.'

'Are you saying that statins can have both positive *and* negative effects on the brain, depending on the statin and the person?' Jasmin queried.

'Yes. Some studies show that statins can impair memory and cognition; other studies have found that people taking statins are less likely to develop Alzheimer's. Fortunately, in people who experience negative brain effects, their cognition returns to normal when the statin is stopped.'

'How can statins have both positive and negative effects on the brain?'

'The effects of a statin are modulated by its specific chemical properties along with a person's age, ethnicity, genetics, microbiota (gut bacteria) and co-existent diseases. Let me draw a table to clarify what researchers have observed to date.

Factors associated with a greater likelihood of reversible cognitive impairment from taking statins	Factors associated with statins lowering the risk of Alzheimer's
Taking statins after the age of 70	Taking statins in midlife (age 45 to 65)
Taking statins that are lipophilic, e.g. atorvastatin, simvastatin and lovastatin	Reducing the risk of heart disease and stroke also reduces the risk of Alzheimer's and vascular dementia.
Taking statins at a high dose	Some studies have found that people with two copies of the APOE4 gene experience greater cognitive benefits from statins than people with APOE2 or APOE3 genes.
Liver disease or taking statins with medications that interfere with statin metabolism by the liver	
Alcohol abuse	
Bipolar disorder or schizophrenia	
Thyroid disease	
Genetic mutations linked to mitochondrial dysfunction	

'There's still more to unravel but at least doctors are now aware they need to carefully assess each person's individual circumstances before prescribing a statin.'

'In some people, statins can also give rise to muscle problems such as pain, spasm, weakness and wasting,' Jasmin added.

'Yes, along with sore joints, abnormal liver function tests, elevated blood sugar levels and an increased risk of type 2 diabetes — exactly the opposite of what you're trying to achieve. That's why it's crucial to closely monitor every patient's individual response to all medications and supplements. There is wide variability in people's responses to statins — both good and bad. Despite sounding like nasty drugs, statins can save lives by reducing cardiovascular disease. And not everyone experiences side effects; many people tolerate statins without a problem.'

'Is heart disease still the leading cause of death in men and women worldwide?' Jasmin asked.

'Yes, about a quarter of all deaths are due to cardiovascular disease.

More women die of heart disease than of breast cancer. And **cardiovascular disease is also a major risk factor for Alzheimer's**.'

'Is that the main reason that high blood cholesterol is linked to Alzheimer's? Because of its association with heart disease and stroke?'

'Firstly, it isn't high cholesterol but high LDL-cholesterol (LDL-C) that has been associated with Alzheimer's. This is an important distinction. Cholesterol is not soluble in water (i.e. it is "hydrophobic") and therefore needs to be attached to one of various proteins in order to move through our blood. These proteins are collectively known as "lipoproteins". One such transport protein is called Low Density Lipoprotein (LDL) and another is High Density Lipoprotein (HDL). Less common cholesterol transporters are Intermediate Density Lipoprotein (IDL), Very Low Density Lipoprotein (VLDL) and chylomicrons.'

Blood cholesterol transporters

Name	Abbreviation	Are they atherogenic? In other words, do they have the potential to lodge in artery walls?	Analogy (this will become clear later)
High density lipoprotein	HDL	no	ambulance
Low density lipoprotein	LDL	yes	car
Intermediate density lipoprotein	IDL	yes	truck
Very low density lipoprotein	VLDL	yes	motorbike
Chylomicron	Chylomicron	no	bicycle

'LDL, IDL and VLDL — but not HDL or chylomicrons — have the potential to lodge in artery walls and are designated as "atherogenic" lipoproteins. You don't hear much about IDL, VLDL and chylomicrons because they don't hang around in our blood for more than a few hours at a time — sometimes only a few minutes. LDL, on the other hand, circulates in our blood for several days and is the major lipoprotein that can embed in artery walls. Hence LDL-cholesterol is colloquially referred to as "bad" cholesterol and HDL-cholesterol as "good" cholesterol. However, this is a misnomer. There is no such thing as "good" or "bad" cholesterol because the cholesterol carried by LDL is the same as the cholesterol carried by HDL, IDL, VLDL and chylomicrons. It's just that LDL gets stuck in artery walls more frequently than other lipoproteins.'

'Got it,' Jasmin confirmed. 'And the problem with LDL-C lodging within artery walls is that it sets off an inflammatory response that can lead to narrowing or blockage of the affected artery. If the artery is one that supplies blood to the heart — i.e. a coronary artery — the corollary is a heart attack. If the blockage occurs in an artery that feeds the brain — e.g. a carotid artery — the result is a stroke.'

'Very well summarised,' I commended. 'The second point is that only people under the age of 70 with high LDL-C have been found to be at greater risk of developing Alzheimer's. **No negative association is seen between LDL-C and Alzheimer's in older people.** In other words, past a certain age, LDL-C no longer predicts Alzheimer's risk.'

'What's the mechanism by which high LDL-C in midlife negatively impacts brain function? Is it purely because high LDL-C contributes to blood vessel injury? And why does the risk disappear as we age?'

'Thousands of research papers haven't yet provided a definitive answer. What you've suggested is one possible explanation. High LDL-C might be a sign that a person is not getting enough blood to their brain. Alternatively, there might be a completely different mechanism linked to LDL-C that we haven't yet discovered.'

'Why is cholesterol circulating in our blood in the first place?' Jasmin continued probing.

'Cholesterol is critical for the survival and functioning of every cell in our body, not just our brain. Only about 25% of the cholesterol in our body comes from what we eat. Cholesterol is found exclusively in animal foods such as meat (especially organs like brain and liver), poultry, egg yolks, dairy and shellfish. The rest comes from what we make ourselves, mostly in the liver and intestines. However, every cell in our body can produce its own cholesterol. If a person eats little or no cholesterol — as is the case with vegans — their body makes more cholesterol to make up for the deficit. We can also recycle cholesterol from our gut by breaking down bile acids.

If cells in a particular organ aren't making enough of their own cholesterol, they overcome the shortfall by obtaining cholesterol from the liver and intestines via the blood.'

'So eating less cholesterol won't make much difference to blood cholesterol levels?' Jasmin looked surprised.

'Correct. Cholesterol exists in two forms: an active form called "free" or "unesterified" cholesterol and a storage form called a cholesterol "ester" or "esterified" cholesterol. About half of the cholesterol we eat is in the storage form, which we are not able to absorb unless enzymes from our pancreas convert it to the free form — a process known as "de-esterification". Before de-esterification happens, most of the esterified cholesterol is excreted in our stools, so we only absorb about half of the cholesterol we eat.'

Two forms of cholesterol

Name	Chemical description	Function	Can we absorb it from the food we eat?
inactive form	esterified	This is the form in which cholesterol is stored.	no — most esterified cholesterol is excreted in stools
active form	non-esterified	This is the form in which cholesterol carries out its various functions.	yes

'Can you repeat that please? I found the unfamiliar terminology hard to follow,' Jasmin furrowed her brow.

'Let me clarify by way of a demonstration. Hold out your hand and show me your open palm. Let's call your open palm the "free" form of your hand because it's free to hold something. Now pick up a pen and wrap your fingers around it. Let's call that the "storage" form of your hand because you're holding (storing) something. You've just illustrated that your hand can exist in two forms: closed (storage form) and open (free form). Which is the bulkier shape —your flat palm or your clenched fist?'

'My clenched fist.'

'Spot on. The same applies to cholesterol. It exists in a free form that is more easily absorbed through our intestinal wall and a storage form that is bulkier and needs to have its load removed before we can digest it. Much of the cholesterol in food exists in the storage form, so our pancreas needs to make enzymes to detach the load (the ester) from the cholesterol molecule. By that time, we've eliminated most of the bulky cholesterol in our stools.'

'Now I understand,' Jasmin looked pleased. 'So why has dietary cholesterol been labelled as a health hazard?'

'**Cutting back on eating cholesterol is outdated advice.** Doctors mistakenly assumed that eating cholesterol raised blood cholesterol. Now we know that, for the majority of people, this is not the case. We made the same mistake in relation to dietary fat consumption. Eating fat doesn't make us fat. Eating sugar and refined carbohydrates makes us fat, damages artery walls and raises our blood pressure and LDL-C, along with increasing our risk of diabetes, stroke and cancer. However, in some people — and I emphasise *some* — eating a lot of *saturated* fat raises their LDL-C. In other people, saturated fat makes no difference to their LDL-C. Once again, we return to the notion that one approach does not fit all.'

'I've heard that we absorb more cholesterol from food as we age. Is that true?'

'Some studies have found that as we get older, men tend to absorb *less* cholesterol, while women tend to absorb *more*, especially after menopause. But this is also influenced by our genes. People with the APOE4 gene appear to extract more cholesterol from food than the rest of the population at any given age.'

'So cholesterol is chauffeured around in the blood on lipoproteins and delivered to whichever organs need it,' Jasmin summed up.

'Yes, great metaphor,' I acknowledged.

'But why does LDL-cholesterol get deposited into artery walls? It's a potentially deadly flaw in the cholesterol transport system.'

'The best way to explain this is to use the analogy of a busy highway that has constant traffic of cars, taxis, buses, trucks, ambulances and other vehicles. [See the diagram.] Each vehicle carries different numbers of passengers — buses can obviously transport more people than cars. Over time, the road can develop cracks, erosions, potholes and other signs of wear and tear. The worse the condition of the road, the greater the risk of traffic accidents. Inclement weather can also lead to more crashes by reducing visibility or making the surface more slippery. Would you agree?'

'Yes,' Jasmin nodded.

'Would you also predict that the more vehicles on the road, the greater the likelihood of accidents?'

'Yes.'

'Therefore, if all the drivers have the same level of skill — and they aren't drunk or distracted by phones — what would be the major factors contributing to road accidents?'

Jasmin was quick with her response. 'To recap what you've just said, the main things leading to collisions would be poorly maintained roads, bad weather and more vehicles on the road.'

'Excellent. Now let's relate this to cholesterol:
- The road represents our arteries.
- The road surface is analogous to the inner lining of our arteries, known as the endothelium.
- The cars, taxis and buses are LDLs of different types — more about this in a moment.
- The passengers are cholesterol.
- The ambulances are HDLs.
- The trucks and motorbikes are IDLs and VLDLs.

'LDLs come in different sizes and carry varying amounts of cholesterol. Some LDLs are like buses, while those with fewer passengers are like cars and taxis. Just for the record, lipoproteins don't only transport cholesterol, they also carry triglycerides and phospholipids, but this doesn't change our story.

'In the same way that road surfaces deteriorate, so can the inner lining of artery walls — known as the endothelium. What specific things can damage the endothelium of an artery?'

Once more, Jasmin answered with confidence. 'Smoking, high

blood pressure and high blood levels of glucose, insulin, uric acid, homocysteine[3] and inflammatory molecules.'

'Right again. So here we have the first reason that LDL-C might get stuck in an artery wall: damage to the wall by sugar, cigarettes or any of the other factors you listed (analogous to cracks and potholes). Sometimes our immune system (analogous to emergency services such as police, tow trucks and road workers) can repair the artery (road) before the situation escalates. This is where HDL enters the picture and gets its "good" reputation. HDL plays a role in removing cholesterol from artery walls. Just as ambulances take casualties to hospital, HDLs deliver cholesterol from artery walls to the liver. HDL does a whole lot more than that, but I don't want to bog you down with too much detail.'

I paused before continuing. 'Unfortunately, there are times when our emergency services can't clean up the wreckage quickly enough, and if LDL remains in an artery wall for a protracted period, the artery undergoes further and further damage.'

'I'm following the analogy,' Jasmin declared enthusiastically.

'Another thing that causes traffic accidents is bad weather. Rain and fog represent chronic major depression and emotional distress, both of which are huge risk factors for heart disease and stroke. In fact, chronic major depression is a bigger risk factor for cardiovascular disease than is smoking.'

Jasmin gasped. **'Depression and emotional stress are worse for our heart than smoking cigarettes?** No way!'

'*Chronic major untreated depression,* not a short spell of mild depression,' I emphasised. 'The more someone smokes, the greater their risk of smoking-related diseases. The worse someone's depression, the greater their risk of heart disease and Alzheimer's. **Our mental health profoundly impacts our physical heath** — a fact that is often overlooked.'

'That's something I'll never forget,' Jasmin asserted.

---

3 High homocysteine levels often indicate vitamin B12 or folate deficiency. For a refresher on homocysteine, refer to Chapter 48 'Vitamins for vitality'.

The cholesterol super-highway

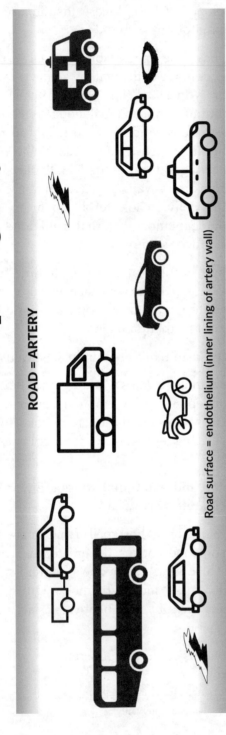

ROAD = ARTERY

Road surface = endothelium (inner lining of artery wall)

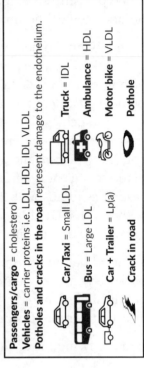

Passengers/cargo = cholesterol

Vehicles = carrier proteins i.e. LDL, HDL, IDL, VLDL

Potholes and cracks in the road represent damage to the endothelium.

Car/Taxi = Small LDL	**Truck** = IDL
Bus = Large LDL	**Ambulance** = HDL
Car + Trailer = Lp(a)	**Motor bike** = VLDL
Crack in road	**Pothole**

Important points:

- Just as a well-maintained road with fewer cracks and potholes leads to fewer road accidents, a healthy endothelium leads to fewer LDLs getting stuck in an artery wall.

- LDLs come in different sizes. Cars, taxis and Ubers represent small dense LDLs and buses represent large buoyant LDLs. Small dense LDLs are more likely to be correlated with heart disease than large buoyant LDLs.

'The third thing we've identified as increasing collisions is the number of vehicles on the road. The more LDL cars and taxis on the road, the greater the likelihood that one of them will knock into an artery wall.'

'What gives rise to having too many LDL vehicles on the road? Genetics or lifestyle?' Jasmin pondered.

'Both. About one in 300 people are born with a genetic mutation that impairs the liver's ability to clear LDL-C from blood. The condition is known as Familial Hypercholesterolaemia (FH) and if it is not diagnosed and treated, the person can develop heart disease at a very young age. If one parent has FH, there's a 50% chance that their children will also have the condition.

'In most people, however, high numbers of small dense dangerous LDLs are due to a combination of factors that include:
- smoking
- too much sugar
- too much stress
- too much alcohol
- too little exercise
- too little sleep
- side effects of certain medications, e.g. steroids
- other medical conditions, e.g. diabetes, chronic kidney disease or an underactive thyroid.'

'Hence we need to measure LDL-cholesterol levels in our blood on a regular basis,' Jasmin concluded.

'Yes. However, there's a very important distinction to make here. Remember that in our analogy, the vehicles are LDL and the passengers are cholesterol. Each LDL vehicle — referred to as an LDL particle or LDL-P — transports varying amounts of cholesterol. Some LDL particles are like buses with lots of passengers, while others are like cars and taxis with few passengers. Therefore, when we measure LDL-cholesterol (LDL-C), we are not measuring the number of vehicles on the road, we are measuring the number of passengers. In other words, we are adding up all the passengers in all the buses, cars and taxis. This does not provide an accurate picture of the risk of traffic accidents. Why?'

Jasmin deliberated before replying. 'High LDL-C could mean you have lots of LDL particles (LDL-P), each carrying only a few cholesterol molecules, or fewer LDL particles, each carrying lots of cholesterol molecules.'

'Precisely! Which is the more hazardous situation?'

'More LDL particles with fewer passengers. More vehicles, not more passengers, are the cause of traffic jams.'

'Exactly. That's why we need to know the number of LDL particles (LDL-P) — NOT the amount of LDL-cholesterol (LDL-C) — in a person's blood.'

'Is there a blood test that tells us the number of LDL-P in our blood?' Jasmin asked excitedly.

'Yes. It's called an Apo B test — short for Apolipoprotein B-100. Apolipoprotein B-100 is a protein found on all LDL particles as well as on IDL and VLDL. Think of IDL and VLDL as trucks and motorbikes that can also cause accidents. Therefore, if you add up all the Apo B proteins, it tells you exactly how many atherogenic (potentially artery-damaging) lipoproteins are in circulation — in other words, how many vehicles are on the road.'

'Why doesn't everyone get an Apo B test? Why are we wasting our time measuring LDL-C?' Jasmin bordered on indignation.

'Because the Apo B test has only recently become available and changing the practice of medicine is a very slow process. In the past, LDL-C was the best approximation for LDL-P that we had. It's not unreasonable to assume that if your LDL-C is very low, you are less likely to have huge numbers of LDL particles floating around. But this is not always the case, especially if you have high levels of triglycerides. Now that the Apo B test is available, it needs to be one of the standard tests for assessing someone's risk of both cardiovascular disease and Alzheimer's.'

'Is it expensive?'

'No. In both Australia and the United States, it costs less than $20.'

'Then that settles it. I'm telling everyone to ask their doctor for an Apo B test!' Jasmin looked triumphant.

'Please do!' I encouraged. 'Many doctors, including cardiologists, are still unfamiliar with the Apo B test so you'll have to explain it to them. And while you're at it, you can tell everyone about one more little-known risk factor for heart disease.'

'What's that?'

'Some vehicles tow trailers that increase the risk of accidents.'

'What do the trailers represent?'

'Have you heard of a protein called Apo(a) — short for Apolipoprotein(a)?'

'No,' Jasmin shook her head.

'About one in five people worldwide have an Apo(a) protein attached to their Apo B protein. Apo(a) + Apo B form an entity called Lp(a) — short for Lipoprotein(a)[4]. Lp(a) is really just an LDL particle with an extra protein called Apo(a) stuck to it — like a car towing a trailer. We still have a lot to learn about Lp(a) but in some people (not in everyone) it can triple their risk of having a heart attack or stroke under the age of 45:

- Car + trailer = more accident prone than a car that is not towing a load
- LDL + Apo(a) = Lp(a) = more atherogenic than LDL alone.'

'Does it run in families?'

'Yes. Lp(a) is genetically determined and does not appear to be influenced by diet or exercise. If you inherit the gene that makes you produce Lp(a) in large amounts, neither a healthy lifestyle nor statins are likely to bring down their number. Your Lp(a) level stays relatively constant throughout your life.'

'So what can someone do to mitigate their risk of heart disease if they have high numbers of Lp(a)?'

'People with high numbers of Lp(a) need to do everything they can to avoid all other risk factors for heart disease — such as chronic stress, sleep deprivation, smoking, high blood pressure, type 2 diabetes,

---

[4] Lipoprotein(a) is pronounced 'lipoprotein little a'.

lack of exercise, processed food and untreated depression. It's what we should all be doing anyway. Lp(a) just makes it more imperative that a person puts health at the top of their priorities. Taking control of lifestyle factors can offset the impact of Lp(a) but, in rare cases, a person can do everything "right" and still have a heart attack.'

'Is there a blood test for Lp(a)?'

'Yes. I recommend the test for anyone with a family member who had a heart attack or stroke before the age of 60. Personally, I think everyone should have an Lp(a) test once in their life regardless of their family history. If you know you have high levels of Lp(a), you're more likely to take symptoms of heart disease seriously and not brush them off as indigestion. Plus, pharmaceutical companies are trialling medications (such as antisense oligonucleotides) that show promise in reducing Lp(a).'

'At what age would you recommend a person has an Lp(a) test?'

'As soon as possible over the age of 20 years. Heart disease, like Alzheimer's, doesn't develop overnight — it takes decades. The sooner you become aware of your personal risk factors, the sooner you can start to live in a way that mitigates those risks. Of course, if you don't intend to be proactive about your health, there is no point in knowing.'

'If your Lp(a) is high, does that mean your Apo B and LDL-C will also be high?'

'No. That's the sneaky thing about Lp(a). All your other blood test results can be perfectly normal. You might have low numbers of LDL particles (i.e. low levels of Apo B) but if a large number of them are carrying the Apo(a) protein, it makes them much more accident-prone. Vehicles towing trailers are dangerous!'

'You've also mentioned "small dense LDL particles" versus "large fluffy LDL particles". Can you elaborate please? It sounds as though small LDL particles (cars and taxis) are more likely to cause damage to arteries than large LDL particles (minivans and buses)? Why would that be the case?'

'This is another divisive chapter in the cholesterol story. To be pedantic, the term "small dense" is tautologous. If the particles are small, they will automatically be dense. While not all doctors are convinced that size matters, I believe there is enough evidence to make me want my LDL particles to be large rather than small. Having predominantly small LDL particles has been linked to a greater risk of heart disease than having mostly large particles. Several reasons for this have been proposed:
1. small particles can wedge more easily in an artery wall than large particles
2. small particles are more likely to be damaged (oxidised).'

Seven subtypes of LDL

Type	Designation	Description	Relationship to cardiovascular (heart) disease (CVD)	Analogy
1	Pattern A	large, fluffy and harmless	lowest risk of CVD	bus
2	Pattern A	large, fluffy and harmless	lower risk of CVD	minivan
3	Pattern B	small, dense and dangerous	higher risk of CVD	Uber
4	Pattern B	small, dense and dangerous	higher risk of CVD	taxi
5	Pattern B	small, dense and dangerous	higher risk of CVD	sedan
6	Pattern B	small, dense and dangerous	higher risk of CVD	hatchback
7	Pattern B	small, dense and dangerous	highest risk of CVD	sports car

'Is there a test that can measure the size of a person's LDL particles?'

'Yes. The test is called "LDL sub-fractions" and it separates LDL particles into seven different sizes. They are numbered LDL-1 (the largest) to LDL-7 (the smallest). If a person has mostly LDL-1 and LDL-2, they are designated as having "Pattern A". If they have predominantly LDL-3 to LDL-7, they are designated as having "Pattern B". All other things being equal, people with Pattern B have a higher risk of heart disease than people with Pattern A.'

'Do you order an LDL sub-fractions test for your patients?'

'It depends on the individual. Knowing a person's LDL sub-fractions is a good idea if the results of other tests are equivocal or if you want to track the effect of lifestyle changes or medications.'

'I can now see why you said that cholesterol was a complex subject,' Jasmin sounded exhausted.

'And we've only just scratched the surface,' I smiled empathically. 'There are also subtypes of HDL, VLDL and Lp(a), plus newer cholesterol-lowering drugs that work differently to statins (such as PCSK9 inhibitors), but we've covered enough to answer your initial questions.'

'Can PCSK9 inhibitors impair memory and cognition like statins?'

'PCSK9 inhibitors do not interfere with cholesterol production and to date there is no evidence that they impair brain function.'

'Phew!' Jasmin exclaimed. 'And all I wanted to know was whether high cholesterol or statins caused memory problems!'

'Since this is a very involved subject, let's recap the main points about cholesterol and Alzheimer's,' I proposed.

'Yes, please!' Jasmin agreed emphatically.

'**Total blood cholesterol is a meaningless measurement.** It doesn't tell you anything about your risk of cardiovascular disease or Alzheimer's. Studies have found a link between high LDL-C in midlife and Alzheimer's in later life, but Apo B (a measure of LDL-P) is a much stronger predictor of risk. Therefore, the blood tests I recommend are:

1. **Apo B** — this tells you how many LDL + IDL + VLDL particles are in your blood — the lower the better.
2. **Lp(a)** — this tells you whether you have a particularly dangerous cholesterol-carrying protein in your blood — the lower the better. You only need to have this test once in your life because the number of Lp(a) does not change over time.
3. **Triglycerides** — we haven't spoken much about these, but triglycerides are the body's storage form of fat. They are transported on lipoproteins along with cholesterol. Having high levels of blood triglycerides is also associated with an increased risk of cardiovascular disease. Hence you want this number to be low. If you have diabetes, high triglyceride levels can also be a sign that your blood sugar is out of control.

4. **HDL-C** — a higher number is generally associated with lower risk of cardiovascular disease.
5. **LDL-C** — this test is not necessary but I usually order it to show patients that high LDL-C does not always correlate with high Apo B. The latter (Apo B) is the important number.
6. **Non-HDL-C** — this blood test is becoming trendy so I mention it for completeness. It's a proxy for Apo B so it isn't necessary if you have the first four tests above. Non-HDL-C is the amount of cholesterol carried by all the lipoproteins other than HDL. In other words, it is the sum of LDL-C + IDL-C + VLDL-C. If this number is high, it's a better predictor of your risk of cardiovascular disease than LDL-C alone. However, it is still not as reliable as the Apo B test. The number of vehicles — not the number of passengers — dictates the number of collisions.
7. **LDL-subfractions** — Pattern A = a lower risk of heart disease; Pattern B = a higher risk of heart disease.

'The purpose of these tests is to give you information relating to your risk of atherosclerotic heart disease. In turn, the health of your arteries is critical to the health your brain. If your test results are unfavourable, it's an indication to do everything you can to turn things around. Unfortunately, most doctors are unfamiliar with Apo B and Lp(a) so they are still ordering outdated tests of LDL-C and total blood cholesterol. LDL-C and total blood cholesterol are useless. Please tell your doctor about the importance of knowing your Apo B and Lp(a) status.

'With respect to statins:
1. In most people they are NOT necessary IF the person improves their sleep, stress management, diet and exercise. Education beats medication every time.
2. If your doctor prescribes a statin because you have a high Apo B count (or because you have other cardiovascular risk factors), ask for a comprehensive memory test before you start taking the medication and monitor for any undesirable side effects.
3. Request a statin that is water-soluble (hydrophilic) rather than fat-soluble (lipophilic). Water-soluble statins are less likely to cross the BBB and exert an unwanted effect on your brain.

4. If the first statin you try doesn't agree with you, there are six more statins to choose from. Just because you experience unpleasant side effects with one particular statin, doesn't mean you won't tolerate a different one. You could also try another class of LDL-P-lowering medications such as PCSK9 inhibitors or ezetimibe.

5. Over the age of 70, high LDL-P is not associated with an increased risk of Alzheimer's.

'Even though the cholesterol story is complicated, the health advice surrounding it is not. **Everything you do to protect your heart will also protect your brain.** Don't smoke, don't drink more than a few standard alcoholic drinks per week, eat real whole foods, exercise regularly, ensure adequate sleep and manage stress. We're constantly looking for the latest health hack but it always comes back to the basics.'

CHAPTER 53

The charms of chocolate

Science never solves a problem without creating 10 more.

GEORGE BERNARD SHAW (1856–1950)

'I'm afraid your dad was trying to convince me that you often give him chocolate Drumsticks for lunch,' Melanie reported when I arrived home one afternoon. 'I've never seen them in your freezer and I can't imagine it's the sort of thing you'd give him. But he was so adamant, I'm sure in his own mind he thought it was true.'

'It *is* true,' I smiled.

Melanie looked dismayed.

'I cook chicken drumsticks tossed in a mix of spices that includes cumin, turmeric, cinnamon and cacao. We call them chocolate drumsticks,' I explained. 'They're delicious.'

'Oh dear, I owe your dad an apology. I feel terrible that I jumped to the conclusion he was having a false memory on account of his dementia. I'm sorry …' she trailed off.

'Why don't you go and tell him I'll make chicken drumsticks for lunch tomorrow?' I suggested.

'I most definitely will!' Melanie strode out to the garden where Dad was admiring our snowflake bush.

She looked appeased on her return. 'Next time he says something that sounds implausible I'll ask him to tell me more,' she reassured herself. 'Speaking of implausible, I constantly hear people saying that dark chocolate boosts brain function and heart health.

'Is that true or is it just wishful thinking?'

'For the time being, it's wishful research. It began with the observation that Kuna Indians living on the San Blas Islands in the Caribbean Sea off Panama have lower blood pressure, fewer heart attacks and strokes, less cancer and live longer than Kuna who live on the mainland (Panama City). So scientists started looking into what was different about the two groups. The first thing they assessed was stress and salt intake, but stress levels were similar, and salt intake actually higher among the islanders. It turned out that those living on the islands ate twice as much fruit, four times as much fish and *10 times more cocoa* than the mainlanders. Since the islands are dry, Kuna islanders need to obtain their water from a mainland river. To ensure that the water is safe to drink, they boil it; to make the water more palatable when it becomes tepid, they add home-grown cocoa powder. Thus, Kuna islanders start drinking cocoa from the time they are weaned and continue to the day they die. Their average consumption is more than 850 mL (30 ounces) a day. They also incorporate cocoa into many recipes. In contrast, mainland Kuna drink much less cocoa and what they use is commercially produced and highly processed.'

'That's a lot of cocoa!' Melanie exclaimed.

'Yes, it's more cocoa than is consumed anywhere else in the world. This led researchers to ask: is there something in cacao that promotes heart health?'

'What's the difference between cacao and cocoa?'

'The words are often used interchangeably but, strictly speaking, cacao refers to the beans (seeds) of the Theobroma cacao tree, while cocoa is the powder that's made from them. To make cacao beans edible, they need to be fermented, dried and roasted. Different cacao companies roast the beans for varying lengths of time to produce distinct flavours. Unfortunately, roasting for long periods reduces the bean's nutritional value. When beans are roasted for only a short amount of time, the products made from them are labelled "raw", even though they are not entirely raw.

'Whether "raw" or roasted, cacao beans are then crushed and

separated from their husk (the outer shell of the bean) to make broken cacao pieces called cacao nibs or "nature's chocolate chips". "Raw" and roasted cacao nibs can be found in many health food shops and larger grocery stores. They have a strong bitter taste and can be used as a seasoning, sprinkled over strawberries or eaten on their own — but it's quite an acquired taste.'

'I'll have to try them,' replied Melanie enthusiastically.

'The fate of most cacao nibs, however, is not to be sold as they are but to be ground into a paste and then melted to form a liquid called "cocoa liquor".[5] Cocoa liquor can be moulded into blocks of "unprocessed" chocolate or mixed with sugar and other ingredients to make regular chocolate.

'Cocoa liquor can also be separated into two components: cocoa solids and cocoa butter.[6] Cocoa butter makes up about half the weight of the cacao bean and is a mixture of healthy saturated (60%), monounsaturated (35%) and polyunsaturated (5%) fatty acids. Cocoa butter is a major ingredient in dark, milk and white chocolate; however, because it is expensive, some food manufacturers have started substituting cocoa butter for cheaper unhealthy oils such as canola, soybean, cottonseed or generic vegetable oils. For a product to be called "chocolate", the European Union stipulates that alternative oils constitute no more than 5% of the total fat content. In the United States, 100% of the fat in chocolate must be cocoa butter. If chocolate contains oils other than cocoa butter, it should be labelled as "compound chocolate". Cocoa butter is solid at room temperature but melts at body temperature (34 to 38 °C or 93 to 101 °F) hence the pleasant texture it produces in our mouth. Because of its temperature attributes, cocoa butter is also used to make suppositories.'

'I didn't need to know that!' interjected Melanie with a grin.

---

[5] Cocoa liquor also goes by the names cacao liquor, chocolate liquor, cacao mass or cocoa mass. Don't confuse chocolate liquor with chocolate liqueur, which is a chocolate-flavoured alcoholic beverage made from whisky or vodka.

[6] Cocoa butter also goes by the name of theobroma oil. Chocolate terminology needs its own thesaurus. Cocoa butter is the only part of the cacao bean used in white chocolate.

'Sorry, I couldn't help myself,' I laughed. 'Cocoa solids, on the other hand, are further pulverised to make cocoa powder, the stuff we mix with milk for a warm drink. At this point, cocoa powder can be sold with no further processing. This is known as "natural" or "untreated" cocoa powder or cacao powder. Natural cocoa powder has a light brown colour and is bitter and astringent. Hence natural cocoa powder is often treated with an alkalising agent to reduce its acidity and bitterness and to make it more palatable to consumers. Alkalising also turns cocoa a darker brown and increases its solubility. This is known as Dutched cocoa or Dutch process cocoa. Dutched cocoa is what's used in most chocolates, drink powders, ice creams and baking. Unfortunately, Dutching significantly lowers the antioxidant content of cocoa, thus removing a lot of its healthful properties.

'To summarise, people often use the term "cacao" in the early stages of processing the bean, and the word "cocoa" after the nib stage. What's important to understand is that **the more a cacao bean is processed, the more it loses any potential health benefits.'**

'What is it about cacao that makes it healthy — apart from providing a base ingredient for suppositories?' Melanie wasn't going to forget that piece of trivia in a hurry.

'Cacao beans contain compounds called flavonoids — especially a subgroup called **flavanols**[7] — that have antioxidant, anti-inflammatory, anti-cancer and brain-boosting properties in the laboratory, but whether this translates into health benefits for humans who consume chocolate has yet to be established. Moreover, many other plant foods also contain flavonoids so it isn't as if cacao is the only source, much as it is one of the richest sources.

'Flavanols in cacao also increase the formation of nitric oxide in the lining (endothelium), of blood vessel walls. This promotes blood vessel relaxation (vasodilation), which lowers blood pressure. However, trials in which people were given flavanol-rich cocoa products only resulted in very small reductions in blood pressure (both systolic and diastolic) — 2 to 4 mm Hg. Other studies investigating a link between cocoa and heart disease have yielded inconsistent conclusions.'

---

[7] See Appendix 5 'What are phytochemicals?' to learn more about flavonoids and flavanols.

'Why do you think the results of human trials have been so underwhelming?'

'For a start, I believe that none of the studies lasted long enough. Remember that the Kuna drink massive amounts of cocoa for their entire lives. Meanwhile, some of the trials on cocoa supplementation lasted only a few weeks. It's a ridiculously short amount of time to expect to see an impact. The response to cocoa is likely to be gradual and cumulative. Other research simply involved people completing questionnaires about what they ate and drank to see if high cocoa- or chocolate-consumers had less heart disease. Not only do we know nothing about the flavanol content of their cocoa products, information collected in this way is highly unreliable because few people accurately recall how much they eat and drink.'

'I guess that means headlines about dark chocolate being a superfood for the brain are hyperbolic clickbait?'

'Yes — with a cacao seed of truth in them. A few trials have suggested that cocoa flavanols *might* be neuroprotective, *might* increase blood flow to the hippocampus and *might* improve certain aspects of brain function. One particularly abundant flavanol in cacao called **(-)-epicatechin** (pronounced "minus epicatechin") supports the growth of brain cells and blood vessels. When pure (-)-epicatechin was fed to snails, mice and rats, it improved their memory and preserved their cognitive abilities as they aged.

'Cocoa flavanols do a great job when it comes to animals that are studied in a controlled environment. However, when humans eat or drink chocolate, the concentration of flavanols is greatly reduced by fermenting, roasting and alkalising (Dutching). Different genetic strains of cacao also contain different amounts of flavanols so it's difficult to know how much (-)-epicatechin we're consuming.'

'Do we know how much (-)-epicatechin is in the cocoa used by Kuna islanders?'

'Great question, Melanie, yes we do. Kuna use both home-grown and Columbian cocoa powder that is high in a number of flavanols including (-)-epicatechin. It's estimated they consume about 1880 mg of flavanols per day. In contrast, the commercial cocoa powder used by the mainlanders is flavanol-poor.'

'I thought the darker the chocolate, the better for my health. I've deliberately weaned myself off white and milk chocolate and only eat dark chocolate with at least 70% cocoa solids.' Melanie was looking at me expectantly.

'All other things being equal, the higher the percentage of cocoa solids, the more flavanols your chocolate is likely to contain. But all other things are not equal. The variety of bean, soil, growing conditions and degree of processing all influence flavanol content. "Raw" cocoa is better than roasted, and natural (non-alkalised) is better than Dutched. One study also found that chocolate made with maltilol (a low calorie sweetener[8]) instead of sugar resulted in lower blood levels of (-)-epicatechin. This suggests that whatever else is in chocolate can interact with flavanols and further modify their effect.'

'What contains more flavanols: cocoa or dark chocolate?'

'Definitely cocoa. Even though the flavanol content can vary dramatically between brands, there are probably 20 times more flavanols per gram of natural cocoa powder than per gram of 60% dark chocolate. Milk chocolate has even less flavanols and white chocolate has none.

'A higher percentage of cocoa also equates to higher amounts of fibre, protein, tryptophan and minerals, including iron, magnesium, manganese, potassium, phosphorus, zinc, selenium and chromium — all of which are salutary.'

'What does tryptophan do?' asked Melanie.

'Tryptophan is used in the production of serotonin, melatonin and vitamin B3 — hence chocolate's reputation as a mood-booster.'

'Why is chocolate poisonous to dogs and cats?' she queried.

'Cacao contains two stimulants called methylxanthines: theobromine and caffeine, which many animals are unable to metabolise or do so very slowly. This leads to theobromine building up to toxic levels

---

[8] See Chapter 71 'You can't fool your brain'.

and causing vomiting, diarrhoea, increased heart rate and eventually heart failure, seizures and coma. Caffeine is also a problem for dogs but there is much less of it in chocolate than theobromine.

'As for humans, the big negatives to watch out for in chocolate are large amounts of sugar, artificial sweeteners, flavourings, emulsifiers and other additives that would undo the benefits of flavanols. Even dark chocolate can contain a lot of sugar and empty calories.

'Don't get me wrong. I enjoy chocolate as much as anyone and would love to find research that proves it's a boon to health. However, the brain and heart benefits appear to come from long-term consumption of "raw" (minimally roasted), natural (not Dutched or alkalised) cocoa powder so I try to use it the way Kuna islanders do:

- add it to warm (not boiling) milk or water because boiling will lower the flavanol content
- add it to a cool green smoothie
- sprinkle it over a bowl of berries
- use it in home-made chocolate or ice cream[9]
- sprinkle it over stir-fried or roasted carrots, mushrooms, beetroot or pumpkin after they've been cooked to preserve the flavanol content — experiment with different vegetables
- I've even stirred cocoa through bolognese sauce at the end of cooking
- if I use it as a seasoning for meat or chicken, I know the flavanol content will be reduced during baking, roasting and barbecuing
- likewise, if you combine cocoa with baking soda (which increases the pH) some of the flavanols will be lost.

'How do you know if the cocoa you're buying is "raw" and non-alkalised?'

'The packaging will usually state that the cocoa is "raw" but as for alkalising or Dutching, I've rarely seen it mentioned either way. If the label says "natural" it *should* mean non-alkalised but some cocoa producers are very lax in their use of the term "natural". I suggest you contact various cocoa companies and ask them if their cocoa is alkalised or Dutch processed.'

'Do you ever buy commercial chocolate?'

---

[9] If you would like the recipe for my home-made ice cream, chocolate or chocolate chicken drumsticks, visit outwittingalzheimers.com/recipes.

'Yes. The healthiest chocolate option is "raw" cacao nibs but they take a bit of getting used to. If I buy regular chocolate I make sure it's at least 70% dark and the only ingredients are cocoa mass, cocoa butter, cocoa powder and a trace of sugar (if any sugar at all). I've emailed my favourite chocolate makers to ask which of their chocolates are made with non-alkalised cocoa. These are the chocolates I buy. If you're going to eat chocolate, choose the best quality, fair-trade, highest cocoa percentage, lowest sugar and least processed you can afford, and really savour it!'

CHAPTER 54

Spice things up

If you have a garden and a library, you have everything you need.

Marcus Tullius Cicero (106–43 BCE)

Turmeric is a flowering plant that belongs to the ginger family. Its official name is *Curcuma longa.* The root (rhizome) of the turmeric plant has been used for at least 2500 years in India and South-East Asia as a dye, cosmetic, spice and medicine. Inside the root is a yellow-orange pulp that is boiled, dried and ground into a powder. It is responsible for the characteristic yellow colour of curry and the robes of monks and priests.

Today it is used in hundreds of food products (because of its colour, flavour and therapeutic potential) including hot and cold beverages (turmeric latte, anyone?), cakes, ice cream, biscuits, popcorn, cereals, sauces and frozen meals. As a food colouring, turmeric is assigned the code E100. The root can also be pickled or used fresh, like ginger.

Turmeric contains compounds called curcuminoids, a subgroup of flavonoids. (See Appendix 6 'What are phytochemicals?') The most widely researched curcuminoid is curcumin, which is believed to be responsible for most of turmeric's medicinal properties. Hence curcumin has been extracted and concentrated in many different supplement formulations. Thousands of scientific papers have demonstrated that curcumin can have anti-inflammatory, antioxidant, anti-tumour, analgesic, heart-protective and carminative (preventing flatulence) effects. It has been used to treat arthritis, depression, anxiety, digestive problems, skin infections, type 2 diabetes, obesity, traumatic brain injury, haemorrhoids and … just about anything — with varying degrees of success.

In relation to brain health, curcumin has been found to counteract many of the processes that contribute to Alzheimer's. In other words, curcumin exerts neuroprotective effects. These include:

1. reduced brain inflammation
2. neutralisation of free radicals (antioxidant effect)
3. enhanced mitochondrial function
4. preservation of synapses (connections between brain cells)
5. clearance of amyloid β (Aβ) plaques
6. prevention of tau tangle formation
7. increased levels of brain-derived neurotrophic factor (BDNF) which promotes the growth and survival of brain cells
8. lowered blood glucose levels and improved insulin sensitivity in type 2 diabetes.

Studies in mice, worms, flies and yeasts show that curcumin increases lifespan and promotes healthy ageing. In rats that suffered a stroke, intravenous infusion of curcumin led to less brain damage and greater survival than was seen in rats not treated with curcumin. Other studies found that curcumin reduced brain impairment in rats exposed to lead poisoning, and improved attention, memory and learning in mice engineered to have Alzheimer's. Curcumin even improved co-ordination and touch sense in worms afflicted with abnormal tau proteins.

A very impressive curriculum vitae. But does it translate to better cognition in humans?

An 18-month trial of a daily curcumin supplement called Theracumin (more on this particular supplement shortly) found that healthy adults taking Theracumin had greater memory and focus, more positive mood, lower anxiety and less Aβ and tau accumulation (seen on PET scans) than the control group receiving placebo pills. Participants in the study were aged between 51 and 84 with no signs of Alzheimer's. Other trials of curcumin in people with and without Alzheimer's have yielded mixed results — some showed brain-benefits while others saw no significant effects. It may be that the unsuccessful studies did not last long enough or used a form of curcumin that was poorly absorbed. In essence, more studies are needed before we can draw definitive conclusions about curcumin's potential in preventing and even treating Alzheimer's.

Unfortunately, Dad and I didn't have time to wait for more trial results. Should we jump the gun and start popping pickled turmeric and curcumin capsules?

To help me come to a decision, I delved into the fine print. Curcumin constitutes only 2 to 3% of turmeric powder and less than half a per cent of curry powder, so we'd need to eat a LOT of turmeric and curry to ingest meaningful amounts of curcumin. Living in India and eating like the locals over the course of a lifetime may conceivably result in sufficient consumption of curcumin to have positive impacts on our health. The prevalence of late-onset Alzheimer's in India is about a quarter the number seen in the US and other developed nations, but whether curcumin can take credit for this is still a matter of speculation. Moving to India was not an option so I turned my attention to concentrated curcumin supplements.

The bad news is that when we consume pure curcumin, it is poorly absorbed from our gut and most of it ends up in the toilet. In medical speak, it has 'low bioavailability'. There are several ways to enhance our absorption of curcumin:

1. Consume curcumin with a compound in black pepper called piperine. This can increase the absorption of curcumin by 20-fold. Hence many curcumin supplements contain piperine. If you use turmeric in cooking, liberally add pepper.
2. Consume curcumin with a meal that contains generous amounts of healthy fats or oils because curcumin dissolves in fat. Think ghee in traditional Indian cooking. Curcumin is better absorbed when consumed as turmeric than when swallowed as a purified supplement because turmeric contains natural oils and other non-curcuminoid components that enhance curcumin's bioavailability. The problem, as already stated, is that Western cooking doesn't use enough turmeric to provide our brain with sufficient curcumin.
3. Choose a curcumin supplement that has been specifically formulated to increase its bioavailability. Three examples are:
   (a) Theracumin (ultra-fine nanoparticles)

(b) Longvida Optimized Curcumin (Solid Lipid Curcumin Particle SLCP formulation)

(c) BCM-95CG (Biocurcumax).

Other scientists have tried to rectify the problem using rectal formulations (I couldn't resist that pun) however these have not taken off.

Do curcumin supplements cause any side effects? Very rarely, and usually only in very high doses, curcumin can produce stomach upset, nausea, dizziness, diarrhoea, headache, skin rashes or liver damage. Curcumin may also affect the metabolism of specific medications but this did not include anything that Dad was taking. Plus, it has stood the test of time in Asian countries. What did we have to lose?

The chemical properties of curcumin, its success in animal studies, and the encouraging trials in humans made it a no-brainer to try. Turmeric and pepper became staples of my culinary repertoire — I added them to almost everything: soups, dips, sauces, stews, steamed and stir-fried vegetables, meat marinades and even our chocolate chicken drumsticks. Dad, Felix and I also began taking a daily curcumin supplement. We chose Theracumin because it had solid research supporting its enhanced bioavailability and positive effects on mood and memory. None of us experienced any side effects and we have now been taking Theracumin for several years.

Did I notice improvements in Dad's cognition? Given that Dad's daily life included many different potentially brain-boosting foods and activities, it's impossible to tease out the relative contribution of each individual intervention. For the most part, Dad's symptoms remained remarkably stable, but whether this was due to luck, genetics, the way we were living our lives, or his particular disease characteristics, I will never know.

In the meantime, I continue to scour the research for more studies on the wide-ranging health benefits of curcumin and how to best consume it for maximal effect. Sign up to my free **Health-e-Bytes** at <u>outwittingalzheimers.com</u> to receive updates.

CHAPTER 55

Ketone crusade

That which we persist in doing becomes easier to do, not that the nature of the thing has changed but that our power to do has increased.

RALPH WALDO EMERSON (1803–1882)

So you've implemented all the dietary suggestions discussed so far in this book but perhaps your brain is still not working as well as it could. Or you're still struggling to overcome a chronic health condition or improve suboptimal blood test results. Or you've been diagnosed with Alzheimer's. If any of these scenarios are yours, you may need to implement one more dietary strategy: **neuro-keto-therapeutics (NKT)**, also known as **ketogenic therapies.** I've hyphenated NKT to indicate its origins. 'Neuro' refers to neuron or brain cell. 'Keto' is short for ketones. Ketones are water-soluble molecules produced in the liver when blood insulin levels are low and our body breaks down fat for energy. I touched on ketones in Chapter 50 'Fast to last'. 'Therapeutics' indicates that NKT is a treatment for a wide range of neurological disorders including (but not limited to) epilepsy, Alzheimer's, Parkinson's, migraines, head trauma, brain tumours and ADHD. NKT has also yielded excellent results in psychiatric conditions such as depression, anxiety, bipolar disorder and schizophrenia.[10]

NKT is based on the finding that **ketones are neuroprotective.** In other words, ketones reduce inflammation, oxidative stress and

---

[10] Visit diagnosisdiet.com by psychiatrist Dr Georgia Ede to learn how people with psychiatric conditions can reduce or eliminate the need for medications by changing how they eat.

amyloid β (Aβ) levels, enhance mitochondrial function, increase brain-derived neurotrophic factor (BDNF) and provide the brain with an alternative fuel source to glucose. Every one of these effects of ketones counteracts the destructive processes that occur in Alzheimer's.

If you've looked into brain nutrition, you may have come across a number of specific diets that have been studied in relation to staving off Alzheimer's. They include:

- the Mediterranean diet
- the DASH diet — an acronym for Dietary Approaches to Stop Hypertension
- the MIND diet — an acronym for Mediterranean-DASH Intervention for Neurodegenerative Delay. This combines aspects of the Mediterranean and DASH diets.
- the DIPLOMA diet — an acronym for Dietary Intervention to Prevent and sLOw Memory loss due to Alzheimer's. This is an individualised approach to food and supplements developed by Dr Richard Isaacson when he was at the Alzheimer's Prevention Clinic at Weill Cornell Medicine in New York. It combines aspects of the MIND and ketogenic diets. I'll explain the ketogenic diet shortly.

All four diets are essentially variations of the real food principles I've been discussing throughout this book and they've been shown to reduce the risk of Alzheimer's by up to 50%. However, they are not potent enough if a person already has signs of cognitive decline. This is where NKT is in a league of its own.

You'll recall from previous chapters that people with subjective cognitive impairment (SCI), mild cognitive impairment (MCI) and Alzheimer's often suffer from **brain glucose hypo-metabolism**, i.e. their brain has a reduced ability to use glucose for fuel. This is known as a **bioenergetic defect** and there are several contributing factors. The most widely studied include the following:

- Alterations in the blood-brain barrier (BBB) prevent glucose from crossing into the brain from the blood.
- Mitochondrial dysfunction. Mitochondria are the site of energy production inside the cell.

- Blood flow to the brain is compromised and therefore not enough glucose reaches the brain in the first place.

These changes lead to brain cell starvation, diminished functioning and ultimately brain cell death. Fortunately, **the brain is able to use ketones instead of glucose for fuel** and thereby restore its energy deficit. Why is it that ketones can get inside brain cells when glucose can't? Ketones do not cross the BBB in the same way as glucose and they improve brain blood flow and mitochondrial function, thus circumventing the problems associated with glucose.

Ketogenic therapies include a number of different dietary and lifestyle strategies (not drugs) that stimulate the liver to produce ketones. The production of ketones is termed **ketogenesis** and, when a person has measurable levels of ketones in their blood (>0.5 mmol/L or millimolar mM), they are said to be in a state of **ketosis.**

Ketogenesis can be achieved through:
- intermittent fasting (see Chapter 50 'Fast to last')
- strenuous exercise that uses up the body's stores of glucose
- restricting carbohydrates — known as a ketogenic diet (KD)
- ingesting what are known as medium chain triglycerides (MCTs)
- a combination of the above methods.

Intermittent fasting and strenuous exercise help a person reach ketosis but they are not stand-alone methods for remaining in ketosis. They need to be combined with carbohydrate restriction.

The three ketones produced in our body are:
1. acetoacetate (AcAc)
2. acetone
3. beta-hydroxybutyrate (BHB) = the primary ketone circulating in our blood.

On a semantic note, ketones produced by our body are called **ketone bodies** or **endogenous ketones,** while ketones produced in a laboratory are referred to as **exogenous ketones.**

Unfortunately, because doctors are not taught about ketogenic diets (more about why this is the case later), they frequently confuse ketosis with ketoacidosis. These are two very different bodily states.

Ketosis is a normal response to low blood glucose levels resulting in blood ketone levels of 0.5 to 5 mM. In contrast, ketoacidosis is a potentially fatal medical emergency that can occur in type 1 diabetes if there is a total lack of insulin. This leads to uncontrolled ketone production and blood levels of over 10 mM. I mention ketoacidosis in case your doctor becomes apprehensive when you mention going on a ketogenic diet. You can reassure them that a ketogenic diet (KD) does not lead to ketoacidosis.

Ketogenic therapies are not a new idea. Using fasting to treat epilepsy was recorded in ancient Greek texts including *The Hippocratic Corpus* as early as 500 BCE. It was also mentioned in the New Testament of the Bible half a century later. In the 1920s, doctors discovered that, like fasting, a low carb/high fat diet could stimulate ketone body production and thus the ketogenic diet (KD) became widely used to treat epilepsy throughout the 1920s and 30s. Despite its success, the KD was phased out in the 1980s when anti-seizure medications took over. Doctors were taught that drugs were an easier option than asking patients to adhere to a restrictive diet. The KD nonetheless remains an effective therapy for children and adults whose epilepsy cannot be controlled by drugs or surgery. Sadly, many doctors neglect to tell patients that dietary management of epilepsy is an option. I can only speculate as to the reasons. Lack of education and lack of time are probably the main barriers. Doctors are not taught to prescribe food or exercise as medicine. Doctors are only taught to prescribe drugs, surgery or radiation. Hippocrates, regarded as the father of Western medicine, taught that healing arose from 'the art of true living and the art of fine medicine combined'. Unfortunately, medical schools have forgotten to convey half of the equation — the art of true living.

Happily, the KD is making a comeback because something that is so effective for so many conditions cannot remain submerged. In 1993, 11-month-old Charlie Abrahams developed intractable epilepsy. He had multiple daily seizures despite brain surgery and medications. Charlie's parents eventually learned about the KD and within one month he was free of his seizures and his medications. He remained on the diet for five years and now eats whatever he wants. He has not had another seizure and currently works as a pre-school teacher. A made-for-TV movie called *First Do No Harm* starring Meryl Streep tells their story.

In 1994, **The Charlie Foundation for Ketogenic Therapies** (visit charliefoundation.org) was founded by Charlie's parents to provide information about diet therapies for people with epilepsy, other neurological disorders such as Alzheimer's, and certain cancers. It details five variations of the KD and explains which diet is best for which situation. It also provides hundreds of free recipes and a list of US health professionals and hospitals that have expertise in ketogenic therapies.

The foundations of a ketogenic diet are:
- very low intake of carbohydrates
- adequate intake of protein based on a person's age, muscle mass, exercise level and individual needs
- high intake of healthy fats.

The KD is NOT a diet that requires calorie restriction. You can enjoy eating to satiety.

Many people (including doctors who have little experience with a ketogenic diet) panic at the thought of a high fat diet. As long as the fats you consume are not trans fats, margarines or vegetable (seed) oils AND you are eating them in the context of minimal carbohydrates, a high fat diet is not unhealthy. On the contrary, you will find that cravings disappear, your appetite self-regulates and you'll restore the health of your brain and body.

If you're keen to dive straight into a ketogenic diet, I recommend any of the excellent programs offered on the following websites. Most of them are free and you will find more than enough information and delicious recipes to keep you on track for the rest of your life. However, if you want further support, you can sign up to one of their paid plans or work directly with an experienced keto practitioner. If you've adopted the way of eating I've been recommending throughout this book, you will already be on your way to transitioning to a ketogenic diet.

Keto Resources

Website	Founder and country of origin	Comment
charliefoundation.org	Jim and Nancy Abrahams (Charlie's parents) — USA	Watch the 10-minute **Keto Crash Course video** and try their amazing FREE recipes.
metabolicneurologist.com	Dr Matthew C L Phi lips MBBS — New Zealand	Download the FREE **Metabolic Strategy Plan** in the Resources section of the website.
tuitnutrition.com	Amy Berger MA (Human Nutrition), CNS (Certified Nutrition Specialist) — USA	Amy is one of the most empathic and keto-knowledgeable practitioners I have come across. She works with clients all over the world. Her brilliant book **The Alzheimer's Antidote** — Using a Low Carb, High Fat Diet to Fight Alzheimer's Disease, Memory Loss, and Cognitive Decline is a must-read.
adaptyourlifeacademy.com	Dr Eric Westman MD — USA	Download the FREE user-friendly e-book **10 Tips for Starting Keto Right**.
dietdoctor.com	Dr Andreas Eenfeldt MD — Sweden (the website language is English)	The Diet Doctor offers **30 days of FREE access to personalised meal plans,** 1200+ recipes, smart shopping lists, progress reports and educational videos. Listen to the **Diet Doctor Podcast with Dr Bret Scher** MD to stay up-to-date with the latest keto research.
ketodietapp.com	Martina Slajerova (creator of the KetoDiet app, blog and 10 cookbooks) — UK	Download the FREE **KetoDiet app** and FREE **Keto Diet Plans**. As with dietdoctor.com this is an information-packed website full of practical resources, articles and recipes. I love her **New Mediterranean Diet Cookbook**.
fabulouslyketo.com	Jackie Fletcher (nutrition adviser) — UK — and Louise Reynolds PhD (paramedic) — an Australian currently based in Thailand	The **Fabulously Keto Podcast** provides a great primer on keto for those with little or no background in science.

Website	Founder and country of origin	Comment
defeatdiabetes.com.au	Dr Peter Bruckner MBBS, OAM – Australia	Dr Bruckner offers a FREE 14-day trial of his program. Although his focus is on reversing diabetes, the same principles apply to reversing cognitive decline. He also provides a directory of low-carb-health professionals in Australia.
ketocookingwins.com	Jennifer Allen aka Chef Jen (retired chef, recipe developer and cookbook author) – North America	Jen began her career in the USA and currently works in Canada. Delicious recipes!
virtahealth.com	Dr Stephen Phinney MD, Dr Jeff Volek MD and Sami Inkinen – USA	Virta was founded in 2014 with the goal of reversing type 2 diabetes in 100 million people by 2025. This will go a long way to reducing the number of people who develop Alzheimer's.

Other sources of information about ketogenic therapies include the following:

Website	Founder and country of origin	Comment
ketonutrition.org	Dr Dominic D'Agostino BS, PhD – USA	This is the most academic of all the websites. I include it for those who want to dive deeper into all things keto.
lowcarbmd.com	Dr Brian Lenzkes MD, Dr Tro Kalayjian MD, Dr Jason Fung MD and Megan Ramos – USA	Low Carb MD is a great podcast aimed at educating people how to use low carb and keto diets to reverse a range of chronic diseases.

I have not listed the websites in any particular order and they are not an exhaustive catalogue of keto resources. Different people resonate with different styles and approaches. Enjoy exploring the approach that works best for you. I have incredible respect for everyone mentioned.

In 2018, a study called The Ketogenic Diet Retention and Feasibility Trial (KDRAFT) published in the journal *Alzheimer's and Dementia* showed that a **ketogenic diet enhanced cognition over a three-month period in people with mild Alzheimer's**. One month after stopping the diet, the improvements disappeared. Another 12-week study published in 2019 in the *Journal of Alzheimer's Disease* also found **significant memory improvements** in participants on a KD. To date, the most robust trial of a KD in Alzheimer's was conducted by Dr Matthew Phillips in 2020 (see metabolicneurologist.com in the previous table) who found that **a KD substantially improved daily functioning and quality of life** in a hospital clinic of Alzheimer's patients. His free downloadable *Metabolic Strategy Plan* allows you to conduct this trial for yourself. It has all the instructions and recipes you need.

When starting a keto diet, some people experience what is referred to as keto flu. Symptoms can include headaches, fatigue, irritability, dizziness, nausea, constipation or difficulty concentrating. It occurs while the body adapts to using ketones rather than glucose for fuel. Keto flu is most common on days three to five but may last up to two weeks. Thereafter you'll have more energy and feel better than you did prior to the diet. Keto flu can be mitigated by ensuring adequate hydration and salt intake. Add salt to taste and drink at least 2.5 L of water per day. Many people find that keto flu symptoms can be nipped in the bud by drinking a glass of water with half a teaspoon of dissolved salt.

One more fascinating chapter in the keto chronicle involves neonatologist Dr Mary T Newport (a doctor who treats newborns) whose husband Steve was diagnosed with early onset Alzheimer's in 2004 at the age of 54. By 2006, Steve (a former accountant) could no longer drive, turn on a computer or use a calculator. In 2008, Dr Newport wanted to enrol Steve in clinical trials of emerging

Alzheimer's drugs. While reading about the risks and benefits of participating in the trials, she came across a study that demonstrated **positive effects of medium chain triglyceride (MCT) oil on memory, cognition and verbal fluency in people with Alzheimer's.** MCT oil constitutes 50% to 60% of the fat in coconut oil, so the following day she bought coconut oil and gave her husband two tablespoons with his breakfast. The previous day he had scored 14 out of 30 in the Mini Mental State Exam (MMSE) and failed to qualify for the trial. A few hours after consuming coconut oil, he was tested again and scored 18 out of 30. This is a notable improvement but Dr Newport didn't know whether it was luck or coconut oil that produced the upswing. She continued giving him coconut oil with every meal and over the next few weeks his memory, energy levels, capacity to converse and overall functioning improved dramatically. Two months later, his MMSE score had jumped to 20 and after nine months he was able to read again. Throughout the next few years, Steve's functioning improved to the point where he was able to do volunteer work. Dr Newport has detailed their story in her book *Alzheimer's Disease: What if there was a cure? The story of ketones.* Since the publication of her book, numerous studies have validated Steve's experience and documented significant cognitive improvements in Alzheimer's patients taking MCT or coconut oil. What is so special about these oils? How do they exert such a striking effect on the brain?

MCTs are composed of saturated fatty acids (SFAs) that are six to 10 carbon atoms long. This makes them shorter than other dietary FAs and gives them unique physical properties. After consumption, MCTs are rapidly absorbed and transported to the liver where they are converted into ketone bodies — the same KBs that are produced when a person is on a ketogenic diet. Therefore MCTs are a way of inducing ketogenesis and providing a starving brain with useable fuel without following a strict ketogenic diet. MCTs also appear to exert direct salutary effects on the brain. The two most abundant and potent FAs in MCTs are caprylic (C8) and capric (C10).

MCT oil extracted from coconut or palm kernel oil is inexpensive and can be purchased from most chemists and health food stores, so why isn't everyone with SCI, MCI and Alzheimer's advised to dose up on it? First and foremost, most doctors — including neurologists and geriatricians specialising in Alzheimer's — are not aware of the research on MCTs. Why? If there is no pharmaceutical company pushing for a drug to come to public attention, it takes several decades for academic research to translate into medical practice. Secondly, most doctors still have an outdated fear that saturated fats cause heart attacks. Thirdly, individual responses to MCTs differ widely and not everyone responds as favourably as Steve Newport. Fourthly, in some people, MCTs can cause gastrointestinal side effects such as bloating, stomach cramps, diarrhoea, nausea or flatulence. The abdominal effects can be ameliorated by 'starting low and going slow'. Try just one teaspoon a day and gradually increase the dose over a period of months to three to six tablespoons per day. Consuming MCTs with food like smoothies, salads, vegetables, eggs, meat or slightly cooled coffee can also mitigate the side effects. Do NOT use MCT oil to cook with; add it when you have served the food on your plate. A small dose of MCTs is better than no dose at all. There have even been anecdotal reports that massaging a person with coconut oil can produce improvements in cognition.

MCTs work better when combined with a low carb or ketogenic diet. However, dietary changes can be challenging for a person with Alzheimer's and burdensome for their care-partner. Do the best you can to reduce sugar and other carbs as much as feasible. Carb reduction can also be a gradual process.

On account of the multiple therapeutic benefits of ketones, scientists have started making edible products known as **exogenous ketones** (e.g. ketone salts and ketone esters) that increase blood ketone levels without the need to adhere to a strict KD. At present, these supplements are largely marketed as weight loss aids or athletic performance enhancers but their effectiveness is context- and person-dependent. Research on exogenous ketones is accelerating faster than I'm able to type and there's a great deal still to learn about them. However, they are showing promise in traumatic brain injury, psychiatric disorders and neurodegenerative diseases. Whilst a KD is inherently therapeutic above and beyond the presence of blood ketones, exogenous ketones may become a viable alternative for people with Alzheimer's who are not able to tolerate or comply with a KD. I eagerly await the results of further research.

Given the ever-growing evidence for the efficacy of NKT, it is wrong to say there is no treatment for Alzheimer's. Even though there is no guarantee of a complete cure, there are definitely strategies that can ameliorate symptoms and slow down decline. Our medical system is based on drug therapies, but drugs are not the only way to treat diseases. Food, fasting and physical exercise are potent therapies for many diseases but they are downplayed — and even disregarded — because they are not packaged in a pill. Ignoring the importance of lifestyle interventions is a limiting approach and denies patients the opportunity to take responsibility for their own health and healing. Ketogenic therapies (fasting, physical exercise, low carb diets and MCT oil) are effective for a wide range of diseases that are deemed 'incurable' by Western medicine. While we don't have all the answers, there is a deluge of published scientific data that supports the use — or at least trial — of a KD in Alzheimer's. To my mind, not offering dietary strategies to people with a metabolic disorder (i.e. any disease linked to insulin resistance) is negligent. As I've highlighted earlier in this book, we mustn't let what we *don't* know stop us from implementing what we *do* know. I take inspiration from the words of Swami Vivekananda (1863–1902): 'The history of the world is the history of a few people who had faith in themselves'.

PART SIX

Dementia is a doorway

You can't run away from trouble. Ain't no place that far.

Uncle Remus

Uncle Remus is a fictional character in a collection of African-American folktales compiled by Joel Chandler Harris (1848–1908).

CHAPTER 56

In search of silence

The quieter you are, the more you are able to hear.

RUMI (1207–1273)

California, summer 2015

Dad and I were attending a weeklong meditation retreat in Monterey. Immortalised in John Steinbeck's novel *Cannery Row*, the town promised stunning coastal walks, elephant seals basking on the beach and pelicans perched on rocky cliffs. I was ready to be rejuvenated by nature and nurture.

Guided meditations and talks on mindfulness took place in an auditorium referred to as The Sanctuary. Upon entry, everyone (other than the presenter) had to abide by a code of silence. Dad forgot the code of silence the minute we were inside, so I had to come up with a speedy solution. During the mindful walking exercise, I mindfully foraged for sticks to which I later attached pieces of paper (like signposts) that I would hold up in front of Dad's face whenever he began talking while we were in The Sanctuary.

I had three signs written in Serbian that pre-empted what I might need to say:
Sign one: *No*
Sign two: *Please be quiet*
Sign three: *Please keep still*

It worked a treat — until Dad looked up from the sudoku puzzle he'd been engrossed in during the lecture. The speaker had just closed his eyes in preparation for meditation. The serene, sun-kissed girl sitting next to Dad adjusted her posture. Before I could intercept with a sign, Dad leaned over to her and announced in a booming voice that resonated through the entire auditorium, 'Ha ha, he's so boring he's put himself to sleep!'

Five hundred pairs of eyes shot open and zeroed in on us.

The girl looked as if she'd been woken from a trance. I pretended I was deep in meditation and hadn't heard a thing. Only the speaker remained unmoved and purposefully struck his Tibetan chime. 'Stay in the present moment and focus on your breathing. Allow any extraneous sounds to wash over you like waves across the ocean.'

As we were leaving, one of the organisers pulled me aside. 'Can I have a word with you please?'

Several words later, I was fervently promising there would not be any more 'inappropriate utterances' in The Sanctuary.

The following morning, we could not find Dad's lanyard and name tag. No one was allowed into The Sanctuary without a name tag. Having achieved notoriety the previous day, I assumed he'd be remembered and permitted entry without it. Just in case, I came up with another ingenious plan. I detached my name tag from my lanyard and safety-pinned it to my jumper. Then I slipped my lanyard around Dad's neck and tucked the other end inside his grey jacket so that no one could see that the name tag was missing. I gave Dad strict instructions to keep his jacket on at all times. This was not unreasonable as the weather was refreshingly cool. 'You look very dapper,' I beamed at him.

It worked a treat — until Dad decided to unbutton his jacket. Before I could intervene, the man ushering us to our seats (the same man who'd had words with us the previous day) noticed the missing name tag. 'Where's your identity tag?' he asked my father. Dad turned to me for inspiration.

'Lost,' I replied.

'Then why the subterfuge?'

'It was easier than having to go through the whole registration process again.'

'Can I have another word with you please?'

Several words later, he handed me a replacement name tag. Just then Dad walked over to us. 'Look, I found my sudoku book!' he announced delightedly. 'It had slipped between our chairs yesterday. Luckily the bookmark is still in place so I can continue where I left off.' He showed me the bookmark. It was, of course, his name tag.

Having managed to evade expulsion from the meditation retreat, Dad and I drove two and a half hours south to magnificent Hearst Castle. Perched on Enchanted Hill overlooking the Pacific Ocean, the palace boasted 130 sumptuous rooms crammed full of eclectic antiques, sculptures, paintings, tapestries and glassware procured from every corner of the globe. Mr Hearst had even bought an entire monastery so he could take it apart and use its architectural elements — as you would, if you owned one of the world's largest collections of ancient Greek vases.

I loved castles and Dad loved history. I immediately booked us on two back-to-back tours — one to explore The Grand Rooms and one to see The Upstairs Suites. In my excitement, I missed the fine print on the brochure that warned we would need to climb 100-plus steps for EACH tour. Dad was ready for a nap by step eight. But I digress.

All tours start with a scenic 15-minute bus ride up the winding cliff face. A recorded commentary explained points of interest throughout the striking countryside. My father, however, was fixated on the whereabouts of our luggage.

'Where did you leave our suitcases?'

'In the rental car.'

'Didn't the bus driver mind about all our suitcases?'

'The bus driver didn't have to deal with our suitcases. Our bags are in the car.'

'Will our suitcases be safe?'

'Yes.'

'How can you be sure?'

'The car is locked.'

'What if someone throws a rock through the car window? There are plenty of rocks around here.'

'San Simeon is a safe little town. It's very unlikely someone would break into our car.'

'Are our suitcases visible?'

'No.'

'If someone steals our suitcases what will we do?'

'No one will steal our suitcases.'

'Where are our suitcases?'

'In the rental car.'

'I can't believe you managed to fit all our suitcases in the car.'

'I can't believe you won't let up about the suitcases.'

Silence for one minute.

'Where did you leave our suitcases?' And so it went on — and on — up the snaking road.

On arrival, we were met by a bubbly smiling tour guide, Stacey. Neither the bubbles nor the smile would last to the end of the 60-minute tour. There were three rules:
Rule one: You MUST STAY on the blue carpet trail and NOT step on any of the Persian rugs or antique tiled floors.
Rule two: You MUST NOT sit on any of the chairs or sofas or lean against the furniture.
Rule three: You MUST NOT touch anything because it takes a troupe of museum curators to adjust the temperature, humidity and lighting in every room to ensure the items do not fade, decay, discolour or degrade.

I was starting to feel timorous.

Even after hearing the warnings, I was not prepared for the maelstrom that ensued. After the first set of stairs, Dad immediately sat down on the nearest chair. 'Oh no, please, sir!' Stacey nervously chirped.

I quickly grabbed his arm and pulled him up. 'But I'm an old man. I'm tired,' he pleaded. Stacey gave him a wan smile and looked at me imploringly.

'I'll look after him,' I reassured her optimistically.

My first tactic was distraction.

'Isn't this an intricate tapestry?' I admired.

'I've seen better tapestries at my mother's house in Belgrade.'

'Isn't this an impressive painting?' I tried again.

'I've seen better paintings in Paris.'

'Isn't this whole castle amazing?' I gasped with genuine awe.

'I've seen better castles in Germany.'

'Look through that window. Isn't that a beautiful beach down there?' I coaxed.

'I've seen better beaches in Sydney.'

'Good — because I'm going to drown you in one of them when we get back.'

So much for the patience I'd cultivated at the meditation retreat. How quickly forbearance goes by the wayside.

The next challenge was keeping him on the blue carpet trail. Every few minutes he would wander off to make a closer inspection of a Vatican-style wall or ornate display cabinet. 'Oh no, please, sir!!' Stacey's chirp became shriller. I tried to inconspicuously hold on to his shirt tails.

'Let go!'

'I need to hold on to you. I'm feeling dizzy.'

'Let go! You're embarrassing me.'

'Don't let me faint.'

'Let go!'

'I'm seriously giddy.'

'I'll sit down with you.'

'No! I'm feeling better now. But please stay within arm's reach.'

Just as I thought he was easing into submission, he leaned towards a delicate Turkish lamp. I grabbed his hand and squeezed it affectionately. 'Isn't this fun?' I whispered.

If I hadn't pre-booked the second tour and we weren't automatically transferred to the next bubbly smiling guide, I would have aborted The Upstairs Suites. Instead, the whole charade repeated itself for the duration of the second hour.

This was not Dad; it was the disease.

As we were boarding the bus to take us back down the hill, an equally cheerful and chirpy security guard greeted us. 'How wonderful that you brought your elderly father to marvel at our spectacular Mediterranean palace.'

'I don't know if your colleagues would share your sentiments,' I responded wearily.

I left him waving at us with a puzzled expression.

CHAPTER 57

Smoke alarm

If not now, when?

HILLEL THE ELDER (110 BCE – 10 CE)

Smoking just ONE cigarette a day increases a person's risk **of having a heart attack or stroke.** Anything that increases cardiovascular disease also increases brain disease. Recognising that what's bad for our heart is also bad for our brain — and reciprocally, what's good for our heart is good for our brain — allows a number of puzzle pieces to fall into place.

Researchers from University College London analysed 141 studies that investigated the differential risks of smoking one, five or 20 cigarettes a day. Smoking one cigarette was associated with a 48% increase in coronary heart disease in men and a 57% increase in women. The risk of a stroke was increased by 30% in both sexes. Given that **one-third of people who have a stroke go on to develop Alzheimer's or vascular dementia**, this does not bode well for smokers.

Smoking *more* than one cigarette a day increases the risk further, but the message is that NO level of cigarette smoking is safe. Cutting down is obviously a positive step, but the goal is to give up altogether. Other benefits of being a non-smoker include a much lower risk of emphysema and a reduced risk of almost all cancers: lung, bladder, cervix, colon, rectum, oesophagus, liver, kidney, pancreas, stomach, larynx, pharynx and breast. Smoking also contributes to erectile dysfunction and decreases fertility in both men and women.

In addition to causing dementia through vascular disease, **smoking**

causes direct injury to the brain. A study comparing cerebrospinal fluid (CSF) obtained by lumbar puncture from smokers and non-smokers, found that smokers had:

- abnormal ratios of Aβ42 and Aβ40 (two subtypes of amyloid β proteins)
- higher levels of damaging proteins such as tumour necrosis factor alpha (TNFa)
- lower levels of protective factors such as brain-derived neurotrophic factor (BDNF), superoxide dismutase (SOD) and nitric oxide synthetase (NOS).

Smoking has also been shown to activate microglia and precipitate brain inflammation. If that isn't enough, smoking disrupts the blood–brain barrier (BBB) thereby making it easier for toxins from other sources to enter the brain and cause further damage. I include this level of detail to demonstrate the precision with which scientists can measure the neurological impacts of smoking. The bottom line is that **heavy smoking** — defined as more than **20 cigarettes a day for over 20 years — doubles the risk of Alzheimer's. However, brain damage begins within one year of smoking 10 cigarettes a day.** The damage is unsurprisingly dose-dependent.

Dad had been a smoker for 40 years until he finally gave up in his mid-60s. He smoked between five and 10 cigarettes a day.

'When I was living in Serbia, in the prime of my life,' he used to explain to Mum and me, 'it was impossible to socialise if you didn't drink or smoke — preferably both. Plus no one knew back then that smoking was harmful. Even doctors were advertising their favourite cigarettes. I was born with an inability to produce the liver enzyme that metabolises alcohol so I can't drink — as little as one sip makes me want to throw up. I had no choice but to light up a cigarette whenever I was in company. It would have been unsociable to do otherwise.'

'That's not the case anymore,' Mum (also a doctor) kept pointing out. 'In fact, smoking is now viewed as *anti*-social.'

'If you've been smoking for as long as I have, is there any point in giving up? Hasn't the damage already been done?' Dad looked beseechingly from Mum to me.

'Yes, there's been damage but it's not irreversible,' we both pronounced compassionately.

'If you give up, half an hour after your last cigarette, your heart rate and blood pressure will drop to a healthier level, and your lungs will be more effective at fighting off infections,' I continued. 'After 12 hours your brain is already getting more oxygen because of decreased levels of carbon monoxide in your blood, and after 24 hours you're substantially less likely to have a heart attack because your blood vessels are more relaxed.' I paused to make certain he was taking in the good news. 'After three days of not smoking, people report that their senses are sharper. Food becomes more fragrant and flavourful.'

'That depends on who's doing the cooking,' he interrupted roguishly.

I carried on undeterred. 'You'll also breathe more easily.'

'That depends on who's in the room with me.' He couldn't resist poking fun at Mum at every opportunity. After she passed away, I took her place as the target of his comic relief. It was his way of expressing endearment.

'How long until I'm completely cured of the effects of smoking?'

'After one year of not smoking you'll slash your risk of heart disease to half of what it was while you were smoking. About 15 years after quitting, you are no more likely to have a heart attack or stroke than someone who has never smoked. And after 20 years, your risk of dying from cancer or other smoking-related illnesses is also pretty much the same as that of someone who has never smoked. Your brain is possibly the only organ that might carry some residual loss of cognitive reserve. I don't know if your blood-brain barrier can fully recover after cigarettes have taken a machine gun to it.'

'Twenty years is a long time. I might have died of something else by then.'

'Or you might be fitter and healthier than ever before. **With each passing year of not smoking, your risk of smoking-related diseases decreases.** It isn't as if you have to wait 15 years to see a benefit. The benefits start immediately and continue to accumulate year after year.'

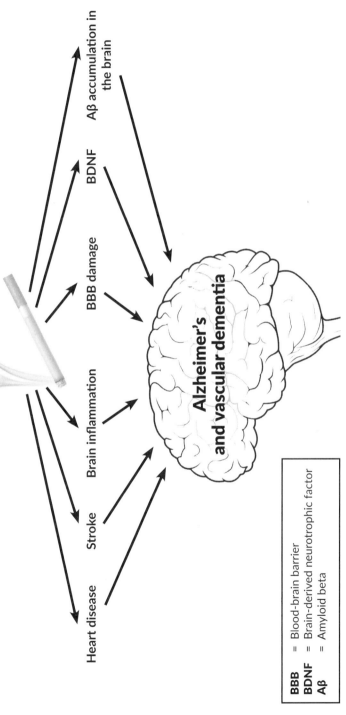

How does tobacco smoking lead to Alzheimer's and vascular dementia?

Heart disease

Stroke

Brain inflammation

BBB damage

BDNF

Aβ accumulation in the brain

Alzheimer's and vascular dementia

BBB = Blood-brain barrier
BDNF = Brain-derived neurotrophic factor
Aβ = Amyloid beta

What about electronic (e-)cigarettes?

E-cigarettes are battery-operated devices that heat a liquid solution to produce an aerosol for the user to inhale. The solution is called e-liquid and the aerosol is referred to as vapour. Hence, using e-cigarettes is known as vaping. E-cigarettes can look like cigarettes, cigars, pens or memory sticks. E-liquids consist of a glycerol (vegetable glycerin) and propylene glycol base, mixed with one or more of 15 000 available flavours and a host of unknown chemicals and contaminants such as pesticides, weed killers (acrolein), cleaning agents and heavy metals. E-cigarettes differ from traditional cigarettes in that they don't contain tobacco. Some e-liquids contain nicotine while others are nicotine-free. As of October 2021, the Australian government ruled that e-cigarettes containing nicotine were illegal without a doctor's prescription.

E-cigarettes have been available since 2004 and are rapidly increasing in popularity throughout the world due to the perception that they are safer than smoking tobacco. China currently has the highest number of e-cigarette users, followed by the USA and Europe. Unfortunately, **e-cigarettes are NOT harmless and the more we learn about them, the more dangers we uncover**.

In January 2022, in the *Medical Journal of Australia* (MJA), researchers from Perth's Curtin University in Western Australia assessed the chemical composition of 65 e-liquids sold in Australia. What they discovered shocked them.

E-cigarettes are also known as:
- vapes
- vape pens
- personal vaporisers
- electronic nicotine delivery systems (ENDS) — if they contain nicotine
- electronic non-nicotine delivery systems (ENNDS) — if they do not contain nicotine
- alternative nicotine delivery systems (ANDS) — if they contain nicotine
- e-hookahs.

All e-liquids contained lung irritants such as benzaldehyde[1] (added to vapes to give them an almond flavour) along with a cocktail of carcinogens including menthol, trans-cinnamaldehyde and polycyclic aromatic hydrocarbons (PAHs). There is no safe level of exposure to PAHs, which have been linked to lung, bladder and gastrointestinal cancers. Meanwhile, the amounts of glycerol and propylene glycol often differed from what was reported on the packaging and several e-liquids labelled nicotine-free nonetheless contained nicotine. The amount of glycerol and glycol is important because they disrupt the functioning of our cells — the higher the dose, the more derangement in cell activity. What's even more alarming is that many of the chemicals in e-liquids had never been tested for toxicity. In other words, we have no idea what they may or may not do to us.

A similar study by scientists at Johns Hopkins University found almost 2000 different chemicals in e-liquids and their resultant aerosols, most of which were either unidentified or known to be toxic. Contrary to what was originally believed, many of the flavourings are also toxic, with cinnamon, vanilla and buttery flavours being the most harmful. Mixing e-cig flavours is more dangerous than exposure to a single flavour.[2]

Even if a flavouring is seemingly harmless when ingested, vaping changes its chemical structure and can turn it into a poison. Add this to the fact that vapes are portrayed as glamorous on social media, and we have a potential health crisis about to explode amongst our youth.

In 2020, a study published in the journal *PLoS ONE* involving more than 880 000 adults over the age of 18 found that **e-cigarette users** (whether or not they had previously smoked tobacco) **reported greater problems with concentration, memory and decision-making than people who had never vaped.**

---

[1] Benzaldehyde impairs the ability of our lungs to fight infections. This is the last thing we need in the presence of COVID-19.

[2] The cinnamon flavouring known as trans-cinnamaldehyde was found in 48 of the 65 e-liquids and is on the Australian Therapeutic Goods Administration (TGA) list of banned flavours.

Even more distressing was a report in the journal *Tobacco Induced Diseases* that examined data from over 18 500 North American high school students and uncovered that e-cigarette users, tobacco smokers and dual-users (those who engaged in both smoking and vaping) were much more likely to have cognitive difficulties such as focusing and remembering than adolescents who had never vaped or smoked. The younger the adolescent when they started vaping, the stronger the association with mental problems.

In addition to cognitive impairment, e-cigarette use has been associated with:
- brain inflammation
- cough, wheeze and exacerbation of asthma
- acute and chronic lung injury
- sudden death due to a condition known as EVALI (E-cigarette or Vaping Associated Lung Injury)
- cardiovascular disease
- disruption of the gut lining leading to chronic inflammation
- DNA damage
- greater likelihood of taking up tobacco smoking than for non-vapers
- passive inhalation of toxins in exhaled aerosols by people in the vicinity of vapers.

Ironically, e-cigarettes have not achieved their original goal of helping large numbers of people quit smoking, even though proponents of e-cigarettes genuinely believe they have the potential to do so. Worse still, many smokers become dual users, thus exposing themselves to an even wider array of toxins than those found in tobacco cigarettes alone.

To summarise, studies to date strongly indicate that people who vape are exposing their body and brain to a dangerous cocktail of chemicals for which no long-term safety data is available. While further research is urgently needed to assess the wide-ranging effects of vaping on human health, there is already substantial evidence that vaping can damage our lungs, heart and brain, as well as potentially cause cancer and sudden death. I have a sad suspicion that e-cigarettes may end up being as harmful to our health as tobacco, albeit via different mechanisms, especially as vaping is being taken up at a much younger age than tobacco smoking. I hope I'm wrong. However, when low-tar cigarettes were introduced in the 1960s, they were also touted as being safer than traditional cigarettes. Later studies demonstrated the claim to be false. Thus, when it comes to e-cigarettes, users are playing Russian roulette with their health.

CHAPTER 58

Listen up!

Life affords no higher pleasure than that of surmounting difficulties.

SAMUEL JOHNSON (1709–1784)

'Your father's going deaf,' Mum announced.

'Your mother mumbles,' Dad countered.

'Your father can't hear what the waiter is saying when we're at a restaurant.'

'Your mother always chooses restaurants that are crowded and noisy. How is anyone supposed to hear anything above the racket going on in the background?'

'Your father has the TV turned up so loud it gives me a headache.'

'Your mother complains so often it gives *me* a headache.'

Every time I visited my parents I was appointed their unwilling adjudicator.

'Dad, why don't you just have a hearing test so you can prove Mum wrong?' I winked at Mum.

'It's a waste of time and effort. Even if my hearing isn't as good as it used to be, so what? Hearing loss isn't life-threatening and it's a normal part of ageing. I hear enough — in fact I hear too much from your mother.' Dad winked at me.

'Why wouldn't you want hearing aids if it meant getting Mum off your back?' I coaxed.

'Then she'd just find something else to complain about,' he bantered.

'Hearing aids are so small, no one would notice you were wearing them,' I persisted.

'But I don't need them.' He remained impervious to my suggestions.

Mum pulled me aside. 'It's exhausting having to repeat myself all the time. And when we're in company, I have to act as interpreter because I can see he hasn't heard what someone said. Not to mention having to field every phone call. His lack of hearing doesn't just affect *him*, it also affects *me* and it's wearing me down. I don't understand why your father is so reluctant to get hearing aids. It's as if he sees them as a sign of weakness or of getting frail. He'd sooner have a tooth out than a hearing test.'

'Do you know anyone who wears hearing aids?' I prompted. 'Dad needs someone to tell him that their quality of life improved when they were able to hear better. He doesn't know what he's missing out on.'

'No one springs to mind, but I'll find someone!'

I was glad to have given Mum a mission. I was equally concerned about Dad's hearing. A study conducted by the American National Council on Aging examined 2300 people with hearing loss and found that those who didn't correct their hearing deficit were much more likely to experience depression, anxiety, social withdrawal and paranoia. **Hearing problems have a profound impact on mental health and can double the risk of depression**.

Other studies have linked untreated hearing loss with headaches, muscle tension and elevated blood pressure. One reason is having to work harder to follow conversations and navigate unfamiliar environments. Poor hearing requires a person to use a great deal of energy simply deciphering what is being said. This leaves them with little energy to *remember* what is actually being said. This can cause a person to think they're developing memory problems when in fact they're having hearing problems. The added strain also leads to stress and fatigue.

Even **mild hearing loss can triple the risk of a fall,**[3] with potentially fatal consequences for older people. I didn't know at the time that **midlife hearing loss was also a significant risk factor for Alzheimer's**. Looking back, I should have connected the puzzle pieces: stress, depression, social isolation and elevated blood pressure all independently increase dementia risk. Therefore, if hearing loss contributes to these conditions, hearing loss will also propel a person towards dementia. Hearing loss can also directly increase Alzheimer's risk because the auditory cortex — the area of the brain responsible for processing sound — is receiving inadequate stimulation and therefore losing synapses (connections between brain cells).

'Dad isn't unique in his unwillingness to have a hearing test. It's common for people to struggle for seven to 10 years before they finally do something. Only 12% of people diagnosed with hearing loss under the age of 69 use hearing aids,' I reported to Mum.

'Why?' She was shocked. 'It's no different to needing glasses when eyesight declines.'

'I don't understand it either,' I admitted. 'I guess when you can't see or read, it has more obvious and immediate impacts on your life. If you don't hear something, you don't know that you haven't heard it unless someone tells you. And if you're really hard of hearing, you won't hear someone telling you what you haven't heard!'

We shared a weak laugh.

It took another 12 months for Mum to finally convince Dad to have a hearing test. He was diagnosed with moderate sensorineural hearing loss, also known as presbycusis. Both are just fancy names for age-related decline in hearing. It was slightly worse in his right ear. He was recommended hearing aids. Rather than being the end of Mum's struggles, it heralded the beginning of a new debate.

'Of course that place is going to tell me I have hearing loss,' Dad scorned. 'The test is free so they have to try and sell me their hearing aids to make their money.'

---

[3] Hearing loss increases the risk of falls because it is often accompanied by problems with balance. The inner ear is composed of two related parts: the cochlea (responsible for hearing) and the labyrinth (responsible for balance).

It remained a subject of contention until she passed away.

Several years later, the headlines started appearing in medical journals:
- Untreated hearing loss is linked to brain changes that compromise memory.
- Even mild hearing deficits are associated with lower scores on memory tests.
- Taiwanese study finds that people whose hearing deteriorated between the ages of 45 and 64 were more vulnerable to developing dementia if they did nothing to rectify their hearing loss.
- US study supports Taiwanese study with a further warning: the greater the hearing loss, the earlier the onset of dementia.
- Hearing aids can reduce falls in the elderly.
- University of Melbourne researchers report that 18 months of hearing aid use led to significant improvements in people's ability to plan, remember and organise information. They also became better at making decisions and solving problems.
- The longer a person delays in getting hearing aids, the longer it takes to get used to them.

Each successive research paper strengthened my resolve to remedy Dad's hearing loss.

'Dad I've found another way to improve your memory,' I began.

'Maybe I don't need to improve my memory. Maybe I'm just selective about what is and isn't worth remembering,' he replied puckishly.

I could never predict Dad's response to the subject of his memory. Some days he wanted to do everything he could to avoid 'being a burden' (his words, not mine). Other days he was in complete denial that there was anything amiss with his brain. You can lead a horse to water but you can't make it drink. I couldn't even lead my horse to water — so I brought the water to him. I found an audiologist who made house calls — complete with testing apparatus to deploy in our living room.

John was a fit, spry 80-something-year-old with a firm handshake and a confident smile. He was accompanied by his niece, Jemma, who he was training to take over his audiology practice. 'But that won't be for another decade or so,' he asserted jovially. The fact that John was a contemporary immediately put Dad at ease.

'Your daughter tells me you were an electrical engineer.' John faced Dad directly when he spoke.

'Yes,' Dad's posture immediately straightened.

'Were you ever exposed to loud noises for prolonged periods of time?'

'No,' Dad replied.

'And you were conscripted into the Yugoslav army?'

'Yes, but I never fired a gun,' Dad announced proudly.

'Did any bombs go off near you?'

'No.'

'Did you spend your youth at roaring discotheques?'

'No. But my daughter likely did.' Dad took every opportunity to deflect attention away from himself.

'Did you now?' John promptly turned to me. 'Most people think that age-related hearing loss is inevitable because 70% of 70-year-olds have a hearing deficit. But repeated exposure to loud sounds is the biggest contributing factor. Some people are more genetically prone to hearing problems, but the most important considerations are: how loud was the noise and for how long were you exposed to it? Noise above 100 decibels isn't recommended for longer than 15 minutes at a time. Most rock concerts hit 120 decibels. Even gym classes can be a hearing hazard because people are exposed to blaring music on a regular basis. I recommend you wear ear plugs whenever you take a fitness class. And don't blast music through your earbuds when you go for a run. I understand that you want to get pumped up, but keep it to a safe volume. The irony is that physical exercise protects against hearing loss.'

My eyes widened. So did Dad's. Mine with glee, his with terror.

It was clear that John was enjoying himself. 'Loud noise causes wear and tear on the hair cells in your cochlea. The cochlea is a hollow spiral-shaped bone deep inside your ear. It converts vibrations into nerve impulses that your brain translates into sound.' He reached into his toolkit and gave Dad a plastic model of a cochlea.

'What am I supposed to do with this snail shell?' Dad looked perplexed.

'Very observant!' John congratulated. 'Cochlea comes from the Latin word for snail shell. Physical exercise stops you losing the hair cells in your cochlea. Sedentary mice lose about 20% of their hearing as they age. Mice that run on treadmills every day only lose 5% of their hearing.'

I was jubilant. Dad turned pale.

'My daughter has set you up to this. She's always looking for excuses to make me exercise.'

'Well, today let's play a game instead,' John effortlessly transitioned to giving Dad a hearing test.

After studying the results, John watchfully addressed Dad. 'I can see that higher pitched tones sound muffled to you. That means you can hear vowels but tend to miss consonants. It's difficult picking out words against background noise, isn't it?'

'Of course it is. That's normal.' Dad became defensive.

'Yes, to a degree it's normal. But we can make it much easier for you. You won't find it so tiring following a conversation. Sometimes people mistake poor hearing for poor memory. It takes so much energy just to listen, they have no energy left to remember anything. Hearing loss takes an enormous toll on older people — physically, mentally and emotionally. Everything they do becomes more stressful. They lose self-confidence, avoid socialising and even fear going outside. When you don't receive auditory cues from your environment, you feel less safe. If you don't hear a cyclist coming up behind you, it gives you a massive fright when they suddenly whiz past. The other problem with poor hearing is that it leads to loss of brain cells. Jemma, tell them about the impact of hearing loss on the brain.'

Jemma had been discreetly taking notes. She suddenly came to life.

'If you don't hear well, the part of your brain that processes sound doesn't receive the stimulation it needs and it starts to shrink. The less you hear, the less you are able to hear, and things start to snowball. **Use it or lose it.** The part of our brain responsible for hearing is also involved in memory and mood. That means hearing loss can also lead to depression and dementia. All this is compounded by the fact that if you withdraw from social activities, it further increases your risk of Alzheimer's. Even subtle loss of hearing when you're young can change the structure of your brain and open the door to dementia. Everyone should get their hearing tested every five years even if they don't think they have a problem. Unless it's due to a specific event such as a viral infection[4] or head injury, hearing loss is gradual so people don't notice that it's happening.'

Now it was Dad's turn to come to life. 'Test my daughter. She's never had a hearing test.'

'I'll be happy to have a hearing test when John and Jemma come to see us again in a few weeks. For now, I want to learn about hearing aids,' I urged them.

John produced a demonstration hearing aid. 'They're so inconspicuous and comfortable you'll forget you're even wearing them.'

'But you said wearing them would improve my memory,' Dad interjected smugly. 'And how is something that blocks my ears going to help me hear?'

John was unfazed. 'Hearing aids make sounds louder. This helps damaged cells in your ear relay the sounds to your brain. Stimulating your brain keeps it in good nick. Hearing aids will bring back wondrous things you've been missing out on. The chirping of birds, a gush of wind, rustling leaves, they're all quite magical. Why don't you give hearing aids a try? If you don't like them, take them out. Think about it and let me know what you decide.'

When the hearing aids arrived, no amount of enthusiasm, explanation or reassurance could penetrate Dad's resistance to wearing them. I flattered, cajoled, bribed and beseeched. I begged, pleaded, urged

---

[4] Viruses such as measles, mumps, chicken pox and HIV can sometimes lead to hearing loss, as can antibiotics like gentamicin.

and implored. I appealed to his logic, pride, charity and conscience. I ended up with a migraine. When I emerged from my throbbing haze, I had an idea. I rang John. A week later, he dropped by with a small white box. Inside were a pair of demo hearing aids. He wished me luck.

The next morning, I began with 'one for me and one for you'.

'What's going on?' Dad demanded.

'This hearing aid is for me,' I announced, and inserted the plastic demo model into my right ear.

'And this hearing aid is for you.' I swiftly placed one of his hearing aids into his right ear.

'And this hearing aid is for me.' I plugged my left ear.

'And this hearing aid is for you.' I slipped the remaining hearing aid into his left ear.

'I don't need hearing aids!' He put his hand to his right ear.

'No, please don't touch! Hearing aids are very finely tuned and very expensive and you mustn't interfere with them. If the volume is too loud, let me know and I'll turn it down.'

He eyed me suspiciously but said nothing. He kept them in his ears for the obligatory few hours and we repeated the process the following day. Soon he was tolerating them all day long and they became an established part of our daily routine. Every morning, I blundered about the house with compromised hearing until it was safe for me to remove my fakes. It was worth it. Over the ensuing months, people started commenting that Dad seemed more relaxed and willing to engage in group activities. He was able to follow conversations involving more than one person and he was noticeably less confused. A win for the cochlea crusaders.

CHAPTER 59

In search of hearing aids

Trust men and they will be true to you; treat them greatly,
and they will show themselves great.

RALPH WALDO EMERSON (1803–1882)

'Wake up! Wake up! My hearing aids have been stolen!' My father's panic-stricken voice broke my slumber.

I reached across to the bedside cabinet and fumbled around for my watch. It was 3.25 am. Exactly the same time as last night. There were times when Alzheimer's felt like an unrelenting Groundhog Day.

'Dad it's okay. Your hearing aids haven't been stolen.'

'Then where are they? They're very finely tuned and very expensive and I don't want anyone interfering with them!' The light from the hallway exposed his bewilderment.

'One of them is hiding somewhere in the house so I put the other one in your cupboard for safekeeping.'

'How did it go missing?'

'I don't know. It's very small and easy to misplace. Let me take you back to bed and we'll find it in the morning. What are you doing up at this hour anyway? Why were you looking for your hearing aids in the middle of the night?'

'I don't know.'

I waited until he'd fallen asleep and tiptoed back to my room.

It was over 24 hours since his right hearing aid had disappeared. I had gone to take them out before his shower — as I did every other evening — but his right ear was bereft of its tenant. He occasionally took them out himself and placed them on his bedside table but it wasn't there. I checked his pockets. Nothing. I scrutinised every surface, searched every cupboard and opened every container. I sifted through the carpet and examined every inch of floor. Still nothing. We had been shopping earlier in the day and I remembered catching sight of them when we unloaded the car so I combed through the car and fridge as well. No joy. Where could it be? Now that Dad was in the habit of wearing them, the last thing I wanted was for him to get *out* of the habit. The thought of having to wean him onto them again was crushing. Wearing only one hearing aid kept reminding him that the other one was missing and it made him fretful and agitated. I resumed the hunt the following morning. Dad's distress was escalating with every passing minute. As was my frustration.

We were interrupted by a knock on the door. Whoever it was would be enlisted to join the search — or at least to distract Dad so he wouldn't drive *me* to distraction. It was Tim — the friendly gardener who mowed our lawn. I forced a smile.

'I was about to start the lawnmower when I saw this hearing aid in the grass.' He held out his hand. 'Does it belong to your dad?'

'Thank you, thank you, thank you!' I was overjoyed.

Sound was reinstalled. Order was re-established. Calm was restored.

CHAPTER 60

In search of a house

*We act as though comfort and luxury were the chief
requirements of life, when all we need to make us really happy
is something to be enthusiastic about.*

CHARLES KINGSLEY (1819–1875)

Dad's house needed ongoing repairs. It was a three-bedroom Federation cottage built by a Scotsman at the turn of the 20th century. My parents had bought it in 1973 and I'd moved back to live with Dad when Mum passed away. It had high ceilings, asymmetric gables and handmade cornices. As a child I'd wondered why the decorative hallway features ended abruptly at the entrance to a second sitting room marked by a curtained archway. The answer was perfectly logical. At the time the house was built, guests were never invited beyond the front parlour. Visitors were entertained in the ornate section of the house while family members went about their business in the no-frills areas. My parents had judiciously kept up this tradition. Also in the front parlour, the once-functional fireplace was now part of a black feature wall that displayed family photographs dating back to my parents' childhoods.

The first thing that required fixing was the terracotta-tiled roof — as evidenced by the buckets we scrambled to line up in the living room whenever it rained. Meanwhile, paint was constantly peeling off the wooden window frames, leaving an exasperating pile of white paint flecks that I felt compelled to vacuum up every evening. It made for my mindfulness practice.

The kitchen linoleum was curling up at every corner but at least it matched the orange flowers that were etched on the cupboard door handles. If a real estate agent was trying to sell the house, they'd undoubtedly describe it as 'a renovator's delight'.

My major concern was the potentially brain-damaging effects of mould. Moulds are a type of fungi that grow on damp surfaces such as bathroom walls, window frames and leaky ceilings. I was also afraid that moisture might be seeping through our concrete foundations and causing mould to build up under the carpet. I couldn't see any obvious black stains or furry outgrowths, but the post-downpour musty odour made me feel uneasy.

Moulds have long been known to increase the risk of allergies, asthma and other respiratory diseases. Recently, a growing body of research also points to **moulds being a contributing factor in a subset of people with Alzheimer's**. Post-mortem brain tissue from Alzheimer's patients — but not from individuals who had no dementia at the time of death — was found to contain fungal material within and around neurons as well as inside cerebral blood vessels. But how does mould cause problems with cognition?

Moulds produce three brain-irritants that we readily inhale without realising:
1. spores
2. fragments of the organism itself
3. biotoxic proteins called mycotoxins.

All these particles can cross the blood-brain barrier (BBB) and lodge inside the brain where they induce oxidative stress and inflammation, interfere with brain cell metabolism and trigger production of amyloid β ($A\beta$), a potent anti-fungal agent. Mycotoxins also damage blood vessels within the brain, thus reducing delivery of oxygen and essential nutrients. Symptoms of a mould-infected brain include depression and difficulties with speech (aphasia), numbers (dyscalculia), decision-making, balance and co-ordination. This is because fungal proteins tend to accumulate in the frontal and parietal lobes, which are responsible for the aforementioned functions. Other people simply report brain fog or difficulty concentrating. The condition is often referred to as inhalational Alzheimer's and the good news is that it can be treated by a specialist physician with medications known as binders or sequestering agents such as cholestyramine (used to lower cholesterol before the advent of statins) and charcoal. Saunas and physical exercise (to promote sweating out of toxins) can also be helpful. Of course, the most critical factor in recovery is removing oneself from water-damaged buildings. High humidity, poor ventilation and carpets all encourage the growth of various moulds.

An argument against mould inhalation as a cause of Alzheimer's is that we're all exposed to mould at one time or another, so why doesn't everyone suffer from cognitive decline? The answer lies in an interplay of genes, underlying health conditions and duration and severity of exposure. We know that smoking causes lung cancer but not all smokers get lung cancer. Moreover, different strains of moulds affect us in different ways.

Seventy-five per cent of people have a robust immune system that effectively gets rid of mycotoxins. Twenty-five per cent of people have a gene variant (HLA-DR/DQ) that increases their susceptibility to autoimmune and inflammatory disorders including mould toxicity. In addition, low blood levels of magnesium, zinc, coenzyme Q10 and vitamins D and B can all impair our body's ability to detoxify and thereby exacerbate the effects of exposure to toxins.

A disturbing study of Polish children found that those exposed to indoor mould for longer than two years had IQ scores 10 points lower than their non-exposed classmates. Exposure beyond two years tripled the risk of having an IQ in the lowest 25%. Children tend to be more sensitive to toxins because their brains and immune systems are still developing.

Diagnosing inhalational Alzheimer's requires a comprehensive assessment of symptoms and sources of mould, along with blood tests, brain scans and neuropsychological testing. Mycotoxins (among other neurological conditions) can also impair a person's ability to see details at low contrast levels. The website VCSTest.com provides a simple online Visual Contrast Sensitivity Test to determine your ability to discern the direction of lines displayed at different levels of contrast. The test is NOT definitive for mould infection because many other diseases can affect our ability to perceive visual contrast.

However, if your results suggest a problem, you may want to see an ophthalmologist or discuss the possibility of mycotoxin disease with a doctor who is experienced in this area.

I wondered whether people who had Alzheimer's due to factors other than mould might become more sensitive to mould because their brain was in a weakened state? Likewise, older lungs are more prone to irritations and infections because they tend to have less filtering power against pollutants. The more I thought about it, the more I felt uneasy about our deteriorating residence.

From the perspective of water damage, almost every room in the house needed an overhaul — for which I had neither time, interest or finances. What to do? Coupled with Dad's intolerance to Sydney's windy winters and ever-increasing traffic, I began toying with the idea of downsizing and moving to warmer climes; to a lighter, brighter, happier house and greener, cleaner, quieter neighbourhood — an all-round more brain-boosting environment. Why hadn't I thought of it before?

Those who have read my prequel *In Search of My Father* will recall that Mum was a shopaholic and a hoarder — a lethal combination. Mum had converted the guest room into her private walk-in-wardrobe-cum-storeroom and neither Dad nor I had ventured inside since she'd died. I was terrified of the emotions we'd both locked behind that door.

I broached the subject with Dad. 'This house takes a lot of work to maintain and it's bigger than the two of us need. How would you feel if we moved to a smaller place by the sea?'

'We need a big house for all of your mother's things,' he contended.

'I think Mum would be happy if we gave away her belongings to people who would appreciate them.' I genuinely believed this to be the case. Mum never missed an opportunity to bestow a gift.

'How about we take her things to our family and friends in Serbia?' he suggested.

'We'd need an entire fleet of planes to carry everything.' I also genuinely believed this to be the case. 'Besides, there are hundreds of local charities in need of donations.'

'Marko's family might like some of her things.'

I did some prompt box breathing and changed the subject.

A few days later I asked Dad again, 'Would you be happy if we moved to a smaller house in a warmer climate?'

'As long as you and I are living in the same house, I'll be happy anywhere.'

With Dad's endorsement, I set the wheels in motion. I soon realised I'd grossly underestimated the enormity of the task. The first step was decluttering. The attempts of Dad and me a few years earlier hadn't made a dent. I was also conscious of the fine line between clutter and clues. By 'clues' I mean that Dad relied on specific objects to reinforce his sense of identity and remind him of what he was capable of. Strategically placed objects cued him to comb his hair, insert his dentures, eat his breakfast, make a cup of coffee, water the garden and sweep the porch. Many of the ornaments I viewed as dust magnets prompted him to talk about life events he was at risk of forgetting. Losing his collection of intimate items could precipitate losing his fragile memories. Being surrounded by familiar objects would be even more critical for maintaining his sense of self and his day-to-day functioning in an unfamiliar house.

Both of us also hated any form of waste and couldn't bear throwing things out, even if we'd never use them. To psych myself up, I read Marie Kondo's eminently practical (and spiritual) book *The Life-Changing Magic of Tidying Up: The Japanese Art of Decluttering and Organising*. Her criteria for keeping something is a single defining question: does it bring joy? If yes, keep it — no other reason necessary. If it doesn't bring joy — even if there are dozens of rational reasons to keep it — give it away. Did Marie have any idea how many times I would need to ask that question? To mask my procrastination, I read the book a second time. Then I had to take the plunge.

We began by painstakingly sorting out what we *probably* didn't want, packed different categories of items into separate boxes, and decided we'd worry about what to do with them later.

What happened next was nothing short of miraculous. My mantra became 'Pack it and they will come'. A friend rang to say her daughter had just bought her first home and had no money left for anything else. Could I spare any basic pieces of furniture or kitchenware? Another friend told me of an inspiring charity called The Footpath Library that distributes secondhand books to people who were homeless; they were always looking for donations of good quality reads. A neighbour mentioned that Stepping Stone House (an organisation providing accommodation, life skills and emotional support for 12- to 24-year-olds at risk of homelessness) was in need of bed linen. And so it went on. Every time I filled a box, someone turned up who either needed it themselves or knew of a charity that was looking for it. I was blown away by the synchronicity.

My own research led me to Fitted for Work (where we donated Mum's clothes, handbags and accessories), Suited to Success (where we donated more of Mum's clothes, handbags and accessories) and the Refugee Council of Australia, which listed all the charities that accept donations of various goods for refugees and people seeking asylum. I lost count of the carloads of homewares we delivered to every suburb of Sydney. It took five months of non-stop effort before we were done.

Then I discovered that we were NOT done. To my horror, a trap door under the house opened to a whole other trove of toys, games, tools, ornaments, furniture, bags and shoes. I spent several days crawling under the house retrieving more and more stuff. Every time I thought I'd come to the end, another hiding place presented itself.

A recurring finding was shoes. Mum loved all manner of things, but what she loved most were her shoes. Shoes from every era and every genre. Casual, classy, chic, cheeky, edgy, elegant, exotic, ergonomic, playful, practical, strappy, sophisticated, saucy, stylish, bold, embroidered, flirty and flamboyant. Shoes with buckles, bevels and butterflies. Yes, patent purple butterflies. Shoes turned up everywhere. Hundreds of them. In cartons, cupboards and drawers. Under beds, sofas and dressing tables. On top of wardrobes, bookshelves and ledges. I started having nightmares about shoes. I spent many a fitful sleep being chased through dark alleyways by disembodied boots. After watching a James Bond rerun, I dreamt

I was dodging a storm of stilettos being fired at me from machine guns. My brain was struggling to process the meaning of so many shoes.

'Do they fit you?' Dad asked as he surveyed the growing mounds of footwear. We kept making new piles to avoid an avalanche.

'Yes,' I sighed, 'Mum had the same shoe size as me.'

'Do you believe in reincarnation?' Dad's question baffled me.

'Why?'

'You'll need more than one lifetime to wear them all.'

The irony was that I was not a shoe person. I owned four functional pairs: black casual, black high heels, trainers and thongs. Why complicate daily decision-making with discretionary footwear? Mum had been indefatigable in educating me about shoes, but to no avail—until now. I suddenly felt that every pair of heels and flats told a story about her. They revealed an aspect of her personality, vivacity and joie de vivre. I couldn't give them all away. I decided to share them with friends, charities, vintage clothes stores, market stalls and Good Samaritan bins. I was still left with over a hundred pairs for myself. I would wear them in Mum's honour. Till death do us part.

The next step was finding a new home. Dad, Felix and I mutually agreed on the Gold Coast.[5] We wanted a quiet, tree-lined street near a lake or park that was close enough to the airport to allow me to continue conference-speaking and running retreats, but not so close as to be under a flight path. We would maintain the same living arrangements as in Sydney: Dad and I would share a single-storey house with a low-maintenance garden while Felix would live in an apartment that was walking distance away. The three of us typed up a list of essentials and desirables and emailed them to a home-buyer's agent. My list comprised 48 essential criteria

---

[5] For my non-Australian readers, the Gold Coast is a sunny subtropical coastal city, 840 km (522 miles) north of Sydney. It's a major tourist destination, best known for its theme parks, nightlife and rainforest hinterland. We were not moving for the razzle dazzle entertainment but the warmer weather, ample green space and relaxed lifestyle — and real estate was much more affordable than in Sydney.

— NO mould, good ventilation, spacious rooms, no steps or trip hazards, walk-in shower, plenty of natural light, open plan kitchen combined with dining and living area, ample storage space, walking distance to a lake or park, no adjacent busy roads, safe tranquil neighbourhood, simple doorbell, no intercom (as Dad wouldn't know how to operate it and it would only serve to confuse him) … along with 35 more entries. I wanted to make certain we were moving into a beautiful, brain-boosting house that would facilitate my father's optimal functioning.

Meanwhile, Felix had eight criteria — he was a low-maintenance man. No wonder we got on so well.

After a dozen video walk-throughs, we narrowed our search to three properties each and flew north for the in-person inspections. Forty-eight hours later, Felix and I had both signed our contracts.

In the meantime, I told our kindly next-door neighbours (Vernon and Hana) of our intention to relocate. They were a hardworking young couple with three primary school-aged children. To my jubilant astonishment, they ended up buying our house! I warned them of the mould but they were undeterred. They promised to organise a formal mould analysis and do what was necessary to get rid of it. Vernon's parents were becoming frail and in need of daily assistance. By moving his parents next door, Vernon and his family would be able to look after them while everyone maintained their independence. I couldn't have wished for a more heartening destiny for Dad's home of 43 years.

CHAPTER 61

Stumbling blocks or stepping stones?

Start by doing what's necessary, then do what's possible,
and suddenly you are doing the impossible.

ST FRANCIS OF ASSISI (1182–1226)

D ad and I spent our first night on the Gold Coast in sleeping
bags on the floor of our empty new home. We awoke to a
warm, welcoming April morning and strolled to our local café for
breakfast. We had just enough time to sample their superb coffee
and perfectly poached eggs before heading back to the house to
meet the removalists.

My first priority was Dad's room. The sooner I surrounded him
with familiar furniture, photos, paintings, ornaments, books and
crumpled Serbian newspapers, the more settled he would feel and
the less strain on his brain to adapt to the onslaught of changes.
I worked feverishly to reduce his disorientation and anxiety by
re-establishing his mealtime, bedtime, grooming, showering and
recreational routines as closely as possible to what they had been.

One of the first neighbours to visit us was lithe and chipper 70-year-
old Henry. 'G'day!' He greeted us with a broad smile and enthusiastic
handshake (it was pre-COVID days). Dad was guarded and taciturn,
which was not unusual for him when he met someone for the first
time. I said nothing about Dad having dementia. We were soon
swept up in Henry's colourful stories of having been a fireman and
… an Alzheimer's care-companion! I couldn't believe our good
fortune. I was so excited I almost dropped the tray of iced water I

was carrying. We didn't yet have anything other than water to offer our guest. Luckily, for all the medical marvels of the world, **water was still the most brain-boosting beverage** available.

'I'm now retired and have grandchildren to fuss over but I really miss the camaraderie of both the fire brigade and the aged care team,' he reminisced. 'And by "team", I include all the extraordinary individuals who make the most of each day despite having dementia. The medical system hasn't a clue what it means to have dementia. Most people think that a diagnosis of Alzheimer's renders a person unable to communicate or contribute. Boy, is that wrong! You just have to provide the right context and an unhurried safe space and you can connect with anyone. *Anyone!*' He repeated the word emphatically. 'Sorry, I'm off on my hobby horse.' He took a satisfied sip of water.

'Not at all, please go on,' I encouraged. 'What do you mean by "providing the right context"?'

'Have a genuine interest in getting to know the person. In the early stages of the disease, ask them about their life growing up rather than what they did yesterday. They might not remember what happened an hour ago or where to find their walking stick or that they even *need* a walking stick, but they often remember the adventures of their childhood and young adult years. Ask about their favourite music, movies, sports and pastimes; their favourite teacher, the time they felt proud of an achievement and the time they fell in love. The more you learn about someone, the more you'll discover how to draw out their stories, wisdom and animating life experiences. If they played a musical instrument, reacquaint them with it. If they enjoyed dancing, play their favourite waltz or folk song. If they followed a particular football team, find relevant memorabilia and place it in their hands. It's like putting new batteries in a flickering lamp. They literally light up. Lack of meaningful stimulation befuddles anyone's brain, dementia or not!'

'What would you do if someone had late-stage Alzheimer's and could no longer remember any of their past or struggled to communicate?'

'Regardless of the severity of someone's dementia, I always **focus on what's strong, not wrong**. For instance, even in the final stages of Alzheimer's, people's response to music remains intact and they recognise familiar tunes and lyrics. Listening to well-known songs can also help people recall personal memories. **In people with Alzheimer's, music is more powerful than photos in bringing back memories.** Have you seen the documentary *Alive Inside: A Story of Music and Memory*?'

'No,' I shook my head.

'It shows how playing music to people with neurodegenerative diseases like Alzheimer's can literally bring them to life. One minute they're completely unresponsive to all stimuli and the next minute their eyes are shining, they're tapping their feet and they're engaging with the people around them. The magic comes from creating a playlist that's specifically meaningful to the individual. The movie won the Audience Award at the 2014 Sundance Film Festival — you have to watch it.'

'We certainly will,' I assured him.

'The other key to connecting with someone who has advanced dementia,' Henry continued, 'is interacting in ways that don't depend on memory. Ask the person how they feel about something or seek out their opinion or advice. Do you think I should buy my wife roses or tulips for her birthday? What colour? Do you like flowers? How do flowers make you feel? Do you enjoy eating birthday cake? What about ice cream? Chocolate or vanilla? I think children eat too much ice cream these days and it's making them fat. What do you think? Should we save cake and ice cream for special occasions or eat them every day? The conversation can take the most fascinating twists and turns. Almost everyone loves giving advice!'

'Especially my daughter.' It was Dad's first input into the conversation.

'Especially my wife,' Henry winked at him.

I loved that Henry shared my philosophy of being a care-companion and care-partner rather than caregiver, care-worker or carer.

'Caregiver makes it sound like the giving only happens in one direction,' he expounded. 'If that's how it feels, you aren't doing it right. I've received so many invaluable gifts from people with dementia. They've taught me how to be a better human being, to let go of grudges and to never give up on someone. I had to learn patience but it certainly paid off.'

I wondered if Henry might like to join Dad's care team? I filed away the question for another day.

'The other thing to remember about Alzheimer's,' Henry declared ebulliently, 'is that **facts fray but feelings stay**. In other words, the person may not remember what you said or did, but they'll remember how you made them feel. My goal was always to make the person feel good — after that, everything else came more easily: eating, showering or getting them ready for an outing. There's nothing more important than creating positive relationships with people. The rest is secondary.'

After Henry had gone, Dad and I ducked out to buy groceries so I could start to prepare dinner.

'What time is it?' Dad asked when we returned home.

'Has your watch stopped? It's almost 6 o'clock.'

'I know it's 6 o'clock but is it 6 am or 6 pm?'

'We're about to have dinner so it's 6 pm,' I was taken aback by his perplexity. People with Alzheimer's can become disoriented with respect to day or night but it wasn't something I had ever experienced with Dad.

'I'm not hungry,' he snapped.

Tetchiness was likewise not a feature of his usual disposition. 'That's okay,' I tried to sound unperturbed, 'I'm hungry enough for both of us. Do you mind sitting with me and keeping me company while I eat?' I knew that by the time we sat down, he'd have forgotten he wasn't hungry and would eat what I placed in front of him.

The minute I turned on the food processor to convert a head of cauliflower into 'rice', he lunged towards me and started shouting, 'Stop all that racket! You'll wake up the people downstairs!'

I immediately turned off the machine. Luckily, it only takes a few seconds to blitz cauliflower.

'What people downstairs?' I asked in bewilderment.

'The mother and her young daughter.'

'What mother and daughter?'

'You know — the ones who live in the house below.'

I foolishly tried to correct him. 'There's no house below us. You must be thinking of somewhere else you've been.'

'But I saw them earlier today.'

My folly knew no bounds as I continued to dispute his assertion. 'There's no one downstairs.' Trying to talk someone out of their delusion only escalates tension on both sides and exacerbates the situation.

'I saw them!' he insisted.

I said nothing as I silently endeavoured to rationalise his confusion. He'd had a very disruptive and exhausting week, he was in a foreign environment, his routine was out of kilter and he was confronted with new faces at every turn. He was suffering from sensory overload and his brain had made a glitch in trying to process everything. He would settle down after a good night's sleep. Come to think of it, I needed a good night's sleep myself.

CHAPTER 62

In search of everything

A life spent making mistakes is not only more honourable,
but also more useful than a life spent doing nothing.

GEORGE BERNARD SHAW (1856–1950)

'Isn't it time for coffee?' Dad prompted as he looked up from his sudoku.

'Sure,' I smiled. I was unpacking the last of the kitchenware. Everything required for a cup of instant coffee was in its rightful place. 'Why don't you make us both a cup?'

He stared at me blankly. 'How do I make coffee?'

I froze. Dad had been making instant coffee all his life, right up until the day we moved. Making a cup of coffee, riding a bicycle, throwing a ball and tying our shoelaces are all examples of what's known as procedural memory. Once we learn how to do these things, the procedures remain in long-term storage and we carry them out without conscious thought, even after a gap of many years. Procedural memory involves a part of the brain called the cerebellum, which is usually spared until the late stages of Alzheimer's. I couldn't believe that Dad had suddenly forgotten how to make coffee — seemingly overnight. What was going on?

'Let's make coffee together,' I changed tack and began talking him through each step. 'Please fill the kettle with water. You don't have to fill it to the top — halfway will do. And while we wait for the kettle to boil, can you get our cups please?'

'Where are our cups?'

'In the left-hand side of the cupboard above the sink.'

He turned around cautiously and opened the cupboard door. 'Why are there so many cups in here?'

'In case we get visitors.'

'We don't need visitors.'

'Having visitors is fun.'

'Visitors are boring.'

'Don't you think Felix is fun?'

He shrugged.

I handed him a teaspoon. 'It's time to put the coffee in our cups.'

He placed a heaped teaspoon of coffee in his cup. Followed by another. And another.

'I think that'll be enough. Can you bring the milk please?'

'Where's the milk?'

'In the fridge,' I responded with exaggerated cheerfulness to conceal my escalating anxiety.

'Where's the fridge?'

'Over there in the corner,' I pointed. While he was preoccupied with the fridge, I transferred the coffee back into the jar and put the appropriate amount in each of our cups. My hand was trembling, my mind was racing and I felt physically ill.

Moving house and having to process an avalanche of unfamiliar experiences in new surroundings on a daily basis must have taxed Dad's brain more than I'd anticipated. I *should* have anticipated it, I thought remorsefully. Everything in his life had changed: where we lived, where we walked, where we shopped, who we encountered and how we spent our time. And rather than purposefully engaging with him, I was preoccupied with unpacking. I had naively thought that as long as Felix and I remained constant figures in Dad's life, the transition would be relatively seamless. In my myopic enthusiasm to create the perfect brain-boosting living arrangements, I'd created the perfect storm of brain-eroding circumstances. How could I have made such a miscalculation? I had never experienced a panic attack but I felt I was close. My chest felt constricted, my heart was pounding and my face was flushed. What had I done to my father? I was overcome by an intense wave of fear. What had I done to this dear trusting man? I gripped the kitchen bench top until the sensation of dread washed over me but I remained weak and wobbly for several more minutes.

Dinner was a distressing replay of the previous evening, only worse.

'Stop banging all the pots and pans! You'll wake up the people downstairs!'

I was not banging the pots and pans. I couldn't avoid the sounds that accompanied meal preparation. Dad had become increasingly sensitive to noise. Was it because he felt anxious and on edge? Was it a symptom of being overstimulated by strange surroundings? Or was it the acoustics of the new house? By now I was struggling to hold back tears.

'The people downstairs have gone,' I responded flatly.

'Where?'

'They've moved away. It's just you and me.'

'But I saw them earlier today!' He stormed off to his room and re-emerged a few minutes later, pacing the hallway and muttering to himself. 'I can't find anything. Everything's wrong. Nothing is where it's supposed to be. No one can help me.'

'I'm here to help you,' I reassured him.

'No, you're not! No one can help me.'

'What do you need help with?' I asked gently.

'I don't know. Something peculiar is going on.'

'Let's sit and watch the swans gliding across the water,' I suggested softly. We were incredibly fortunate to have our back garden bordered by a soothing lake. Our home-buyer's agent had excelled in fulfilling all our property requirements. Dad found the swans calming and we managed to get through dinner without mention of the people downstairs.

After he'd gone to bed, I set about labelling every door, wardrobe, cupboard and drawer in the house. *Pantry, microwave oven, laundry, toilet, bathroom, Helena's room, guest room.* I had already hung Dad's favourite photo of himself on his bedroom door. *Cups, plates, bowls, glasses, serviettes, cutlery.* On second thoughts, I divided the cutlery drawer into thirds and stuck the words *spoons, forks* and *knives* in line with each item's location in the drawer. To the front of the fridge, I attached the sign: *Milk is in here. Look inside the door. Coffee, salt* and *pepper* also had separate labels on their designated cupboard doors. In the morning I would add signs for *socks, underpants, handkerchiefs, belts, short-sleeved shirts, long-sleeved shirts, trousers, jumpers, sudoku, jigsaw puzzles, dominos and newspapers* to all the drawers and wardrobe doors in Dad's bedroom. At least he would now be able to find things. It was also time we started a jigsaw puzzle. In the rush to unpack, it was a constant I had overlooked.

I collapsed into bed exhausted, but couldn't fall asleep. What if I'd caused irreversible worsening of Dad's dementia? **Stress exacerbates the symptoms of Alzheimer's and drives disease progression** by inducing chronic inflammation and increasing production of amyloid β (Aβ) and tau tangles. In turn, worsening cognition makes day-to-day functioning more difficult, thus further increasing a person's stress and creating a vicious self-perpetuating cycle. A disturbing example of the brain-damaging effects of stress is seen in war veterans. Those who are diagnosed with PTSD are twice as likely to develop dementia in their latter years. Other research followed more than 2200 US civilians (with an average age of 48) for eight years. Participants underwent assessments of their memory and thinking skills, together with blood tests to measure cortisol (stress hormone) levels and MRI scans to measure their brain volumes. Those with the highest levels of cortisol (indicative of the greatest levels of chronic stress) had the lowest scores on neuropsychological testing and the smallest brain volumes.

'Have I told you about the night I spent on the moon?' Dad posed the following evening. By now I was ready to howl. This was not my father talking. An alien had taken over his brain.

'I went with two scientists,' Dad continued.

I didn't want to listen. I wanted to run out of the house. I wanted to wind back the clock to when we were living in Sydney and having coherent conversations, even if repetitive. 'Tell me about your time in France,' I tried to steer him onto something that was uplifting and grounded in reality. While he was relating his adventures in Paris (all of which I could recount word for word myself), I had an idea. As soon as he finished his story, I started playing his favourite Édith Piaf CD. The French singer was one of his all-time idols and I could see the songs immediately transporting him to a safe and familiar place. Might music bring my father back?

Over the ensuing weeks, I started to recognise a pattern: in the late afternoons as shadows emerged and daylight dissipated, a Jekyll to Hyde-like transformation took place. Dad became aggravated by the slightest noise, took to pacing the corridor and kept checking the contents of his manbag. If I dared enter his room, he briskly stuffed the bag under his pillow and eyed me suspiciously.

'What do you want?' he demanded.

'I came to see if you wanted to choose our dinner music,' I said brightly.

'You choose,' he ordered.

'Would you like to help me with the puzzle?' I asked optimistically.

'No!' he snapped.

The phenomenon of evening agitation, irritation and confusion is known as sundowning — so called because symptoms emerge as the sun goes down. It occurs in up to 50% of people who have Alzheimer's, usually in the middle stages of the disease. Several causes of sundowning have been proposed. Sunset precipitates a rise in the hormone melatonin and a drop in the neurotransmitter dopamine. These biochemical changes prepare our body for sleep. People with dementia often under-produce melatonin, which can disrupt a range of bodily processes and lead to restlessness, disorientation and the aforementioned behaviours. Giving people a small afternoon dose of **melatonin (0.5 to 5 mg) often mitigates sundowning** but do not start anything without consulting your doctor. Side effects of melatonin are uncommon, but include depression, dizziness and stomach cramps.

Medication was always my last resort so my first priority was to identify any sundowning triggers and create a soothing afternoon ambience using soft music and scented candles while prompting Dad to tell stories of his childhood. I also made lunch his biggest meal and kept evening meals lighter.

Many factors other than melatonin dysregulation can contribute to sundowning. I compiled a list and tried to control for as many of the following as I could:

- having had a poor night's sleep
- lack of exposure to daylight, especially in the morning
- insufficient indoor lighting during the day
- lack of physical exercise
- the presence of shadows (which can add to a person's disorientation and confusion about their surroundings)
- feeling fatigued as the day wore on (this applied to both of us because Dad often mirrored my energy levels)
- being in an unfamiliar environment
- not having a regular routine for meals, activities, showering and going to bed
- a disruption to usual routine
- being over- or under-stimulated
- pain or discomfort
- tooth decay or ill-fitting dentures
- being unable to express unmet needs.

Retrospectively, it was little wonder that moving house had brought on sundowning and unravelling of Dad's functioning. I felt simultaneously heavy and hollow. I wanted to throw my arms around him and sob. I wanted to apologise for ripping away the props that had held together his frangible world. How was I to undo the damage I had unwittingly done?

CHAPTER 63

How many colours in a rainbow?

Everyone wishes to reach old age but nobody wishes to be old.

Bernardino of Siena (1380–1444)

Sun-speckled beads of rain were trickling down our living room window when I noticed a vivid rainbow diving into the lake behind our house.

'Hey Dad, come and see the rainbow!' I called out to him.

'Where?' he looked around, not knowing where to focus.

'Over there to the left,' I pointed, 'Isn't it stunning?'

He gazed at it for a long time before commenting, 'Yes, those three colours in the sky are lovely.'

'*Three* colours?' I queried.

'Yes — can't you see three beautiful colours?'

Rainbows consist of a continuous spectrum of colours but the human eye usually perceives seven: red (the outermost band), orange, yellow, green, blue, indigo and violet (the innermost band). What did Dad mean by *three* colours?

'What three colours do you see?' I probed.

'Red, yellow and blue.'

'What about green?'

'Do you mean the grass?'

'No, I mean can you also see a band of green in the middle of the rainbow?'

'No. There are only three colours in the rainbow. Red, yellow and blue.'

'What about orange?'

'There's no orange.'

I was taken aback and deeply saddened. Alzheimer's is known to affect visual pathways in the brain but exactly what this means in terms of a person's visual capabilities is not fully understood.[6] I quickly searched the internet for images of rainbows and showed my father a high-resolution photo of a rainbow with seven easily distinguishable colours.

'Dad, take a look at this picture. How many colours do you see?'

'Three,' he responded again.

'How many colours is a rainbow supposed to have?' I implored him to remember.

'I don't know.'

I choked back my tears as I recalled getting frustrated with him a few days ago for not being able to find his watch among a pile of objects on the table.

'Your watch is right there in front of you,' I had muttered in exasperation. 'Take a proper look, will you?' There is nothing more piercing than the pain of guilt. The world was fading from him, and I feared he was fading from me.

The relationship between Alzheimer's and changes in eyesight is an accelerating area of research. When people with mild to moderate Alzheimer's are asked to read letters on an eye chart, their vision is usually no worse than people without Alzheimer's. However,

---

[6] A specific type of dementia known as Visual Alzheimer's (VA) or Posterior Cortical Atrophy (PCA) selectively affects the visual processing region of the brain. This was not what was happening with my father.

when tested on more complex aspects of visual perception, their ability to detect contrast, movement and spatial relationships is significantly compromised. The lower their score on visual tests, the lower their score on memory tests.

In 2013, researchers from Georgetown University Medical Center, Washington, USA, and the University of Hong Kong observed that the retina (the light-sensitive layer of cells lining the inner back wall of the eye) was up to 49% thinner in mice who had Alzheimer's than in healthy mice. This finding prompted scientists to compare the retinas of three groups of people:

- those with a diagnosis of Alzheimer's
- those with a genetic history of Alzheimer's
- those with no Alzheimer's in their family or themselves.

Using new eye scanning technology called optical coherence tomography angiography (OCTA), people with a diagnosis or genetic history of Alzheimer's were revealed to have thinner retinas and fewer tiny retinal blood vessels compared with people who had no Alzheimer's and no genetic history. Subsequent brain scans found that retinal thinning correlated with a smaller hippocampus (the brain's learning and memory centre). The retina is an outgrowth of our brain, so it is not surprising that **our eyes are a window to our brain.**

In August 2017, there was another breakthrough in Alzheimer's and eye research. Scientists from the Cedars-Sinai Medical Center in Los Angeles identified amyloid β (Aβ) and tau proteins on the retinas of people with Alzheimer's.

Furthermore, a five-year study published in 2018 in the journal *Alzheimer's & Dementia* examined 4000 people over the age of 65 and found that those who had diabetic retinopathy, macular degeneration or glaucoma were 40% to 50% more likely to develop Alzheimer's than people with no eye problems. This is not to say that eye diseases *cause* Alzheimer's, but that eye diseases and Alzheimer's may have a common origin. Moreover, eye diseases are likely to exacerbate Alzheimer's because they lead to suboptimal stimulation of the visual cortex and subsequent brain atrophy (shrinkage).

The good news is that **people aged 65 and older who had cataracts and underwent lens replacement surgery were 30% less likely to develop dementia** compared with people who did not have their cataracts removed. A convergence of several factors is likely to contribute to the reduction in dementia:

- Better vision encourages greater participation in brain-stimulating activities.
- Cataract surgery restores stimulation to the visual cortex, with a corresponding increase in grey matter volume.
- Cataracts produce a yellow tinge that reduces the amount of blue light entering our eyes. You'll recall from Chapter 51 'Good timing' that this can interfere with our circadian rhythms and contribute to a host of diseases including Alzheimer's. Cataract surgery can thus restore our circadian rhythms and reduce sundowning.

These findings open possibilities for early screening of Alzheimer's using non-invasive eye scans — akin to a mammogram for breast cancer, but performed much more quickly and comfortably, and without the need for radiation. It also means that **people with degenerative eye diseases need to be proactive about their brain health** because the underlying disease process affecting their eyes may also be affecting their brain. In addition, deteriorating eyesight may reduce a person's involvement in mentally, physically and socially stimulating activities. It's imperative that we continue to do as much as we are capable of and seek out new ways of staying mentally agile. Withdrawing from intellectual, creative and social pursuits only accelerates cognitive decline.

I was left pondering three questions:

- Do Aβ and tau proteins distort a person's vision in ways we haven't yet detected?
- What was Dad *not* seeing that I assumed he was?
- Could the changes in Dad's vision be having a domino effect on other areas of his functioning?

CHAPTER 64

Dare to care

*We are each of us angels with only one wing
and we can only fly by embracing each other.*

LUCRETIUS (CIRCA 99–55 BCE)

'Give him time,' Felix tried to raise my spirits, 'your dad will recover his former level of functioning. Everyone finds moving house ridiculously stressful. All three of us are still getting used to the changes. This is your father's adjustment phase. Resist the temptation to judge the situation — or yourself — as problematic. Your dad instinctively picks up on your mood and state of mind. If *you* feel distressed, so will he — even if you try and hide it. What do you need to relieve some of the stress *you're* feeling?'

'I need to assemble a care team.'

'Then let's do it.'

The first person I approached was Henry. He was delighted to come on board and he and Dad were soon playing pool at the local surf club, browsing around Bunnings or having a game of darts, dominos or quoits on our back deck. They even tried their hand at fishing from the edge of our lake.

Given that I could no longer leave Dad at home alone, I also registered our care requirements with <u>findacarer.com.au</u> and crossed my fingers that a warm, fun-loving individual with experience in dementia care would want to spend time with 'a charming, sprightly 84-year-old gentleman who enjoyed cappuccinos, classical music and all things French'. Within 72 hours I received 21 keen responses.

How to decide who would be the best fit? I began by sending each applicant the following email.

Dear Applicant's Name,

Thank you for offering to assist Dad in achieving the best quality of life possible. I prefer to use the terms 'care-partner' or 'care-companion' rather than 'carer', 'caregiver' or 'care-provider' to emphasise that your relationship with Dad will be an equal partnership. Although Dad has Alzheimer's — which limits his capabilities in specific areas of his life — he is still fully mobile and able to:

- *dress, bathe, shave and feed himself*
- *express his preferences*
- *make simple decisions*
- *connect with others in meaningful ways*
- *contribute to his community*
- *engage in creative pursuits*
- *sing, dance and appreciate music — especially classical, opera, ballet, cabaret and André Rieu*
- *experience joy.*

His particular interests (things that animate him and make him smile) include:

- *all things French*
- *ancient Greek history and mythology*
- *astronomy*
- *soccer and tennis*
- *sudoku*
- *question him to discover more.*

*As stated at the outset, Dad's and my goal is for him to have the best quality of life available to him. This can mean different things to different people so here is a checklist of our specific needs. All begin with **S** so they're easy to remember.*

1. ***Safety*** *— Please ensure that Dad is not only physically safe and takes his medications as prescribed, but that he also feels mentally and emotionally safe. I prepare all his medications so all you need to do is **Supervise** him taking them.*

2. **Stimulation**
    (a) *Physical* — take a daily walk or equivalent
    (b) *Mental* — keep his brain active through games, excursions or creative activities
    (c) *Social* — have conversations that encourage him to share his thoughts and opinions
    (d) *Natural* — spend time in nature and sunshine if weather permits

3. **Sustenance** — Please follow the dietary requirements I'll email to you in due course. This will not be complicated. The bottom line is no junk food, fast food or soft drinks.

4. **Support** — This entails a fine balance between helping/prompting Dad when he needs assistance, while allowing him to do as much for himself as possible. You'll work this out through observation, trial and error. Support also means paying attention to any positive or negative changes in his behaviour and working out what might have brought about the observed changes. If the change is positive, let me know so that we can do more of the good stuff. If the change is negative, don't assume 'it's the disease taking a bad turn' or sundowning or 'he's just playing up'. Most negative behaviours are an expression of distress, discomfort, pain, tiredness, fear, uncertainty or something that Dad is unable to coherently communicate. The most important thing in this situation is to **Soothe** him in whatever way you can. Speak to him softly and slowly and make him feel safe. Ask if he is in pain. You may not always be able to establish a cause, but you can always respond in a way that de-escalates his distress. Also observe if there is a pattern/ time of day or a consistent trigger for a particular behaviour. This will help us mitigate similar scenarios in the future.

I appreciate that I may have presented a daunting picture of care-partner. I simply want to establish whether you share the philosophies of our household and feel excited by the role I've outlined. If you're still interested, please let me know a time that you'd like to meet us.

Kind regards

Helena and Ika

Dad was adamant that he didn't need anyone around when I went to work, so I truthfully told him that I was the one in need of assistance. Knowing that he considered washing, cleaning, ironing and cooking to be 'women's work' I gave him a choice. 'Would you like to do chores around the house while I'm out or will we employ someone? I won't manage to look after this house on my own.'

The matter was quickly settled. 'Of course you should find someone to help you,' he insisted.

'Okay then. Since we both have to feel comfortable with the person, I'll invite them here to meet us before we make a final decision.'

'Naturally,' he replied matter-of-factly.

My email scared off only four applicants so the next step was to meet each of the courageous 17 in person. Thus began two weeks of meeting a new potential friend for an hour every day. I made certain they came in the morning when Dad was at his best and brightest. He never spoke about his trip to the moon until the moon came out at night. Nor should I have been concerned that he wouldn't want to socialise, as he always rose to the occasion when we had female visitors. I'm convinced there's a region of the brain dedicated to flirting that remains untouched by Alzheimer's. Dad was so enamoured of all our female 'neighbours' (they introduced themselves as living in the neighbourhood) that I was tempted to keep the interviews going indefinitely. After several more weeks of trial outings with the care-companions Dad seemed most at ease with, we asked Linda and Sophie to be part of our care team and invited them to a home-cooked meal. They already knew each other from having job-shared in the past, and between them they could cover all my working hours. Before they left, I handed them both the following 'onboarding' document. They had been good-naturedly warned that this was coming.

* * * * *

CARE-PARTNER ORIENTATION DOCUMENT

Dear Linda and Sophie,

Thank you so much for taking the time to meet Dad, Felix and me. We're thrilled that you'd like to join our care team. As promised, here is a detailed description of Dad's day-to-day activities. It isn't as complicated as it looks and you'll soon become familiar with things.

Dad's name is Ilija (pronounced ee-lee-ya) but everyone calls him by his nickname, Ika (pronounced eeka).

DAD'S MORNING ROUTINE

When you arrive, please see that Dad has followed his morning routine as outlined below. It seems like a lot, but most of it is self-evident. Apart from inserting his hearing aids, you don't need to do anything except make sure that he has done the following for himself.

1. *Dad inserts his own upper and lower **dentures** every morning. He takes them out before bed and keeps them in a cup of water in his bedroom overnight. I get him to tip the water out of the cup in the bathroom sink in the morning so that he has to put fresh water in the cup every evening. I clean the dentures with a special toothbrush after he goes to bed. Once or twice a week I dissolve a cleaning tablet in the water with the dentures. You won't have to do this as I'll take care of his dentures when I get home.*

2. *If he runs out of denture glue (Polident) while I'm away, I always keep a new tube in the top drawer in the bathroom. I hide it under the shower cap so he doesn't see it, otherwise he'd start a new tube every day! If he asks for new denture glue and you know that he has enough in the old tube, please reassure him that he won't run out and that you have a new tube to give him when required.*

3. *Similarly, I keep a plastic box of disposable **razors** in the second drawer in the bathroom under the blue denture brush. You'll see it in the left-hand side of the drawer. Dad usually shaves himself in the morning. Please check that he has done this. He doesn't have much facial hair so each razor lasts about one week.*

4. *Dad chooses his* **clothes** *for the day. I have labelled in Serbian all the cupboards and drawers where his shirts, jackets, jumpers, trousers, socks and underwear are kept. If you ever need anything, ask him to tell you what the labels on the cupboards mean. He'll be happy to teach you his mother tongue. No doubt he'll also explain why it's called mother tongue: 'because the father never gets a word in!' Be sure to laugh heartily every time!*

5. *If it's a cold morning, sometimes Dad puts his clothes on over his night-shirt. If I discover he has done this, I coax him into taking off his sleepwear and putting on a proper shirt and jumper. Please do the same. If he objects, feel free to play 'good cop, bad cop'. In other words, tell him I'll be upset with you if he wears his night-shirt all day. He won't want you to get into trouble.*

6. *Please allow Dad to put on his* **watch** *without assistance, even if he takes a considerable amount of time to do so. He prides himself in doing things for himself and I can see his sense of achievement whenever he is able to complete a task on his own.*

7. *Please insert Dad's* **hearing aids.** *He will tell you he doesn't need them so you'll have to cajole him into wearing them. If he continues to refuse, it isn't the end of the world if he goes for a day without them. See below for details about where they are kept and how to insert them.*

8. *Dad then eats* **breakfast.** *He starts with a cappuccino (full cream milk), which I make using the coffee machine. Please sprinkle raw cacao over the froth otherwise it's not a real cappuccino. Instructions for the coffee machine are in the drawer immediately under the machine. The cacao and the fine sieve are in the cupboard above the coffee machine. Later in the morning he is happy to drink instant coffee. Ask him which type of coffee he'd prefer. If instant, allow him to tell you how much milk to add. No coffee after 1 pm or it will disrupt his sleep. When I'm home, I cook a three-egg omelette with feta cheese and spinach or scrambled eggs with stir fried mushrooms and home-made low carb bread. If I need to leave the house before he's ready to eat, I boil two eggs (exactly nine minutes) and place them on a plate with a few slices of tomato, cucumber and aforementioned bread. Please butter the bread for him because 'food-preparation is women's work'. I always respond with a list of famous male chefs but I haven't managed to shift his view.*

Pre-Alzheimer's, he always did a fabulous job whenever we had a BBQ but he no longer remembers this.

9. *After breakfast, Dad rinses his plate, cup and cutlery and takes his morning medications. I always re-wash his breakfast dishes when he's not looking. Please do the same as he never uses detergent.*

10. *After Dad has taken his medications, please check the **blue pill organiser** to make sure one of the tablets hasn't remained stuck in the box as this occasionally happens. He might ask you why he needs medications. Please tell him they keep him strong and healthy. He might tell you that he doesn't need to take them. Tell him that his daughter thinks it's important so he'd better take them or you will get into trouble!*

11. *After he has taken his medications, put the blue pill box wherever you find space in the wine fridge (which has everything in it except wine). The wine fridge came with the house, which is ironic given that both Dad and I are allergic to alcohol — yes, such a condition exists. If Dad sees the medication box, he will keep checking to see if he has taken his medications. Take it out of the fridge while he is eating dinner and place it next to his plate when he has finished eating so that he is prompted to take his evening dose.*

12. *When you go out, please make sure that Dad is wearing appropriate **outdoor shoes** and takes a jumper or jacket. He is very sensitive to the cold and it's one of the reasons we moved from Sydney. He did not tolerate Sydney winters and all he wanted to do was stay in bed with the electric blanket on all day. Inside the house he only wears slippers so please help him choose whichever shoes are best for the day.*

13. *If it is sunny, please take his **cap**. There are lots of caps hanging on the large wooden hat rack in the front passage. He can choose whichever cap he wants.*

14. *Dad likes to take his **reading glasses** everywhere he goes. He has had bilateral cataract surgery so his distance vision is excellent. He only needs his glasses for reading fine print but he wears them around his neck for security. He also likes to carry his **glasses case** with him in his right trouser pocket wherever he goes. If he doesn't have the glasses case with him, he will panic that he has lost it.*

15. *I recommend you encourage him to leave his black man bag at home. If he has it with him, it serves as a constant distraction and he is likely to fret and fiddle with it all day long.*

16. *Please check the mailbox with him and bring in the mail. Put it on my desk otherwise Dad will leave it somewhere and forget about it and I may never find it.*

DAD'S HEARING AIDS

HEARING AID INSERTION

1. *After breakfast, please insert Dad's hearing aids into both of his ears. They are marked R (right) and L (left).*

2. *You will find the hearing aids in the Hearing Aid Dehumidifier. This is a small white jar in the yellow box on top of the fridge. Please always put the box back on the fridge.*

3. *When you have taken the hearing aids out of the container, insert the battery into the slot and close up the battery compartment. The battery fits snugly with the smooth side facing outwards.*

4. *Hold the hearing aid with your thumb and index finger on the outer edges of the flesh-coloured plastic part.*

5. *Insert the narrower clear part into his ear. The red R (right) and L (left) stickers need to face the front.*

6. *Rotate the hearing aid slightly backwards for a snug fit. Do NOT push it hard into his ear.*

7. *If he objects, tell him he only needs to keep them in for half an hour. Tell him these little instruments will help keep his hearing sharp.*

8. *If he continues to object, change the subject and distract him. If he resists wearing them, tell him to keep them in for just a few minutes and start talking about something else. He will forget he has them in. I don't think you will have any issues because he has become accustomed to them and accepts them as part of his routine.*

9. *While you are with him, make sure he NEVER takes them out. If he does, reinsert them immediately so that he doesn't lose them. They are very expensive.*

10. I will make sure there is always a fresh battery in each hearing aid so you won't need to change them. However, if Dad tells you that he hears a voice saying 'change battery' please change the battery. He is not hallucinating! The device tells the wearer when the battery is due to be changed! The new batteries will be in a packet in the same box as the hearing aids on top of the fridge.

HEARING AID REMOVAL

1. The hearing aids must NOT get wet. Please take them out before Dad has his shower.

2. Once the hearing aids are out, gently wipe them with the black cloth.

3. Carefully open the battery compartment so that the battery is no longer touching the internal machinery of the hearing aid.

4. Place the hearing aids into the white jar on top of the foam pad.

5. Close the lid securely and place the jar back in the box on top of the fridge ready for the morning. I will, of course, show you everything. It isn't as complicated as it sounds.

DAD'S EVENING ROUTINE

Please check the indoor plant and the two plants in the red pots at the front of the house to see if they need watering. This is Dad's job. Fill the **blue watering can** with cold water and ask Dad to give an equal amount of water to each of the three plants.

6 pm (or earlier if he starts pacing and wanting to go to bed):

1. Please give Dad **dinner** at the glass table. I will label all his meals and place them on the top shelf of the fridge. All you need to do is heat up the appropriate plate. He will often tell you he is not hungry or that he has already eaten or that the meal is too big, but if you put the food in front of him, he will finish his plate. Sometimes I need to distract him with opera music or an André Rieu video. Sometimes he needs more coaxing to eat than at other times. Do your best to ensure he receives adequate nutrition.

2. Feel free to eat dinner with him. You are welcome to any of the prepared meals in the freezer or you can bring your own. Do whatever you prefer.

3. Make sure that Dad takes his **evening medications.** Please check that he gets all four tablets out of the pill organiser because sometimes one of them gets stuck. It's important that he does as much as he can for himself so that he doesn't lose his skills. Even something as seemingly simple as getting pills out of a box can cause frustration when the disease starts impairing a person's dexterity.

4. After dinner, Dad takes a **shower.** This is part of his bedtime routine but occasionally he'll tell you he's already had a shower. It is his memory playing tricks on him. The best thing is not to disagree with him but to try to encourage him to take a shower nonetheless. You might like to suggest that he will sleep better, which is genuinely the case. If he continues to refuse, bring him back to the living room and work on the jigsaw puzzle or play some music and try the shower again in a few minutes. If he remains immovable, let him go to bed without a shower. Hopefully this will not happen, but I want you to be aware of all possible scenarios. Once he is in the shower, he is fine. You might even hear him singing! **Sometimes people with dementia develop very sensitive skin and find it painful when water emanating from the shower hits their body.** If you think this is the case, please let me know and I'll find a gentler alternative.

5. I don't know why Dad always asks if there's hot water in the shower. The answer, of course, is yes. However, he tends not to turn the hot tap far enough so you'll need to turn it on for him and tell him to wait. It takes a while for the hot water to arrive because it is heated by solar panels on the roof.

6. **BEFORE he takes a shower, please take out his hearing aids.** They must NOT get wet. Place them in the little white plastic jar on top of the fridge. The rest of the hearing aid instructions are written above.

7. While Dad is taking a shower and has his back to the door, please grab his underpants and throw them in the tall white laundry basket. Try not to let him see you sneak into the shower because he doesn't like to be seen naked (understandably) and he doesn't think his underpants need washing every day.

8. Dad will get clean underpants from the underpants drawer in his room after he gets out of the shower. The drawer is labelled 'Tatine čiste

gaće'. His underpants fill the top two drawers in his bedroom so he will never run out of clean underwear. Please let him do this for himself.

9. *Also while Dad is in the shower, go into his room and get the clothes he wore that day and place them in the laundry basket.*

10. *After he has had his shower and put on his white night shirt, please* **stick the medication patch to his back.** *The patches are kept in a small pink box in the wine fridge (of course). The name of the medication is Exelon or Rivastigmine. It helps to slow the progression of Alzheimer's disease. Cut open the seal with the scissors in the kitchen drawer and peel off the clear plastic from the back of the round patch. Stick it in a fresh place on his back after removing the old patch from the previous day. You can stick it high up near his neck so he doesn't have to lift his white night shirt. Sometimes the old patch falls off in the shower.*

11. *After he has gone to bed, go to the* **calendar** *stuck on the kitchen bench top and place an X through the day that has just gone so that when Dad wakes up he can see what day it is. This helps him take the medications for the correct day. Use the thick black marker pen on the kitchen bench top.*

12. *This is the routine every evening.*

I also included:
* A list of emergency contact numbers
* Suggested activities and outings.

* * * * *

A few months after the move, I was booked to lead a three-day retreat on the outskirts of Melbourne. Dad was still not back to his pre-move self and I was hesitant to leave him for almost four days — flights and car hire added half a day of travel in each direction. 'He'll be fine,' promised Felix. 'Between Linda, Sophie, Henry and me, your dad won't even notice you're gone. Besides, we've re-established a regular routine and he's much more familiar with the new house. He rarely experiences sundowning anymore and you didn't even need to resort to melatonin.'

I reluctantly boarded the plane.

Dad and Felix were waiting to greet me at the airport on my return. As I approached them, I could see Felix wrapping Dad's hands around a bunch of flowers. 'No!' Dad protested, 'she doesn't deserve flowers. She abandoned me.'

CHAPTER 65

Care conundrums

Being deeply loved by someone gives you strength, while loving someone deeply gives you courage.

LAO TZU (6TH CENTURY BCE)

I was broken.

I felt gutted, guilty and grief-stricken. I'd sought out the perfect brain-boosting house but I'd forgotten the human being who'd be living inside it. How could I have made such a colossal mistake?

'I should have kept him in his home of 43 years and just fixed what needed fixing,' I wailed to Felix.

'You made the decision we both felt was best for him. It wasn't just the house that needed fixing. Every time you drove somewhere, he became distressed by the traffic. Every winter you struggled to get him out of bed. There were no green spaces within walking distance of your home and life was inherently more hectic. Moving here offered an ideal environment for your dad to thrive.'

'It was too big a change for him.'

'Right now, that's how it seems. But he might have become just as unsettled if you'd repaired the old house. Tradespeople, noise, having areas that were off limits, moving furniture to accommodate the work — the place would have been a mess and so would your dad. Nothing in life ever remains static — especially a disease like Alzheimer's.'

'I can't seem to do anything right for him. Everything I try, I'm met with rejection or indifference.'

'It isn't our mistakes that define us, it's how we deal with them. Haven't you always said, "**There's no such thing as failure, there's only feedback**"?'

'I don't know what to do with the feedback. I don't know how to reach him anymore.'

'Hang in there. Continue being kind and loving. Doing small caring acts, day in and day out, will make a difference in the long run. It's like going to the gym and lifting weights. You won't see any difference after the first session. Nor after several sessions. You might even be in pain for a while. But if you keep going, you'll inevitably get stronger. So will your relationship with your dad.'

'It took a long time to build our relationship in the first place. It's heartbreaking seeing things sliding backwards again. It's hard just getting through each day at the moment.'

'**Hard doesn't mean bad.** When things are hard, we discover who we really are and what we're capable of. Popular culture leads us to believe that happiness comes from lack of hardship and achieving success. It doesn't — or only fleetingly. Lasting happiness comes from working towards something bigger than ourselves; from the *pursuit* — not the attainment — of worthwhile goals. Think about it. The minute you achieve something, you're looking for the next challenge. Well, here it is.'

'I didn't want a challenge of this magnitude.'

'We don't always get what we want. But we always get what we *need* in order to grow and learn. When things are easy, we become stagnant; we don't stretch ourselves. It doesn't mean we *want* things to be hard, but hardship is the price we pay for a more meaningful life. Hardship enables us to connect with each other more deeply and authentically because it strips away the piffle. Hardship lets us see what truly matters. It can bring out our strengths or expose our weaknesses. What will it be? It's entirely your choice.'

'Where do I start?'

'Let go of the notion that hard equates to bad. And stop thinking you can control the outcome of your actions. You can't. You can only control *how* you act, not the *results* of your actions. At the moment, your actions don't seem to be delivering what you want them to. Maybe it isn't action that's required. Maybe you just need to be patient and empathic. Release your expectations about how things should be. Let go of having to fix everything. Allow your father the space to find his own way. Just stay true to who you want to be: a loving daughter. He doesn't expect any more from you than that.'

I sighed.

'Do you remember Henry's motto?'

'Focus on what's strong, not wrong,' I recalled.

'So tell me what's strong, not wrong. What do you appreciate about your father? What are you grateful for? What strengths does he still have?'

'Dad loves his new friends: Linda, Sophie and Henry. He loves watching the ducks and swans. He can still communicate in both Serbian and English. He even remembers some French. He's physically fit, he dresses, showers and shaves himself, he eats without assistance and he derives great joy from playing with our neighbour's puppy.'

'Haven't you just listed the most important things in life?' Felix proposed cheerily. 'What's more important than playful connections with people and puppies?'

CHAPTER 66

In search of blood

We often discover what we WILL do by finding out what we will NOT do.

Samuel Smiles (1812–1904)

My conversation with Felix inspired me to dust off our Gratitude Box and place it where I would see it every day. Whenever Dad, Felix or I experienced something we felt profoundly grateful for, we'd write it on a piece of paper, fold up the note and place it in our colourfully decorated Gratitude Box. Conversely, if one of us felt down about something, we'd reach into the box and pull out one of the folded papers. Whatever we read always put the current issue into perspective and lifted our mood. We also celebrated World Gratitude Day every year with an extra special home-cooked dinner followed by taking it in turns to read all the bits of paper we'd amassed in our Gratitude Box during the preceding 12 months. It was my favourite day of the year, made all the more soul-stirring by the fact that **World Gratitude Day and World Alzheimer's Day were on the same date: 21 September.**

Reminding myself of things to be grateful for didn't change the immediate situation, but it lifted my spirits and re-energised me. Feeling grateful generated an optimistic filter through which I perceived life. What I found most challenging was *not* trying to fix things. My knee-jerk response to any obstacle or unwanted turn of events was to do whatever it took to rectify the situation. In the current circumstances, the best thing to do was to accept that Dad was struggling and to keep things as simple as possible. I needed to resist the urge to judge the situation as negative. To quote Hamlet,

'There is nothing either good or bad, but thinking makes it so.' Who knew where our present quandary might lead us? What new ideas, conversations, people or solutions might it bring to our lives? Staying open-minded, curious and supportive was the most healing thing I could do.

If my emotions started getting the better of me, I escaped to medical journal surfing. (Doesn't everyone?) I binge-read article after article on the latest Alzheimer's research being conducted in every corner of the globe. That's when I came across a 2017 Stanford University trial called PLASMA — an acronym for **Pl**asma for **A**lzheimer's **S**ymptom **A**melioration.

Eighteen patients with mild to moderate Alzheimer's were randomly assigned to one of two groups.
- Group 1 received a weekly infusion of blood plasma[7] for four weeks, from young donors aged 18 to 30 years.
- Group 2 received a weekly infusion of placebo saline solution.

After a six-week break (known as 'the wash out period') those who'd received plasma switched to placebo and vice versa. Neither doctors nor patients knew which infusion the participants were receiving (referred to as a 'double-blind' study). Did the plasma confer any benefits? Yes! Not only was it safe and well-tolerated, patients receiving plasma saw improvements in their day-to-day functioning such as cooking, following conversations, remembering to take medications and paying bills.

The PLASMA trial was inspired by experiments in which old mice infused with blood plasma from young mice became better at learning new skills and remembering their way through a maze. This was accompanied by regenerative changes in their brains such as formation of new neurons, stronger connections between existing neurons and reduction in brain inflammation. In another series

---

[7] Plasma is the straw-coloured liquid component of blood that remains after red cells, white cells and platelets have been removed. Plasma consists of 92% water, 7% proteins and 1% hormones, vitamins, mineral salts, fats and sugars. Proteins in plasma play critical roles in blood clotting, fighting infections, transporting substances from one organ to another, and regulating blood pressure and body temperature. Plasma transfusion is not a new concept. It is used to restore blood loss following trauma or to replace missing proteins in people with genetic clotting disorders.

of experiments, old mice were injected with blood plasma from 18-year-old humans. Once again, the older mice produced new cells in their hippocampus and showed improvements in learning and memory.

What was it about young blood that rejuvenated old brains? If plasma was subjected to high temperatures, its brain-boosting effects were lost. Heat disrupts the structure of proteins, therefore it was likely that a protein or collection of proteins might be responsible for plasma's ability to restore mental capacity. As we age, proteins in our blood undergo a number of changes so it's plausible that receiving young proteins could heal ageing organs including the brain. To find out which of the hundreds of proteins in blood might be the silver bullet, scientists will need to compare blood from young and old donors, separate out the proteins, and see which proteins change or decline the most as we age. Then they'll have to test the proteins individually and in combination to elucidate their functions. Eventually, the winning proteins could be packaged into a pill or injection and given to people with Alzheimer's. One of the lead researchers in the early mouse transfusion studies, Stanford professor of neurology, Tony Wyss-Coray PhD, has co-founded a Californian biotechnology company called Alkahest to do just that. Several protein candidates have already emerged. They go by the names of GDF11 (daily shots of this protein increased muscle size and strength in mice), osteopontin (a protein that invigorates our immune system) and TIMP2 (a protein obtained from umbilical cord plasma that makes old mice smarter).

But I didn't have time to wait for years of painstaking research to come up with answers. I needed Dad to receive a dose of young plasma NOW. I already knew that Dad and I were the same blood type, so I wrote a proposal to donate my plasma to Dad (citing the studies that supported my case), emailed it to a progressive haematologist, and made an appointment to see him. I didn't bring Dad with me to the consultation because, first and foremost, I had to establish the feasibility of my plan.

Dr Matthews welcomed me into his office with a warm smile. 'I must say, this is the first time I've had such an interesting request,' he opened our conversation. 'It's certainly a rapidly advancing area of research but there's still so much we don't know about plasma transfusions for people with Alzheimer's. For a start, it's never been done outside a clinical trial.'

'I understand that. I was hoping you might consider taking us on as a case study?'

'It isn't only up to me,' he explained. 'The TGA (Therapeutic Goods Administration) hasn't licensed the use of plasma for treating Alzheimer's so the blood bank is unlikely to come to the party.'

'We don't need the blood bank to be involved if I'm the donor,' I pursued.

Dr Matthews leaned back in his chair and twirled his pen. 'I think your father would be at serious risk of transfusion-associated graft-versus-host disease (TA-GVHD) if he received your plasma.'

'I thought GVHD only occurred with bone marrow transplants, not with plasma transfusions,' I impugned.

'As you know, GVHD occurs when a bone marrow donor's lymphocytes (white blood cells) attack the recipient's skin, liver or gastrointestinal cells. This can cause a range of symptoms from fever, rashes, diarrhoea and liver inflammation to potentially life-threatening infections. It can happen because — despite being a match in terms of blood type — donors and recipients are not an exact genetic match when it comes to every single protein on the surface of their cells,' he paused to put down his pen. 'You're correct in assuming that blood or plasma transfusions don't usually cause GVHD because the recipient's immune system destroys the donor's hostile lymphocytes. However, if you and your father are not an exact match for specific proteins called HLA antigens, his immune system might identify your cells as similar enough not to mount an attack. In contrast, *your* lymphocytes might still regard *his* cells as foreign and start attacking not only his skin, liver and intestines but also his bone marrow. Attacking his bone marrow would be fatal. This is especially likely to occur with a female donor and male recipient, or when the donor is a family member. You tick both boxes.'

What is graft-versus-host disease (GVHD)?

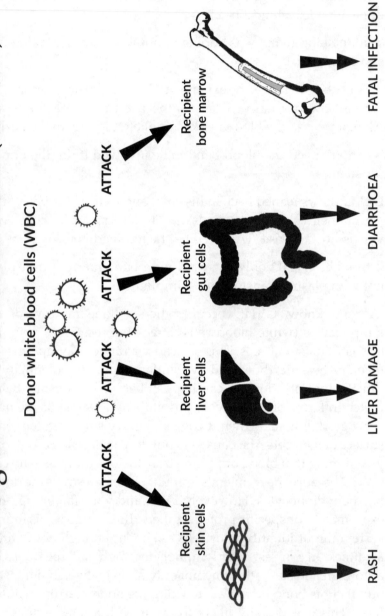

Donor white blood cells (WBC)

ATTACK → Recipient skin cells → RASH

ATTACK → Recipient liver cells → LIVER DAMAGE

ATTACK → Recipient gut cells → DIARRHOEA

ATTACK → Recipient bone marrow → FATAL INFECTION

'I still don't understand why this would happen with plasma transfusions since all my lymphocytes should have been removed,' I persisted.

'Yes, in theory they've been removed. Unfortunately, plasma can still be contaminated by residual blood cells of all types: red, white and platelets,' Dr Matthews explained patiently.

'Wouldn't blast-freezing plasma kill any residual cells? Isn't that why plasma usually comes in the form of fresh frozen plasma (FFP)?' I wasn't ready to give up.

'We used to think so, but experiments have since shown that lymphocytes can survive and function even after freezing and thawing.'

'What about irradiating my plasma before giving it to Dad? Isn't gamma irradiation a way of preventing GVHD?'

Dr Matthews shook his head as he continued apologetically. 'Even in the absence of GVHD, trials in which plasma transfusions improved brain function used donations from young people between the ages of 18 and 30. Your blood would not be young enough to exert the desired effect, even though you're fit and healthy.'

'I had the same reservations,' I confessed, 'but the rate at which our brain processes information is just as fast in our 50s as in our 20s. The outdated belief that mental agility starts to decline in our 20s has been overturned. Our decision-making skills only begin to slow down in our 60s and only to a small degree. I thought that being under 60 might still qualify me as a donor. As it turns out, my age is irrelevant in light of the possibility of GVHD.'

'According to the research, donor age is critical. Frail old mice receiving plasma from similar-aged healthy mice don't show any benefits. Meanwhile, young mice transfused with plasma from old mice *decline* in physical and mental functioning.'

'The studies made it sound so safe and simple,' I sighed.

Dr Matthews shook his head. 'TA-GVHD is much less common with pooled plasma from unrelated donors, but there are other risks associated with plasma transfusions. These include transfusion-associated acute lung injury (TRALI), transfusion-associated circulatory overload (TACO), allergic transfusion reactions (ATR) and transmission of infections such as HIV. We also have no idea how long any brain-benefits might last. Would your father need to have monthly transfusions to maintain his brain gains? Would repeated transfusions increase his risk of developing an autoimmune disease or cancer? If this really worked, how would we keep up with the demand for young plasma? I'd have grave concerns about the emergence of a black market for young blood. There are still so many unknowns associated with this. Some scientists suggest that we don't just need to give old people young proteins, we also need to remove old proteins that are causing damage. Reversing brain degeneration through manipulation of blood components is likely to involve a complex interplay between hundreds of different compounds. A start-up company called Unity Biotechnology is developing a device similar to a dialysis machine that passes a person's blood through a filter to clear out harmful compounds before re-infusing the blood back into their body. This would eliminate risks of GVHD because you're receiving your own blood. The idea makes me feel more comfortable than relying on donors, but the process wouldn't be pleasant and is still years away from human trials. I'm sorry to disappoint you.'

I left Dr Matthew's office feeling utterly deflated.

* * * * *

Although my hopes for Dad to receive youthful plasma did not materialise, scientists continue to search for brain-boosting ingredients in blood. In December 2021, a fascinating experiment was published in the prestigious multidisciplinary science journal *Nature*. Stanford University researchers placed mice in one of four groups:

- Group 1 were allowed to run on an exercise wheel whenever they wanted for one month.
- Group 2 had their exercise wheel locked for one month.
- Group 3 were also kept sedentary and then received a blood transfusion from Group 1 (the exercising mice).
- Group 4 were kept sedentary and received a blood transfusion from Group 2 (the non-exercising mice).

What were the results?

The exercising mice increased the size of their hippocampus (the brain's learning and memory centre) and performed better in tests of brain function. The sedentary mice experienced no increase in brain volume and were not as smart as their exercising compatriots. However, the mice who received a blood transfusion from the exercising mice also became smarter!

What was going on?

Physical exercise stimulates the production of hundreds of different proteins, many of them involved in reducing inflammation and stimulating brain cell growth. A blood transfusion allows the transfer of anti-inflammatory brain-healing proteins from one mouse to another. A protein called clusterin (CLU) was found to be particularly potent. Was this something that only pertained to mice or did the same thing happen in humans? When 20 veterans with mild cognitive impairment (MCI) were put on an exercise program three days a week for six months, they had higher levels of clusterin (CLU) in their blood and performed better in memory tests. Does this mean blood transfusions from athletes could make us smarter? Or will clusterin become available as a medication one day? Maybe, but I'd rather just do some exercise myself.

PART SEVEN

Education is more powerful than medication

To be what we are, and to become what we are capable of becoming, is the only end of life.

ROBERT LOUIS STEVENSON (1850–1894)

CHAPTER 67

Let music be your medicine

Where words fail, music speaks.

Hans Christian Andersen (1805–1875)

After my appointment with the haematologist, I took a break from medical journal surfing and turned my attention to shoe arranging. The Japanese have made flower arranging into an art (ikebana), so why not shoe arranging? For all the anguish of dealing with my mother's hundreds of pairs of shoes while decluttering and packing up the old house, they now became a source of solace. Sorting and organising them in our new home was soothing and meditative. My first task was to buy individual transparent plastic boxes from a discount variety shop to store them in. I bought all 112 boxes in the emporium and promised to return when they received more stock. I then spent several days debating how to categorise the shoes: by season, style, colour or era? Summer sandals through to winter boots, or casual loafers through to killer heels? What about making each row of shoes a colour of the rainbow? Topped and tailed with a row of white and a row of black. No, that didn't work because there were many more black shoes than white shoes. I also needed a dedicated row of crazy shoes — shoes with macrame butterflies, bouncing baubles and diamanté buckles. The most ridiculous aspect of the endeavour was that I didn't care about shoes. But I did care about Mum. That's what it was all about.

One blustery evening, Dad and I snuggled down on the couch to watch *Alive Inside* — the documentary about music and memory that Henry had recommended. Dad was still not back to his level of functioning prior to the move, but at least I was keeping the

Moon Men away. From the opening scene of the film, I was blown away by it. The story follows Dan Cohen, a social worker who was bringing music to nursing home residents. The film begins with Dan asking a 90-year-old long-time occupant, 'What was life like when you were a little girl?'

Her response is dolefully apologetic. 'I'm very sorry, I don't remember. I've forgotten so much. I've forgotten what I used to do after I became a young lady. If I could remember, I would tell you, but I can't remember.'

Dan then gently tells her he wants to try an experiment. He places headphones over her ears and says, 'I want you to try and let the music take you back into your memories, back in time. Where does the music take you?' The song is Louis Armstrong's rendition of 'When the saints go marching in'. The 90-year-old woman correctly identifies the music and suddenly her memories come flooding back. She relates intricate details about her school dance — 'Mama told us not to go and listen to him but we would sneak off at night and bring back pictures' — and discusses the various places she worked, what she did during World War II, and the date of her son's birthday. Her speech is fluent, her vocabulary is rich and her demeanour is animated. Her concluding remarks are punctuated by laughter: 'I didn't know I could talk so much!'

She is not an isolated case. The movie introduces us to countless other nursing home residents, all of whom are transformed by music that has personal significance for them. Pre playlist, their posture is stooped, their eyes are half closed and they are angry, agitated or minimally responsive. Within minutes of listening to their favourite songs, they straighten up, their eyes are wide open and they start singing, dancing or tapping their feet. Their songs enable them to recapture their identity, history and connection with others. When a hitherto incognisant elderly man is asked 'What does music do to you?' he replies with new-found coherence and enthusiasm, 'It gives me the feeling of love. I feel the band of love and dreams. God gave me these sounds.'

The healing metamorphoses must be seen to be believed. Like a caterpillar that no longer needs its protective cocoon, those who are touched by music spread their wings and reveal their true colours. When a person's selfhood is peeled away by Alzheimer's, music can restore it — at least temporarily. Music can draw people out of themselves and reach those who seem unreachable. Familiar music transports them to a world they know. It reconnects them with who they were and who they remain at their core. Music shows people that joy and love still reside inside them. Music coaxes out their vital spark. I recommend everyone watch *Alive Inside* (aliveinside.us) — it is simultaneously heartbreaking, heartwarming and eminently inspiring.

Music is inseparable from emotion. Music can heal trauma by allowing us to experience our feelings. This is where **a qualified music therapist can facilitate deep healing**. The therapist begins by playing music or singing a song that matches the mood of the listener and validates how they feel. Gradually the therapist transitions to an uplifting melody, slowly guiding the patient to a more joyous state. Music is an invisible hand that can lead us out of despair. This is but one example of music therapy — the science-based use of music to achieve individualised goals related to psychological or physical illness, injury or distress.

We're all moved by music. A study of 220 people published in the journal *Psychology of Music* found that when we're sad, listening to what we personally identify as beautiful music (not necessarily upbeat or happy music) is a reliable way of lifting our mood. When we listen to familiar, appealing music, we feel empowered, we stop struggling and we allow the harmonious sounds to carry us to a fond reminiscence, a future hope or a dance floor. At the most basic level, **by lowering stress, music automatically increases a person's ability to function**, especially when they're living with a disease like dementia.

We instinctively know there's something magical about music. Why? How does music exert its manifold effects? What makes music so powerful? How does music revive dormant memories and despondent souls? In Alzheimer's, why is our memory for music not only spared, but brings a tapestry of memories along with it? Many musicians also retain the ability to play their instruments (referred to as implicit procedural memory) even in advanced stages of Alzheimer's. If someone you know has Alzheimer's and previously played an instrument, dust it off and encourage them to start playing again. You might both be pleasantly surprised at the beautiful music they're still able to produce.

No doubt the fact that we listen to our favourite songs over and over helps to cement them into our brain's architecture. Likewise, a musician practises daily for decades. However, repetition doesn't hold up in Alzheimer's when it comes to remembering how to cook, dress or find our way home. Something more complex is going on in the brain when it comes to music. Seeking answers to these questions led me down another research rabbit hole.

Dan Cohen speaks about music as a back door to the brain. Music is not merely a right hemisphere function nor is there a 'music centre' in the brain. Rather, **music is a super-stimulus that activates vast and varied regions of our brain**, depending on the type and familiarity of the music. If one area of the brain is compromised, there are other pathways through which music can reach us. In addition, fMRI and FDG-PET scans show that brain areas involved in encoding long-term musical memory remain preserved in people with Alzheimer's, even when other regions of their brain show shrinkage and impaired glucose metabolism.

Not only can our favourite music unlock our memories, research has demonstrated that **music is as powerful as medicine** (in some cases more so) in a wide range of contexts and conditions.

As early as 1991, Dr Deforia Lane, music therapy consultant based in Cleveland Ohio USA, published a study of 40 hospitalised children between the ages of six and 12 years. Half of the children were randomly assigned to an experimental group and the other half to a control group. The experimental group engaged in 30 minutes of singing and playing musical instruments. The control group were allowed to spend 30 minutes in whatever activity they chose, such as reading, playing games or talking on the phone. Before and after the activities, all children gave a sample of saliva to be tested for salivary immunoglobulin A (IgA) — a protein that neutralises toxins and protects us from infections. The children in the music group demonstrated an increase in IgA levels while the children engaged in other activities did not. **Music strengthens our immune system** after a single 30-minute session.

Music can also mend minds. A personalised playlist is more effective than any Alzheimer's drugs currently available. Nursing homes that create individualised selections of music for their residents to listen to on a daily basis have much less need for antipsychotic medications. Antipsychotics are drugs used to manage acute distress, delusions, hallucinations and paranoia, but in elderly populations their effect is minimal and they do more harm than good. Antipsychotics can cause muscle spasms, restlessness, tremor or rigidity as well as dose-dependent brain shrinkage. In other words, the higher the dose and the more often the drugs are given, the greater the reduction in brain volume. For someone with dementia, this is adding insult to injury. Any measures that reduce the use of antipsychotics should be eagerly embraced, especially something as simple to implement (with no negative side effects) as music.

In facilities where music is part of standard care, staff report that residents are friendlier, happier and more co-operative. This boosts staff morale and improves quality of life for both staff and residents. There are several mechanisms through which music can exert remedial effects. Familiar and much-loved music promotes relaxation, reduces anxiety and elicits positive emotions that the listener has previously linked to the music. It can also be a form of self-expression and encourages social interaction through sharing, singing along and talking about the music. In some instances, patients who were unresponsive prior to hearing their favourite song suddenly recognised a relative and began engaging with them. Even after music stops, brain activity can remain heightened for 20 minutes to several hours.

Taking things a step further, researchers from the University of Helsinki in Finland studied the effects of musical activities in 89 pairs of dementia patients and their care-companions. One group took part in a 10-week singing program. The second group focused on listening to music. A third group were given standard care without any musical activities. After nine months, those in either the

singing or music groups showed improvements in concentration, memory, mood and reasoning ability, compared to the group that only received standard care. Singing produced the greatest benefits in people under the age of 80 with mild dementia, while music-listening was best for those with more advanced forms of dementia. Depression was alleviated equally well in both groups. It didn't matter whether or not a person had previous musical experience; they benefitted either way.

In another study, researchers from Iowa State University in Ames, USA, demonstrated that in people with Parkinson's disease, singing could improve their ability to control their breathing and swallowing, increase the volume of their voice and enhance their ability to be understood. Singing also lowered stress, anxiety, blood pressure and symptoms of depression. An unexpected corollary was reduction in their tremors, easier use of their upper limbs and steadier gait. The scientists described the participants as 'having a spring in their step' whenever they finished a singing session. Subsequently, the concept of *ParkinSong* has spread throughout the globe. Local groups of Parkinson's patients regularly meet with a music therapist to sing together and learn skills that preserve their speech. Our vocal cords are like any other muscle — they can be strengthened through targeted exercise.

There are various reasons for the therapeutic effects of singing, many of which are still being discovered. Singing stimulates the production of oxytocin (the calming and bonding hormone), reduces inflammation and enriches connections between brain cells. Singing in a choir unites and energises us.

In 2011, a study at McGill University in Canada found that when people listened to music, they produced the neurotransmitter dopamine, which boosts motivation, makes us feel good and enhances fluidity and control of our movements. Hence people with Parkinson's can often dance more easily than they can walk. Next time you get a sugar craving or feel the urge to comfort eat, listen to your favourite piece of music and allow yourself to become immersed in it. Chances are, your urge to self-soothe with food will dissipate. If you're prone to bouts of low mood or depression, find a variety of songs and musical pieces that trigger happy memories or simply make you feel better. Then listen to them frequently – not only when you're depressed, but every day. It's like taking medication — you don't just take one dose and expect to be cured. Administer your musical medicine several times a day, and your depressive symptoms are likely to reduce in frequency and severity.

An analysis of 72 trials involving over 7000 surgical patients revealed that listening to music after their operation reduced anxiety, pain and discomfort to the extent they required significantly less pain medication than patients undergoing the same procedures who did not listen to music. The greatest pain relief was seen in patients who were allowed to choose their own song list. Music played prior to surgery can even lead to lower requirements for anaesthesia!

One of the ways in which **music relieves pain** is by triggering the production of endorphins (endogenous opioids) in the pituitary gland of the brain. The primary role of endorphins is to block pain signals and induce a state of euphoria. Even in people with severe fibromyalgia, music was found to improve movement and lessen pain and fatigue.

Stroke patients are also benefitting from the use of music. Listening to two hours of music every day enhances not only their mood but also their concentration and ability to remember words and abstract concepts. In stroke patients with speech difficulties, a technique known as Neurological Music Therapy (NMT) is being used to help them regain lost language skills.

I soon became buried in study after study on the use of music as medicine. The overarching message is that music — in particular a personalised playlist created specifically for the individual with dementia — is an under-utilised, inexpensive, easy to implement and effective therapy for anxiety, agitation, apathy, aggression, depression, sundowning, low energy, lack of motivation, withdrawal, pain, discomfort and movement disorders. It can also boost memory, alertness and social engagement. Just because it doesn't come in a pill, potion or lotion doesn't mean it is any less potent. In many instances, music is *more* potent and doesn't have harmful side effects. It also comes with a bonus: healthcare workers and care-partners report that giving the gift of music lifts their own spirits and makes their job easier.

It was time to give Dad a dose of music. I'd instinctively been playing calming melodies to ameliorate his sundowning and to accompany mealtimes, but I hadn't compiled a dedicated playlist to aid Dad's functioning in other contexts, or to improve his general quality of life. I had several hundred of his and Mum's CDs crammed into battered boxes, so I started playing each of them in turn and asking for his feedback. Research published in the *Journal of Multidisciplinary Healthcare* revealed a 'reminiscence bump' between the ages of 13 and 19, when music embeds itself most deeply into our psyche. Other studies found that our 20s are also significant times for music and memories to become entwined. Dad was born in 1931 so I focused on music from the mid 40s through to the early 60s. He had no hesitation expressing his preferences and telling me the stories that belonged to 'his' songs — the first opera his mother took him to see when he was eight years old (*La Traviata*), sneaking out with his aunt to visit a fortune teller, dancing in the streets of Paris, serenading Mum at their favourite restaurant in Skadarlija, Belgrade ... His transformation overwhelmed me. Sometimes I'd just play a CD and observe his reaction — a smile, a tear or an animated conversation would ensue. Sometimes he would grab my hand and start waltzing me around the living room. Music took him to a place inside himself where he felt safe and self-assured. I realised that playing his special music wasn't about entertaining or distracting him, it was about reconnecting with him on an emotional level. Nothing, but nothing, was more important than that.

Music brought him back from the moon and gave him moments of clarity. In fact, it was more than mere moments — the effect of a handful of songs could last for hours. Each song was like a stepping stone to his former effervescent self.

Playing his happy songs was particularly helpful at shower time — a 'chore' he frequently objected to. After a few verses of *Singing in the rain*, he'd forget that he didn't like showering. Getting ready to visit the dentist or ear-cleaning clinic was aided by *We're off to see the wizard, the wonderful Wizard of Oz*. Any time I needed to transition him from one activity to another that he wasn't keen on, music was my go-to aid. I encouraged all his care-companions to play his favourite songs when in the car or to simply spend a few unhurried hours at home exploring his musical past.

With all the established benefits of music that have been unfolding since the 1940s, it begs the question: why aren't personalised playlists part of standard care for all elderly people in aged care residences and in their own home? Why isn't music used therapeutically in hospitals? Pre and post surgery, for pain management, stroke, brain injury, anxiety — I can't think of a condition in which carefully chosen music would not facilitate healing. As soon as I typed the words, I could hear the protestations by decisions-makers in healthcare. 'We don't have the time or resources to ask patients or relatives about their preferred music and special songs. Or to figure out from their age and cultural background, the type of music that would provide the greatest comfort. Then there's the issue of administering music. Staff are already overworked as it is. Who would create the playlist and load it onto an iPod? Where would we get headphones? It all takes time and money.'

Of course it does, but it would save time and money in the long run. Pharmaceutical costs and length of hospital stays would go down, while staff morale would go up. Music enhances balance, co-ordination and basic bodily functions such as swallowing. This translates to fewer falls, less choking and a reduction in aspiration pneumonia. The benefits would more than compensate for the set-up costs. We all want to make a positive difference to our fellow human. **The problem is not a lack of resources, but a lack of belief that anything other than pharmaceutical products constitutes medicine.**

Music would be easy to implement in aged care facilities if we had the will to do so. The website musicandmemory.org provides free guides for care-partners and health professionals to bring therapeutic music to older people.

If you're a care-partner, visit:
musicandmemory.org/resources/#loved-one
— *How to Make a Personalised Playlist for a Loved One at Home.*

If you're a care professional, visit:
musicandmemory.org/resources/#free-guides
— *Making the Case for Personalised Music: A Guide for Care Professionals*.

At the time of writing, the *Music and Memory Program* was in 650 nursing homes across the United States … and counting.

Family and friends visiting their loved ones report that music removes the awkwardness of their visit. Music offers a shared experience, a topic of conversation and an alternative means of communicating with people in advanced stages of dementia. Music can loosen the grip of dementia, at least temporarily.

Countless other websites offer therapeutic music programs (live and virtual) for individuals, families and healthcare facilities. Visit: outwittingalzheimers.com for a comprehensive list that I update on a regular basis.

Music is a means through which anyone can help outwit Alzheimer's. You don't need to be able to sing or play music yourself. Encourage your parents, grandparents or elderly neighbour to join a choir. Volunteer to create a playlist for someone living in an aged care residence; donate an iPod and headphones; sit with an older person and listen to their chosen music with them. If you *do* play music, take your violin, guitar, flute or voice to your local aged care facility and play a tune. Your gift will come back to you in ways you couldn't imagine. Changing one person can change an entire room. This is truly one area in which anyone can contribute.

For people with dementia, **music is not a desirable, it's an essential.**

The magic of music inspired me to borrow a song from *The Sound of Music* and adapt it to our situation. Instead of *How Do You Solve a Problem Like Maria?* I sang: *How Do You Solve a Problem Like* **Dementia?** If you'd like to sing along, my version is shown overleaf:

*How Do You Solve a Problem Like **Dementia**?*

Dementia makes me feel perplexed
About what's going on
I don't remember people's names
And when I do, they're gone
And underneath **my friendly smile**
I feel that life's a con
I even **wonder what's the date tomorrow?**

I'm often lost and muddled
I do not know what is real
I don't remember how to plan
Or cook a healthy meal
I hate to have to say it
But I very firmly feel
My brain is not an asset to **my body**

I'd like to say a word **on my** behalf
Poems make me laugh

*How do you solve a problem like **dementia**?*
How do you catch a thought and pin it down?
*How do you find a word that means **dementia**?*
A memory glitch! A brain under siege! A dare!

Many a thing I know **I'd like to tell you**
Many a thing **I** ought to understand
But how do **I concentrate**
When I am in this state?
My brain no longer follows my command

Oh, how do you solve a problem like **dementia**?
How do you hold a **memory** in your hand?...

See Song 3 at the end of the book for the complete lyrics.

CHAPTER 68

Education prevents stagnation

Anyone who stops learning is old, whether at twenty or eighty.
Anyone who keeps learning stays young. The greatest thing in
life is to keep your mind young.

HENRY FORD (1863–1947)

Music is not only therapeutic after someone has developed dementia; learning to play a musical instrument can help stave off dementia in the first place.

The importance of lifelong active learning, mental challenges, intellectual pursuits and creative thinking cannot be overstated. There is no shortage of research showing that **the more we engage in mentally stimulating activities throughout our lives, the less likely we are to develop Alzheimer's** or experience cognitive decline. Even after cognitive decline begins, mental stimulation can slow further deterioration, especially if combined with other brain-boosting pursuits.

What then constitutes mental stimulation? Does a mentally demanding job serve as a buffer against Alzheimer's? Yes — as long as it doesn't push us into chronic stress, depression or burnout. Are some forms of mental activity more beneficial than others? Is it better to learn a musical instrument or a foreign language? Take up drawing, painting, writing, calligraphy, pottery, basket weaving, archery, cooking, carpentry, photography, chess, drama or ancient history classes? Learn to sing, dance, juggle, crochet, embroider, memorise poems or play mahjong? Join a book club, environmental action group, debating team or Toastmasters? Visit museums, art galleries, wildlife sanctuaries or foreign lands? What about crosswords, sudoku, Wordle, bridge, boardgames, darts, dominos, origami, orienteering, meditation, reading Shakespeare or online brain training? Is it more valuable to attain mastery in one thing or to engage in a variety of activities and reach a modest level of skill? Jack and Jill of all trades or master of one?

Any and all of the above. Learning to play a musical instrument or speak a foreign language top the charts in terms of their brain-boosting power. Crosswords and sudoku, while better than watching TV, have a much weaker effect.

In 2013, researchers in Barcelona, Spain, recruited men and women aged 60 to 84 years with no prior musical training and taught them to play the piano. They had one group lesson per week, complemented by 45 minutes of individual daily practice. They were also educated in music theory and sight-reading. An age-matched control group participated in other activities such as painting, philosophy and computer lessons. After four months, those in the piano-playing group showed dramatic improvements in attention, processing speed, short-term memory and quality of life, along with less depression and lower stress levels. Those in the control group also saw improvements but to a lesser extent. Perhaps, given enough time, the painters and philosophers would have caught up with the piano players in terms of brain-benefits? Unfortunately, the study only lasted four months so the question remains unanswered.

Another study called The Synapse Project conducted at the University of Texas, USA, in 2014, differentiated between what they termed *productive* (active) and *receptive* (passive) engagement. *Productive engagement* refers to learning novel information or new skills that require active participation, decision-making and use of short- and long-term memory. In contrast, *receptive engagement* involves familiar activities, relying on existing knowledge or passive observation. Productive engagement obviously puts more demands on our brain than receptive engagement. To drill down further, over two hundred 60- to 90-year-olds were randomly assigned to one of six groups, each of which spent 16 hours a week for 14 weeks in one of the following structured activities:

- Group 1 were taught digital photography including the use of photo-editing software.
- Group 2 were taught how to design and sew quilts.
- Group 3 learnt both photography and quilting, splitting their time between the two activities. This means their learning involved more variety but less depth than Groups 1 and 2 because they could only spend half as much time on each activity.
- Group 4 participated in organised social activities including cooking, watching movies, reminiscing, playing luck-based games and going on themed field trips.
- Group 5 were provided with a range of home-based activities including word games, crossword puzzles, documentaries, DVDs, CDs and magazines such as *National Geographic* and *Reader's Digest*.
- Group 6 were asked to make no changes in their lives. They simply completed a weekly checklist of their daily activities.

Groups 1 to 3 comprised productive engagement while Groups 4 and 5 spent their time in receptive engagement. Group 6 were the controls.

All participants completed extensive tests of memory, concentration, processing speed and visuospatial skills (the ability to distinguish between different objects and hold a mental image of them) before and after the 14-week study. What would you predict was the outcome?

All five groups involved in doing something improved their test scores. However, those who learned digital photography (the most demanding of the activities for the 60- to 90-year-olds), either alone or in combination with quilting, had the most dramatic improvements in what is known as episodic memory. Episodic memory refers to memory of recent and past everyday events such as what you ate for breakfast yesterday or the details of your wedding day 30 years ago.

The message is that **any mental activity is better than no mental activity, and the more demanding the better. Use it or lose it. Train it and regain it.** From a lifespan perspective, more years of education (both formal and informal) and higher occupational attainment lead to greater protection against Alzheimer's through building what is known as **cognitive reserve.** The term cognitive reserve originated in the 1980s when autopsies revealed that many people with no symptoms of dementia nonetheless had physical brain changes consistent with advanced Alzheimer's. Likewise, a stroke causing the same amount of physical damage in two people can produce profound impairment in one patient but minimal symptoms in another.

This indicates that the brains of some people are able to continue functioning in spite of structural damage because they've developed backup pathways to compensate. Cognitive reserve is like having a second income stream. If you lose one job, you still have the funds to keep your life going. Similarly, if we lose one circuit in the brain, we can use alternative pathways to accomplish the same cognitive task. Cognitive reserve is built up through lifelong learning, problem-solving, mentally demanding work, seeking out new experiences and all the other proactive measures discussed in this book. **When the going gets tough, the resilient brain keeps going.**

Receptive engagement alone is not enough. **Stretch yourself as much as you can by doing as many different things as you enjoy.** Just as we regularly exercise our body to stay physically fit, we need to regularly exercise our brain to keep mentally fit. And just as we need different exercises for different body parts (squats, chest press, bicep curls, etc.) we need different types of brain training for different mental functions. The process of learning — including discovering new cultures and exploring unfamiliar neighbourhoods — is what matters most because it increases brain blood flow and BDNF levels. The more taxing you find something (without it being so hard that you give up) the better. **Our brain doesn't stop learning because we get old. Our brain gets old because we stop learning.** There is no age at which we are unable to learn new things, including languages.

A study from Michigan State University, USA, found that Nobel Prize-winning scientists are almost three times more likely (2.85 times to be precise) than the average scientist to have an artistic or craft-related hobby such as painting, poetry, dancing, photography, glassblowing, acting or playing music. This suggests that brain function is enhanced by engaging in diverse pursuits. Art and science are not mutually exclusive; they are cross-training for the brain. Leonardo da Vinci is the quintessential example: he was as much an inventor and philosopher as a brilliant painter and sculptor.

Whenever we learn a new skill or engage in something that is stimulating and challenging, we form new brain cells (neurogenesis) and new connections between them (synaptogenesis). Regularly practising the new skill or using the new information strengthens those connections, thus making the task easier. If you continue to find an activity challenging, it will continue to boost your brain. Once we get good at something or start finding it effortless, it's time to find another challenge. By all means, keep up the old activity if you find it enjoyable. But to continue boosting our brain, we need to continue extending ourselves. What matters is that *you* find it stimulating. Older people with minimal computer experience benefit far more from computer-based activities than young people for whom computers are second nature. **Boredom, monotony and sameness are poison for our brain.** Choose a new holiday destination every year. Don't get stuck in a rut.

If the activity also happens to be social or physical, it will boost our brain even more. This is another reason why playing music, dancing and foreign language-learning seem to be particularly effective in enhancing brain function. Learning a musical instrument involves a vast number of different brain regions. It requires careful listening, keeping time, reading a new language and practising co-ordinated movements with our hands, feet or mouth. Musicians are subsequently better than the rest of us at remembering spoken information and discerning speech in noisy environments (an increasing challenge as we age).

Dancing is not only physically and socially engaging, it requires us to listen, balance, keep time, make judgments, synchronise our limbs and memorise steps. It's also a source of fun and laughter. An interesting corollary of dancing with other people is that it makes us prosocial. When toddlers are bounced in time to music, they are more content and co-operative than if they are bounced out of time with the beat. Similarly, studies in adults have shown that moving in flow with others makes us more caring, sharing and generous. It worked a treat with Dad. Whenever he didn't want to come shopping, weed the garden or hang out the washing with me, I'd put on Mozart's *The Marriage of Figaro,* and after swinging me around the living room for a few minutes, he was ready to follow me out the door.

Bi- and multilingualism also confer specific brain-benefits. Being able to speak more than one language sharpens our ability to focus on what is relevant and to ignore distractions. The bilingual brain is also better at switching from one task to the next, and more resilient to cognitive decline and Alzheimer's — even in people who are illiterate.

If you haven't yet learnt a second language, it's not too late to start, regardless of your age. In addition to being a complex intellectual activity, learning a foreign language facilitates social engagement and ignites interest in different cultures, thus fostering overseas travel and exposure to novel environments — a domino brain-boosting effect.

If you find language-learning intimidating, scientists have found a way to make remembering new words easier. Adults learning Hungarian were divided into three groups. The first group were taught to speak Hungarian phrases just as they would in ordinary conversation. The second group were asked to sing the phrases, while the third group had to repeat the phrases in a rhythmic fashion. When they were later tested, those who had sung the phrases remembered them more easily and with greater accuracy than either of the other two groups. So give your brain a double boost by learning to sing songs in a foreign language.

Our individual needs often dictate which mentally stimulating activities provide us with the greatest benefits. People who have had a stroke might beat on drums to improve gross motor movements or do embroidery to regain fine motor skills. Memorising facts, figures and grocery lists leads to a better memory and a bigger hippocampus. Contrary to public opinion, **we are able to memorise a list of words just as well in our 50s as in our 20s.** In fact, the current generation of 50-plus-year olds are probably better at memorisation than 20-year-olds because they didn't have mobile phones in their adolescent years and therefore had to remember phone numbers and other facts now stored on handheld devices.

There are infinite possibilities for giving ourselves a mental workout. To get started, use the following questions to guide you:

- What is something you've always wanted to do / learn / study / explore but never had the chance?
- What fascinates you?
- What excites you?
- What are you passionate about?
- What are you a little fearful of trying?
- What are you curious about?
- What would you find fun?
- What would bring you joy and fulfilment?

Go and do it.

Go and study it.

Just give it a go!

Are you afraid of not being talented enough or smart enough? Of being too old or too slow? None of that matters. Getting good at something isn't what brings the greatest benefits. Making a concerted effort to learn something challenging is what matters. Feeling uncomfortable — but not overwhelmed — is a sign that you're changing your brain for the better. Exertion is what it feels like to build up our brain. If it's a breeze from the get-go, it isn't boosting your brain. I have never had any musical training so one of my goals is to stimulate my brain in a completely new way by learning to play the piano.

Teaching others is another terrific brain-booster. Teaching not only stretches our thinking, it brings purpose and meaningful social interactions into our lives. Is there something you could volunteer to teach at your local kindergarten, primary school, community college or University of the Third Age (U3A)? It doesn't have to be something of an academic nature. You could pass on your knowledge of how to make paper aeroplanes, grow herbs, knit scarves or cook traditional meals. Or perhaps you could coach a child who is struggling with reading, writing or basic arithmetic.

What about teaching adolescents and adults how to change a car tyre or use a sewing machine? The opportunities to help or teach others are endless if we seek them out. The very process of planning, deciding and organising how to incorporate more mental challenges into our lives is itself a brain-booster.

Here is another song I've adapted from *The Sound of Music* to stimulate ideas of your own.

My **Brain-Boosting** Things

Singing and dancing and **stroking my** kittens
Learning a language and **knitting new** mittens
Playing piano or plucking harp strings
These are a few of my **brain-boosting** things

Cherries and berries and crisp apple **slices**
Helping my neighbours and **cooking with spices**
Reading and drawing, admiring paintings
These are a few of my **brain-boosting** things

Walking in nature and soaking up sunlight
Flossing my teeth before sleeping the whole night
Nurturing friendships and swimming in springs
These are a few of my **brain-boosting** things

When **I get lost**
When **a wound** stings
When I'm feeling sad
I simply remember my **brain-boosting** things
And then I don't feel so bad

Singing and dancing and **stroking my** kittens
Learning a language and **knitting new** mittens
Playing piano or plucking harp strings
These are a few of my **brain-boosting** things ...

CHAPTER 69

Neurobics

Education is the kindling of a flame, not the filling of a vessel.

SOCRATES (CIRCA 470–399 BCE)

Have you ever thought about *how* you think?

Do you think critically about what you hear or read in the media, or do you take things at face value?

Do you reflect on the status quo and consider how things could be done more efficiently?

Do you perform routine chores on autopilot or do you try to devise ways to make them more interesting?

Do you have lively discussions with people whose opinions differ from yours?

Do you seek to learn from unwanted situations or do you blame misfortune?

Are you able to:
- prioritise your most important tasks for the day?
- stay focused on the task at hand?
- sift through information and extract what is relevant to your current needs?
- weigh up the pros and cons of taking on a new role?
- think on your feet when faced with an unexpected obstacle?
- consider an issue from different perspectives?

The way we organise our thoughts, analyse information, make decisions, entertain divergent viewpoints and approach problem-solving can serve as mental gymnastics that keep our brains performing at their peak. In other words, **we can learn to think in ways that energise rather than drain our brain.** This is sometimes referred to as **neurobics** (akin to aerobics for the body): practising ways of thinking that make us smarter, sharper and more resilient to Alzheimer's.

The previous chapter discussed the importance of lifelong active learning — referred to as productive engagement. This chapter outlines the importance of **lifelong active thinking** — which I refer to as **productive reflection.** Without having to step outside our heads, we can increase our capacity for learning, generating new ideas and managing whatever mental challenges life throws our way. Productive reflection leads to greater productivity in all areas of our lives and helps build cognitive reserve. A sharp memory is not the only measure of a healthy brain — the ability to focus, ignore distractions, make plans and come up with new solutions to old problems are all important measures of a robust brain.

Productive reflection is a mental skill that improves with age if we practise it because of our accumulated years of knowledge and life experience. Productive reflection strengthens the functioning of our frontal lobes — the seat of our deepest thinking, reasoning, understanding and goal-setting. Productive reflection is a buffer against boredom and leads to wisdom and insight. Productive reflection will lead us out of current world problems including Alzheimer's.

What, then, does productive reflection entail?

Refer back to the quote by Socrates at the beginning of this chapter.

How would you explain the meaning of the quote? Consider your own answer before reading mine.

Here is my interpretation: a flame, once ignited, continues to draw on surrounding fuel and becomes self-sustaining. In the same way, true education ignites the fire of curiosity and stimulates ongoing learning — not only for the purpose of acquiring knowledge, but for the sheer joy of learning. The word 'educate' stems from the Latin *educere* meaning 'to lead out'. The aim of education is to make us more resourceful and bring out our innate love of learning, not to fill our minds with rote-learned facts.

The process of extracting multiple meanings from a quote, poem or story is an example of productive reflection. So is implementing the suggestions implicit in the questions at the beginning of this chapter:

- Think about how you think.
- Critically evaluate what you read.
- Consider how things could be done more efficiently.
- Devise ways to make routine chores more interesting.
- Have lively discussions with people whose opinions differ from yours.
- Seek to learn from every situation and person you meet.
- Prioritise your most important tasks for the day (no more than three — preferably two).

I'll leave you to extrapolate the rest.

When you habitually practise productive reflection, your brain power will soar.

In addition, take the following five breaks on a regular basis:

1. **Take a break from constantly needing to be busy or attached to technology**. It's just as important to **still the mind** as it is to stimulate the mind. This means engaging in doing nothing that requires or arouses thought. Take a hot bath, a garden walk or simply sit in the sun (with a hat). Don't read, listen to music or even meditate — simply enjoy being and allow your mind to drift nowhere in particular. Taking five-minute brain-breaks five times a day dramatically increases clarity of thinking, creativity and productivity, while reducing mental fatigue and burnout.

2. **Take a break from your dominant hand**. Spend five minutes a day (or longer) doing everything with your non-dominant hand or foot; for example, opening doors, turning on taps, brushing your teeth, combing your hair, using your computer mouse, holding a cup or stirring a pot.

3. **Take a break from your usual routine.** Shop at a different grocery store, take a different route to a regular destination, try a new

recipe, wear your watch on the opposite hand and listen to music you've never heard before. Then reflect on what you did and didn't like about the new experience.

4. **Take a break from your calculator and GPS.** Add up the cost of your meal or grocery items in your head as you shop. Look up a map and work out your route before setting off to a new destination.

5. **Break free from the belief that you can't remember names.** When you initially meet someone, play a game in your head that will prompt you to retain their name. First and foremost, pay attention when you hear their name and repeat it out loud. Secondly, think of a word that rhymes with or starts with the same letter as the name and link the word to an image of the person you create in your mind. For instance, if you've just met Paul, you might immediately conjure up the word 'ball' and picture Paul with a big ball on his head. The more absurd the image, the easier it will be to remember. Thirdly, replay the image and the name in your mind. Simply going through the process of trying to remember a name is a form of mental gymnastics and will enhance the likelihood of recall. This is just one example of a name game. Feel free to make up your own.

Small daily tweaks such as these stop us from living on autopilot and trigger electrical activity along dormant brain pathways.

There's one more huge brain-drain we need to eliminate from our daily lives: **multitasking.** The research on multitasking is unequivocal. Regardless of how effective at multitasking a person *believes* themselves to be, they are more likely to make mistakes, miss important information, feel stressed, take longer to complete the task and do a suboptimal job. This is because our brain can only focus on one thing at a time. Thus, multitasking requires our frontal lobes to rapidly switch back and forth between two stimuli. During this toggling, information gets lost and we become less capable of blocking extraneous distractions.

Multitasking is a far less efficient way of getting things done and generates superficial rather than deep thinking. Multitasking increases brain cortisol levels, which erode our memory and contribute to brain cell decay. If your employer encourages you to multitask, either explain the research on multitasking or keep quiet and do things one at a time, knowing you will be more efficient. When people around you start noticing that you're more effective and less stressed than your co-workers, you can tell them your secret: **mono-tasking.**

Many people believe they thrive on multitasking simply because they haven't discovered the joys and rewards of mono-tasking. Give it a go. You'll find yourself in flow and on a productivity high. Hence the importance of identifying your top two tasks for the day and giving them your full attention for 20 to 50 minutes at a time. Then take a five-minute brain-break and either return to the task at hand or start something different — giving it the same undivided attention you gave the first task.

If you reflect on the previous three paragraphs about multitasking, it might occur to you that many activities incorporate multitasking by their very nature: driving a car or cooking a meal are two examples. With driving or cooking, even though we might need to do two or more things concurrently, each action serves the same end. In the case of driving, the end is safely reaching our desired destination; with cooking, the end is a delicious, nutritious dining experience. Hence our attention is not divided in the same way as it would be if we were following a recipe and simultaneously listening to a podcast.

Another situation in which we are able to multitask is if one of the activities does not require conscious thought — for instance, hanging up the laundry or washing dishes. Most people can conduct a coherent conversation while performing menial chores. The message is that if two tasks require thinking, do them one at a time. If one task does not demand concentration, attending to something else at the same time will not be a problem. If you'd like to practise mindfulness however, doing even the simplest tasks with your undivided attention is the way to go.

What about online brain-training programs? Are they an effective way to boost brainpower and ward off Alzheimer's? Some are, some aren't. I know of at least three online brain-training companies that have been fined millions of dollars for misleading consumers about the purported benefits of their programs. To date, my top two recommendations for computer-based brain-training that is backed by decades of sound scientific research are brainhq.com and centerforbrainhealth.org.

Developed by an international team of neuroscientists led by Michael Merzenich (a trailblazer in the field of neuroplasticity), **BrainHQ** provides exercises to improve memory, attention, navigation, processing speed, intelligence and even people skills. Their website provides links to research conducted by independent investigators on the specific benefits of various mental workouts.

The Center for BrainHealth is a neuroscience research institute at the University of Texas in Dallas, USA. Founder and chief director Sandra Bond Chapman PhD leads a team of scientists and clinicians dedicated to helping people create a better brain, better life and better world through **The BrainHealth® Project.** The project is a free, online, self-paced, interactive program that teaches brain-healthy habits to incorporate into daily life. After completing a **BrainHealth Index,** you will receive a breakdown of the areas in which your brain is functioning well, alongside areas that may need improvement. Based on your results, you will receive tools and strategies tailored to your individual cognitive needs. Every three months you can have an online meeting with your **BrainHealth coach** to keep you on track and answer any questions. Every six months you can repeat the BrainHealth Index to monitor your progress.

BrainHQ and The BrainHealth Project offer different programs that complement each other. I encourage you to try them both.

To close this chapter, here is one more exercise in productive reflection. Examine the front cover of this book and answer the following questions:
- What messages does the cover convey to you?
- What is the significance of the puzzle pieces?
- Why are the puzzle pieces grey and white?
- Why are certain letters in the title bold?
- If you were designing the cover, what would you do differently?

CHAPTER 70

Friends for life

A man's feeling of goodwill towards others is the strongest magnet for drawing goodwill towards himself.

LORD CHESTERFIELD (1694–1773)

Chris was a master of creating meaning. He was a professional window cleaner and twice a year he brought sparkle to our windows and sparkle to our day. He was the only person I knew who whistled while he worked. Yes, like the seven dwarfs. Dad followed him warily from window to window. Paranoia was a corollary of memory loss. As Dad became increasingly forgetful, his world became increasingly sinister. When he couldn't find something, his conclusion was that someone had stolen it. When a person he no longer recognised greeted him with unexpected familiarity, Dad was immediately suspicious: 'Why is this stranger pretending he knows me?' Making sense of a world in which large chunks of time are randomly missing becomes increasingly difficult.

Chris was unperturbed by his chaperone. 'You're making sure you get your 10 000 steps today, aren't you?' He gave Dad a nod of approval.

'You obviously enjoy what you do,' I commented.

'What's not to enjoy? I have the best job in the world — I light up people's lives,' Chris winked. 'Who was it that said, "If you love what you do, you'll never work a day in your life"?'

It was a rhetorical question because he didn't wait for an answer. 'Everyone likes clean windows. Looking through grimy glass is depressing. It reminds you of all the other chores that need doing.

And humid weather encourages the build-up of mould along window frames so it's important to stay on top of it.'

I winced at the mention of mould.

'If you expose yourself to bright natural light every morning,' he asserted, 'you'll sleep better at night. Morning light helps regulate your internal body clock, which in turn boosts your mood and strengthens your immune system.'

He knew his stuff.

'But d'you know the most important aspect of what I do?' he asked.

I shook my head.

'I talk to people. For some of my clients, I'm one of their few social contacts … and last year I took a punt and played matchmaker.'

'What do you mean?' I was intrigued.

'One of my clients is a quick-witted elderly widow in Varsity Lakes. Another is a well-read 75-year-old widower in Robina. Two adjoining suburbs, two lonely people. I asked the gentleman if he was interested in female companionship — just someone to have coffee and conversation with. He said yes. I told him I couldn't promise anything but I had an idea. I then asked the lady the same question with regard to male companionship. She was more hesitant but accepted the man's number and indicated she'd consider calling him. Three months later she finally plucked up the courage to ring his number. They've become close friends and she tells me her world has expanded in ways she never anticipated.'

'How wonderful!' I exclaimed.

'As I see it, each day is an opportunity to figure out how you can help someone. But you have to think outside the box — or, in my case, the window.' He gave Dad another grin. 'I feel sorry for people who've forgotten that money is a means, not an end. If you start by asking yourself what makes you happy and how you can contribute to someone else's happiness, you might find you don't need as much money or as much stuff as you thought. If a big pay packet means making sacrifices that make you unhappy, is it worth it? I asked my kids what they wanted: more stuff or more of me. They thought I was crazy for asking. They'd much rather I go bike-riding or camping with them than buy them fancy gadgets and spend the weekend at work. I'm not saying you can't have a well-paid job and also be happy. But from what I can see, a lot of people are making themselves miserable in pursuit of a so-called "better" life. That doesn't make sense to me.' He paused reflectively before continuing. 'Are you aware of Japan's grey crime wave?'

'No.'

'An increasing number of over-65-year-olds living in Japan are shoplifting or committing petty crimes in order to receive a jail sentence. Japan has a harsh justice system and you can be locked up for two years just for stealing a bunch of grapes. One reason for the crimes is the high cost of living — the pension is insufficient to cover an individual's ongoing expenses — but an even bigger driver of geriatric crime is loneliness and boredom. Japan's family structures are no longer what they used to be and young adults are less likely to live with and look after their ageing parents. Social isolation can lead to desperate measures. Loneliness is painful. I've seen the pain in people's eyes and bodies; in the way they walk and in the way they talk.'

Chris's observations were consistent with experiments showing that feeling rejection activates the same parts of our brain as does physical pain. (If any budding neurologists are reading this, the specific brain regions in question are the dorsal anterior cingulate cortex and the anterior insula.) Loneliness also diminishes the quality of our sleep and affects our genes and immune system — it lowers production of antiviral compounds called interferons and activates genes that promote inflammation.

Extraordinary as it seems, **loneliness** even **reduces the effectiveness of vaccines**. Eighty-three university students were asked to list up to 20 members of their social circle whom they contacted at least once a month. Those who recorded the fewest friends and felt the loneliest produced the lowest antibody response to a flu vaccine. Similar results were found in another group of students in relation to receiving a hepatitis B vaccine: those who could name at least one confidante and felt they had a strong social support network had a better response to the vaccine. The same is true for seniors. People in happy marriages have stronger natural immunity to coughs and colds and receive better protection from influenza after getting the vaccine compared with seniors in unsatisfying relationships.

These findings mean that loneliness is quite literally deadly. **Chronic loneliness can damage our health to the tune of smoking 15 cigarettes a day** and is more harmful than obesity, high blood pressure and lack of physical exercise. It also makes people more likely to develop depression, heart disease, stroke, metastatic cancer and dementia. In fact, **feeling lonely and yearning for meaningful social connections doubles the risk of developing Alzheimer's** even when other predisposing factors have been ruled out. In short, **loneliness causes brain damage.** Conversely, a review of 148 studies involving more than 300 000 people found that feeling socially connected reduces premature death by 50%. In the early days of HIV, physicians noted that gay men who feared being spurned and ostracised and had not come out about their sexual orientation died much more quickly than men who were open about their sexuality.

A study in the *New England Journal of Medicine* December 2019 recorded brain size, BDNF[1] (brain-derived neurotrophic factor) levels and various aspects of cognitive function in five men and four women who lived at the German Neumayer III station in Antarctica for 14 months. Extreme environmental conditions meant that all nine individuals were subjected to prolonged periods of social isolation. MRI scans at the start and end of their secondment revealed a 7% reduction in the volume of the dentate gyrus in their hippocampus — an area of the brain critical for memory formation. Several other grey matter regions had shrunk by 3% to 4%. These physical changes were accompanied by a decrease in BDNF and a drop in their spatial processing and selective attention. A comparable group of subjects who did not experience social isolation saw no such brain changes. **Social deprivation leads to a smaller brain and diminished mental functioning.**

---

[1] BDNF acts like a fertiliser for brain cells. It stimulates the growth of new neurons and increases the number of connections between them. More BDNF equates to better learning and memory.

It's important to distinguish between feeling lonely and being alone. If you enjoy time by yourself and don't feel that your life is lacking by having limited social contacts, your choice to have fewer friends is not necessarily harmful. For some people, one confidante is enough. However, if you're anxious or unhappy about being socially isolated, your body produces stress hormones such as cortisol, which interfere with memory and immune function. Loneliness is a biological drive akin to hunger and thirst. Like physical pain, loneliness is a signal to act and relieve the discomfort. Feeling lonely is our brain telling us to seek out companionship.

A study of 1138 men and women with healthy brains and an average age of 79.6 years were followed for up to 12 years. After adjusting for the effects of socioeconomic status, physical exercise, emotional wellbeing and overall health, those who were the most socially active experienced 75% less cognitive decline (as assessed through 21 annual tests of brain function) than those who were the least socially active. Countless other studies involving hundreds of thousands of people in their latter years have likewise found that limited social networks are associated with increased risk of developing dementia, while **high social engagement reduces cognitive decline and protects against Alzheimer's.** Stronger relationships lead to a stronger heart which leads to a stronger brain. (Yes, you can die of a broken heart.[2]) Stronger and more satisfying relationships also have a direct positive impact on our brain.

Many researchers describe positive social interactions as our brain's most potent vitamins and minerals. There are several mechanisms by which relationships nourish our brain.

- Social interactions are a mental workout. We need to pay attention, listen, assimilate and evaluate what is being said and formulate an appropriate response. This process is often contingent on the

[2] Dying of a broken heart was first described in Japan in 1990 and is known as takotsubo cardiomyopathy. The word 'takotsubo' comes from the name of an octopus trap used by Japanese fishermen. When someone develops takotsubo cardiomyopathy, the left chamber of their heart (ventricle) develops a narrow neck and distended round base, making it look like an octopus pot. It is caused by a massive rush of adrenaline that constricts blood flow, leading to a heart attack. The condition is rare but was diagnosed in more than 20 people during the week following the 2011 Christchurch earthquake in which 185 people died. The population most at risk are women after menopause.

memory of previous conversations so as to contextualise what the person is saying. Sometimes this also entails complex decision-making, such as 'Will I challenge this person's perspective and engage in a friendly debate or is the issue too trivial to bother?' Most of the time we take these mental manoeuvres for granted but they all depend on the smooth operation of complex neural networks. Thought-provoking conversations with people of different ages, backgrounds and viewpoints activates many different regions of our brain.

- Exchanging ideas with other people broadens our interests and is a form of learning. We're also more likely to find solutions to problems, especially if we're open-minded and engage in meaningful discussions.

- Feeling supported greatly reduces stress levels, as measured by blood tests, brain scans and psychological questionnaires. Feeling less stress benefits all our bodily functions including our brain. When we feel that we have people we can count on in our lives we perceive our surroundings as less threatening — friends make us feel the world is a friendlier place. When people are asked to rate the difficulty of a task or judge the steepness of an incline, they rate things as harder and steeper when they are on their own versus when they are asked to bring a companion — even if the companion is not permitted to help and is standing several metres away, facing in the opposite direction.

- Being involved in the lives of others provides a sense of meaning, purpose and validation, all of which are powerful brain-boosters. This is one of the reasons that **volunteering or assisting at intergenerational schools has a very positive effect on young and old alike.**

Intergenerational schools, play groups and initiatives such as *Old People's Home for Four-Year-Olds* and the AARP Foundation Experience Corps (a North American intergenerational program that trains older adults to become literacy tutors for struggling students) are starting to gain ground throughout the world because of the huge benefits for all involved. Elderly citizens — including those with dementia — are given the opportunity to assist young children with reading, crafts or gardening. In secondary schools, the elderly are invited to share their life experiences with teenagers and engage in lively question and answer sessions. In all cases, mutual respect and heartwarming friendships have ensued with unexpected gains for elders. Not only do they experience greater joy and purpose in their lives, doctors have noted remission of depression and anxiety, fewer aches and pains, and improvements in hand grip strength, balance, mobility, memory, cognition and energy levels. These findings have been supported by fMRI scans that showed increases in brain volume in regions vulnerable to dementia such as the hippocampus. In another instance, when a group of seniors was told that new safety rules no longer permitted those with walking frames to assist at the school, the great majority of volunteers suddenly found they could function without their walking aids — such was their desire to continue interacting with the children. Where there's a will, there's a way — regardless of age or apparent disability. I believe that meaningful social connections produce the strongest will of all, and that love always finds a way.

What matters more: quantity or quality of social relationships? The larger and more diverse our social circle, the more stimulating it is for our brain. Engaging with people of various ages and opinions broadens our perspective and challenges us to entertain divergent points of view. All this provides excellent mental gymnastics. However, **the most crucial factor is the quality of our relationships.** Interactions that promote anxiety or leave us feeling stressed and unvalued erode both physical and mental health. Even one negative encounter with someone important to us impairs our immune system. Forty-two married couples aged 22 to 77 participated in a study that measured the speed of wound healing. Each couple agreed to have a blister induced on their forearm on two occasions. On the first occasion, the couple were guided through a positive interaction; on the second visit, they were asked to talk about a disagreement. To the amazement of doctors and nurses, the blisters healed more slowly following conflict than after a pleasant interaction. Couples who were more hostile to each other during both visits healed at 60% the rate of happier couples. This means it took them nearly twice as long to heal. In addition, blood levels of inflammatory proteins were elevated in hostile couples the following morning. Over the long term, hostile relationships can contribute to developing chronic diseases by interfering with our immune system.

Another study found that wound healing took an average of nine days longer in women experiencing a high degree of stress while caring for someone with dementia compared with women who had little stress.

These findings are remarkable. They indicate that health professionals and policy makers need to take loneliness and poor social relationships as seriously as smoking and excessive drinking. Healing our relationships is a key step in improving our health on every level. Sometimes when I found myself caught up in the bustle of attending to Dad's daily needs, I had to pause and remind myself that the most important aspect of his care was ensuring he felt loved and supported — not insisting he ate broccoli or wear his hearing aids. Those things mattered of course, but not more than our relationship. Unsurprisingly, when I focused on validating his feelings and simply being a reassuring presence, he was more likely to eat his broccoli and wear hearing aids without objection.

Given that we're facing a worldwide epidemic of loneliness, what can we do to bring about positive change?

We can begin by spreading the word about the importance of feeling socially connected. Telling people about the noteworthy studies I've documented in this chapter is a great conversation starter.

Secondly, ask not what others can do for you, but what you can do for others (with apologies to JFK). In a British study exploring what promotes happiness, volunteers were given either £2.50 or £10 and instructed to spend the money on themselves or someone else. Which group felt happier afterwards? Regardless of the amount of money, those who spent it on someone else felt happier than those who spent it on themselves. We get a buzz from being kind and doing things for others — as long as we don't feel used or taken for granted. The key is to give willingly and to see the positive difference we can make to someone.

I'm reminded of the philosophy of Chris, our friendly window cleaner: 'Each day is an opportunity to figure out how you can help someone'. Now that you understand how just talking to someone can improve their physical and mental health, take every opportunity to speak to as many people as possible. Have a conversation with your postal worker, barista, supermarket attendant and the person standing next to you in a queue. It doesn't have to be a long discourse — a simple and pleasant exchange of words is a great start. If someone doesn't respond, don't let that stop you trying again with someone else in the future. People often imagine that others don't want to be approached or that random conversations with strangers would feel awkward. Behavioural scientists Nicholas Epley and Juliana Schroeder did a series of experiments to test this very hypothesis.

Commuters on trains and buses were randomly assigned to one of four groups:
- Group 1 were asked to have a conversation with a stranger.
- Group 2 were told to keep to themselves and enjoy 'me-time'.
- Group 3 were asked to do whatever they would usually do on public transport.
- Group 4 were asked to predict which of the above three groups would have the most pleasant journey.

What would *you* predict?

Most people in Group 4 predicted that those who rode in solitude would have the most pleasant trip, while those speaking to strangers, the least positive experience. The result was the exact opposite. People enjoyed conversing far more than they expected. The same results were obtained when people in a taxi were asked to speak with their driver. In another experiment, participants who were spoken to by a stranger in a laboratory waiting room reported just as favourable an experience as the person instructed to strike up the conversation.

It's sad that we've created a culture of 'stranger danger'. I'm not suggesting you seek out someone in a dark alley, but when we find ourselves in non-threatening environments, having brief and authentic conversations can build a sense of belonging and community. Moreover, lots of little conversations throughout the day contribute to physical and mental wellbeing by increasing our levels of the anti-stress hormone oxytocin (also known as the cuddle hormone). Scientists refer to frequent friendly interactions as a measure of social integration. A seven-year study by professor of psychology Julianne Holt-Lundstad at London's Brigham Young University found that the higher a person's level of social integration, the longer they lived. **Social integration was in fact the strongest predictor of a long and healthy life.** In other words, social integration was more important than not smoking, maintaining a healthy body weight and exercising. (This is not to endorse going outside for smoko with your workmates! By all means, go outside with your mates but support each other in *not* having a cigarette.) Who would have guessed that having a chat could lengthen our lives?

The second most important ingredient for great health and longevity was having close friends we could depend on. These can include a spouse, sibling, cousin, co-worker or bestie from primary school. Given the frantically busy lives we've adopted, if we have more than two people who fall into this category, we're doing well.

In case you were wondering, not smoking was the third most important ingredient for longevity. I keep bringing up smoking to emphasise the superior power of positive relationships.

From a young age and throughout our entire lives, we need to prioritise building and maintaining relationships. We need to be there, care and share. We need to have authentic conversations, allow ourselves and others to be vulnerable and create small and large supportive communities. Relationships don't just *add* meaning and purpose to our lives, relationships *are* the meaning and purpose of our lives. If you take away all the people I care about, you take away the meaning of my life. What do my goals matter if they don't in some way bring peace, joy, beauty, healing or comfort to others?

Thus, what happens when COVID-19 drives the world into lockdown? It's even more critical that we stay in touch through whatever means are available to us. Any form of pleasant contact is better than no contact. Anything we can contribute to others is better than no contribution at all.

Prior to COVID-19, research showed that real life conversations provide greater improvements in brain function than phone or digital communication. Nonetheless, a study of 80-year-olds found that 30 minutes of conversation every day for six weeks via a computer produced improvements in tests of complex thinking.

Another study demonstrated that spending as little as 10 minutes discussing social issues boosts performance on tests of memory and processing speed immediately after the interaction, compared to simply sitting with someone and watching TV. The take-home message from all the aforementioned research is that **positive social interactions are more powerful than any currently available medications or supplements in keeping our brains sharp and our bodies healthy.** The most effective way to reduce depression, anxiety, stress, heart disease and dementia is for governments at all levels to address homelessness, fund organisations such as Lifeline, promote community groups, and facilitate greater social engagement between all its citizens.

In the meantime, how can you strengthen your social connections? Is there a community project, book club, team sport, card game, choir, shared interest group or volunteer organisation you'd like to get involved with? Is there a neighbour you can get to know? Is there someone whose day you can brighten through a kind gesture, a thank you note or a caring conversation? Take a break from reading and do so now.

CHAPTER 71

You can't fool your brain

We are generally the better persuaded by the reasons we discover ourselves, than by those given to us by others.

BLAISE PASCAL (1623–1662)

I arrived home to find Dad and Sophie sitting on our back deck pouring the last of a can of diet soft drink into their respective glasses. Sophie was pointing to our resident kookaburra.

'In the old Tarzan movies you can hear kookaburras laughing in the background,' Dad was telling her.

'I didn't know there were kookaburras in Africa,' Sophie looked puzzled.

'There aren't — it was simply a recording to make the jungle sound alive. No one watching would have questioned what animal was producing the noise.' Dad's long-term memory for trivia remained remarkably robust.

'That's very funny!' Sophie exclaimed before turning to greet me. 'We saw you on TV today,' she announced.

I'd been interviewed about a study showing how chronic stress could shrink our brain and increase the risk of dementia.

'It was fascinating,' Sophie squeezed Dad's hand. 'We learnt a lot, didn't we?'

'Yes, we did,' Dad nodded. 'We learnt that we shouldn't turn the TV on in the afternoon. There's no escaping your lecturing even when you're not home.'

'You're so cheeky!' Sophie wagged her finger at Dad playfully. All three of us chortled.

How to segue into a conversation about artificial sweeteners without ruining the moment?

'It's great that you're avoiding sugary drinks,' I observed. 'Unfortunately, artificial sweeteners are probably no better. A 10-year study published in the medical journal *Stroke* found that **people who frequently drank artificially sweetened beverages were three times more likely to have a stroke or develop dementia**. The researchers tracked more than 4000 people, and after ruling out other risk factors such as smoking, poor diet, low educational attainment and lack of exercise, the more diet soft drinks they consumed, the more likely they were to suffer a stroke or Alzheimer's.'

Sophie looked aghast. 'I had no idea!' she exclaimed.

'I'm sorry if I come across as a killjoy, but I thought you'd want to know so you could make informed choices about what you consume,' I stammered an apology. 'I don't expect you to take my word for it. I can send you a pile of research papers so you can review the evidence for yourself. I make no judgement about what you choose to eat or drink — I strongly believe in freedom of choice — but, equally so, I feel that people have a right to know the repercussions of their choices.'

'You don't need to apologise,' Sophie reassured me. 'It's your job to keep people healthy and I appreciate the advice.'

'But it's unsolicited advice.'

'I want to know,' she reiterated.

'I don't,' Dad gave me a wry smile as he walked into the house. 'I think I'll go and read the newspaper. Call me when the lecture is over.'

'I enjoy your daughter's lectures,' she affirmed. 'So what's the story behind sweeteners? I must admit, I've wondered whether artificial sweeteners were any healthier than sugar. In the end I decided they were probably the lesser of the two evils. And I guess not all sweeteners are the same?'

'The various sweeteners have similarities as well as differences. There are three categories of non-sugar sweeteners — also referred to as sugar substitutes or simply sweeteners — and the way our brain and body respond to them is complex and variable.'

'I've heard there's also potential bias in studies on sweeteners — it depends who provides money for the research, doesn't it?'

'Yes, very much so. Studies funded by sweetener companies almost always report no harm in consuming their products. Meanwhile, research funded by the sugar industry — which has a vested interest in people *not* using sugar substitutes — usually results in adverse findings about sweeteners. So you have to read everything with a skeptical eye. For historical interest, ancient Romans used lead acetate as a sugar substitute because of its sweet taste. It wasn't until centuries later that people discovered it could cause lead poisoning and it became illegal. It often takes humans a long time to realise that what we're consuming is a health hazard.'

'Sometimes I think **our love affair with processed food is one big human experiment,**' commented Sophie.

'I couldn't agree with you more,' I pronounced.

'What are the different types of sweeteners?' she asked.

'The three categories of sweeteners are:
1. **zero-calorie or non-nutritive artificial sweeteners (NNS)** — these have negligible calories hence the designation non-nutritive. They are intensely sweet — hundreds of times sweeter than sugar.
2. **low-calorie or nutritive sweeteners** — these provide some calories but much less than sugar. Most of them are sugar alcohols or polyols because they're made from sugars by a process called hydrogenation. They aren't necessarily sweeter than sugar so they're often combined with NNS in diet products. They're used because they add bulk and texture to foods, without adding many calories.
3. **natural sweeteners** — derived from plants such as stevia and monk fruit — which are not as natural as the name suggests. They resemble non-nutritive artificial sweeteners in that they are several hundred times sweeter than sugar and have zero calories.'

'What are examples of zero-calorie artificial sweeteners?' Sophie pursued.

I pulled out my phone so I could look up the list to show her.

'The most common zero-calorie artificial sweeteners are:
1. Acesulphame potassium or Ace-K (additive number 950)
2. Alitame (956)
3. Aspartame (951), e.g. Equal and Nutrasweet
4. Cyclamate (952)
5. Neotame (961)
6. Saccharin (954), e.g. Sweetex and Sweet 'N Low
7. Sucralose (955), e.g. Splenda.

'Sometimes they aren't listed in product ingredients by name but by number, so make a note of the numbers and check the label on everything you buy.'

'Using numbers is sneaky!' Sophie uttered disapprovingly. 'Does the same apply to sugar alcohols?'

'Yes,' I produced another list. 'Sugar alcohols include:
1. Erythritol (additive number 968)
2. Lactilol (966)
3. Maltilol (965)
4. Mannitol (421)
5. Sorbitol (420)
6. Xylitol (967).

'Bear in mind that sugar alcohols can cause bloating, wind and diarrhoea, especially in large doses, and they're often used in chewing gum. Anything that plays havoc with our gut sets off alarm bells for other diseases because gut health is linked to everything from diabetes and depression to Parkinson's and Alzheimer's.'

'Good to know,' she stated. 'And does stevia have a number?'

'Yes. Stevia is E960. Unless you're eating the stevia leaf itself, what you're consuming is not natural. To transform a green leaf into a white powder requires solvents and ion exchange resins so you're still exposing yourself to industrial chemicals. Nonetheless, stevia is likely to be safer than other types of sweeteners.'

'What about monk fruit extract? That's the Buddha fruit isn't it? I've heard that it's rich in antioxidants and has been used in Chinese medicine for centuries.'

'Yes, all of that is true. It's also called luo han guo and it contains antioxidants called mogrosides. The mogrosides are what make it several hundred times sweeter than sugar. It's likely to be the least processed and least harmful sugar substitute. The sweetener is made by removing the skin and seeds, crushing the remaining fruit to extract juice and then drying the juice to yield a concentrated powder. Because it's so intensely sweet it's often mixed with sugar alcohols to tone it down. It was only approved in Australia in 2018 and I haven't found any rigorous studies relating to its health benefits or otherwise. But here's the critical thing: our brain evolved to associate sweetness with calories. All sweeteners teach our brain the opposite — that sweet foods don't necessarily provide energy. The brain then needs to recalibrate, and it responds by ramping up our hunger so that we eat more to make up for the caloric deficit in the artificially sweetened food. Over time, people can end up consuming more calories than if they'd eaten sugar in the first place. That's one reason sweeteners can lead to weight gain. Another problem is that sweeteners stimulate insulin release, however because there is no glucose for the insulin to work with, blood sugar regulation is thrown into disarray. Insulin is a hormone that tells our body to *store* fat rather than *burn* fat, so sweeteners — whether they're labelled artificial or natural — can mess up our metabolism if consumed in large amounts,' I paused for breath. 'That's another reason sweeteners have been shown to contribute to obesity, diabetes, heart disease and fatty liver — because of metabolic derangements. In some people, artificial sweeteners can also disrupt sleep and cause insomnia.'

'What an irony,' Sophie remarked. 'People use sweeteners because they want to consume fewer calories but their brain compensates by driving them to eat more.'

'Not everyone experiences an increase in appetite, and people often don't realise they're eating more. But whether we're aware of what's happening inside us or not, scientists have identified the brain pathways that are affected. In addition, there's one more casualty of artificial sweeteners.'

'What's that?' Sophie was intrigued.

'Our gut microbiota — the trillions of bacteria that live in our digestive system. Artificial sweeteners modify the chemicals produced by our bacteria, leading to inflammation. Chronic inflammation amplifies the risk of heart disease, diabetes and dementia even further.'

'What about cancer? Aren't certain artificial sweeteners linked to bladder cancer?'

'I haven't found enough scientific evidence linking artificial sweeteners to cancer. In 50 years, more data may be available. However, robust research involving tens of thousands of people substantiates the increase in obesity and diabetes.'

'I used to look after a man whose family claimed he could not have aspartame because it gave him seizures. Could that be true?' Sophie looked dubious.

'He must have had a rare genetic disorder called phenylketonuria in which a person is unable to metabolise the amino acid phenylalanine. Phenylalanine is a breakdown product of aspartame. For the general population, phenylalanine is an essential dietary nutrient. But for someone with phenylketonuria, phenylalanine can be toxic. He must also have avoided other foods containing phenylalanine such as soy, eggs, beef and chicken.'

'Yes, that's right. I remember the family being very careful about his diet. As for me, I'm off all sweeteners for good,' Sophie resolved.

'You won't miss them. In fact, you'll find that you enjoy your food more.'

'How so?'

'**Sweeteners change the way we taste food.** We lose our appreciation for natural foods because they aren't as sweet as additives. Fruit and vegetables become bland or bitter because they can't compete with the intensity of artificial chemicals and extracts. Sweeteners increase our desire for sweet foods and reduce our intake of vegetables.'

'That sounds like an unhealthy marriage.'

'There's also a behavioural component. If something is labelled as a diet product, we unconsciously tend to eat more of it. Or we think that if we're saving calories in the drink department, we can afford to order dessert.'

'What about using sweeteners for the sole purpose of weaning myself off sugar? Like a nicotine patch for smokers, or methadone for opioid addicts? I imagine artificial sweeteners aren't as addictive as sugar and would be easier to give up,' she suggested.

'I'm not so sure about that. When rats are given the choice of cocaine or saccharin they usually choose saccharin. And regardless of the sweetener, soft drinks erode tooth enamel because all carbonated drinks are highly acidic. Diet soft drinks don't do your teeth any favours either. Even plain sparkling water erodes tooth enamel because of its acidity, but it's infinitely better than flavoured drinks.'

'Have you had to give up sugar or have you never had a sweet tooth?' Sophie wanted to know.

'Twenty years ago I couldn't imagine drinking coffee without sugar. I used to add two teaspoons to every cup. Fortunately, I only drank one cup a day. But when I learned about the hazards of sugar, I decided to give it up. I couldn't go cold turkey so I reduced the dose to one and a half teaspoons per cup. After a few weeks I dropped down to one teaspoon. Every few weeks I kept reducing the dose by half a teaspoon until I reached zero. Now if someone accidentally puts sugar in my coffee I can't drink it. I literally feel sick. So you won't miss sweetness once you're off it — especially in drinks. I did the same with Dad. He used to be addicted to sugary soft drinks. He would drink a litre every day. So I started diluting them with sparkling mineral water — just a little at a time so he wouldn't notice. It took about six months for him to switch to plain mineral water — no sugar, no sweetener and no flavour. Our taste buds are highly adaptable.'

'What are your tips for giving up sugar and sweeteners in foods as opposed to drinks?' Sophie was ready to take notes.

'Assuming you're fit and healthy, aim for less than six teaspoons of added sugar a day. This includes the sugar in sauces, salad dressings, marinades, baked beans and ready-made meals. However, if you have pre-diabetes (insulin resistance), type 2 diabetes, high blood pressure, heart disease, cognitive impairment or any other chronic inflammatory condition, zero added sugar would give you the best chance of reversing the disease. The poison is in the dose — and the dose differs for each individual. When you want something sweet, eat fresh whole fruit or make or buy the best quality dessert/ice cream/chocolate you can afford and really savour it. If Dad wants ice cream or custard, I make it with a bit of monk fruit sweetener because I think it's the safest option. The more you taste, smell and appreciate every mouthful, the less you'll need to feel satisfied. It's also helpful not to label sweets as treats. If you tell yourself you're depriving yourself of something pleasurable, you'll find yourself wanting it all the more. Adopt the attitude that your body deserves the most nutritious fuel you can give it, not toxic edibles that lead to disease.

'Another important strategy is to schedule non-food treats into your day — **find ways to feed your spirit**. What are things you enjoy doing? Listening to music, reading a novel, having a massage, hiking in the mountains, taking a bath or learning to paint? Reward yourself with fulfilling experiences and you'll find that you stop craving processed sweets. And, of course, be patient while your tastebuds recalibrate and you notice that real food starts becoming more flavourful. Strawberries and blueberries are much tastier than lollies. Or try a handful of raw nuts — they're delectable when we eat them slowly enough to notice. And raw nuts are excellent brain food — with an emphasis on raw. There's a world of mouthwatering delicacies to be discovered when we switch to unprocessed food. People are afraid they'll miss out on pleasure if they give up sweets. The opposite will happen. That's the big paradox: **life is sweeter without sweets because our senses grow sharper and we derive more pleasure from other sources** — not just from other foods but from other activities and hobbies. Experiments have shown that feeding sugar to rats reduces their interest in playing and having sex. When the rats were weaned off sweets, they became more active and enthusiastic about life again. So will we.'

CHAPTER 72

Mental floss

Your living is determined not so much by what life brings to you as by the attitude you bring to life.

KAHLIL GIBRAN (1883–1931)

Dad's dentures had started clicking and rattling every time he ate. The cacophony was not a pleasant accompaniment to mealtimes. He was unperturbed, but I was losing my appetite and my composure so I booked an appointment with our dentist, Dr Elizabeth.

'I don't see why I need to visit the dentist when I have no teeth left,' Dad protested as we sat down in the waiting room.

'The dentist still needs to check that your gums are healthy and your dentures fit properly.'

'Of course they fit properly. I glue them into place every morning.'

'Yes, you do a great job with them. But over time your gums can shrink and your dentures can wear down. Besides, you told me that you liked Dr Elizabeth.'

'Mr Popovic!' called a mellifluous voice.

Dad didn't move. I resorted to the tactic of 'one for me and one for you'.

'I need a check-up too,' I tried to encourage him.

'Then ladies first,' he insisted resolutely.

I sighed. 'Okay, I'll go first, but please come in with me.'

He hesitated before realising he would be left on his own in the waiting room. Reluctantly, he shuffled along behind me and immediately made his way to the furthest corner from the dentist chair.

'Your father's such a gentleman,' complimented Dr Elizabeth. Dad betrayed a flicker of a smile.

'Do you have any pain or sensitivity in any of your teeth?' Dr Elizabeth turned to me.

'No.'

'Do you floss every day?'

'Yes,' I replied proudly.

'Excellent. It's essential that you maintain good dental hygiene because gum disease can lead to many other problems: heart disease, rheumatoid arthritis, Parkinson's, Alzheimer's — the list goes on.'

I'd only recently become aware of the link between gum disease and Alzheimer's so I was keen for Dr Elizabeth to elaborate. 'Please tell us more about the connection between gum disease and Alzheimer's,' I urged her.

'For a start, **Parkinson's and Alzheimer's tend to be more common and more severe in people with gum disease**.'

'Why? What's the mechanism?'

'Gum disease incites our immune system to ramp up production of cells called neutrophils. The neutrophils circulate throughout our body and trigger widespread inflammation in multiple organs, including our brain, joints and colon. Meanwhile, one of the bacteria responsible for gum disease — called *Porphyromonas gingivalis* — can travel directly to the brain and damage areas involved in planning, learning and memory. The hippocampus and cerebral cortex seem to be the regions of the brain that are most affected.'

'How do the bacteria cause brain damage?'

'*P. gingivalis* produces two protein-digesting enzymes (proteases) called gingipains, which it uses to feed on human tissue. These gingipains have been found in 99% of brain samples from people

How can gum disease lead to Alzheimer's?

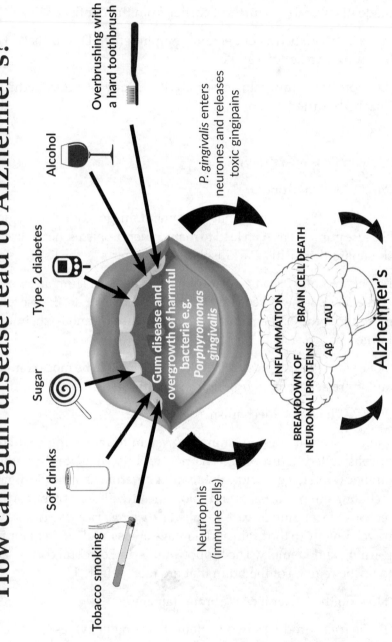

who died with Alzheimer's. The more severe the dementia, the more gingipains in their brain. And these gingipains appear to trigger production of amyloid β (Aβ) and tau tangles — the two hallmarks of Alzheimer's. Meanwhile, the bacterium itself has been found in spinal cord fluid (CSF). When mice were infected with *P. gingivalis*, they developed dementia, and when the gingipains were blocked, their brain damage was reversed.'

'Why aren't gingipain-blocking drugs being offered to everyone with Alzheimer's?' I wondered.

'Drug trials are underway as we speak, but it's a tricky situation. Some people *without* Alzheimer's were also found to have gingipains in their brain, albeit at lower levels.'

'That makes perfect sense. Alzheimer's is multifactorial. Gingipains alone are probably not enough to cause the brain changes that lead to Alzheimer's. But if you add a large dose of gingipains to an insulin-resistant, sleep-deprived or otherwise compromised brain, you could conceivably tip someone into dementia. What about taking antibiotics to kill the bacteria before they get a foothold in the brain?'

'That's also harder to accomplish than it sounds,' Dr Elizabeth explained patiently. 'The first problem is that gum disease is probably the commonest of all diseases but few people regard it as an actual disease. Somehow dental issues are seen as separate from the rest of the body — as if our mouth were part of a parallel universe. Everyone is obsessed with gut health but forget that gut health includes oral health. Good gut health starts with good dental health. How can it not? Everything we eat, drink, swallow and smoke enters through our mouth and affects the health of our teeth and gums. Our mouth is like the canary in the coal mine.'

'I know about canaries in coal mines,' piped up Dad. I was so absorbed in what Dr Elizabeth was saying, I'd almost forgotten he was still standing in the corner. 'Coal miners take canaries down into the mines with them. The purpose of the canary is to provide advance warning of carbon monoxide poisoning.'

'Precisely!' Dr Elizabeth was jubilant. 'The fact that canaries are much smaller, breathe faster and have a higher metabolic rate than humans means the birds will succumb to the poisonous gas before the miners, thereby giving them time to act. In many cases, our mouth does the same for us. Every time you drink a glass of water, you swallow millions of bacteria.'

'Yuk!' Dad grimaced.

'That isn't a bad thing,' Dr Elizabeth reassured him. 'Our mouth is home to more than a thousand species of bacteria and most of them are our friends. However, they are very finicky about where they live. The bacteria on our front teeth are different from the bacteria on our back teeth, and the bacteria on the front of a tooth are different from the bacteria on the back of the same tooth! Some bacteria protect our teeth, while other bacteria contribute to decay. The good bugs keep the bad bugs in check. But if harmful bacteria overgrow in our mouth — as a consequence of eating too much sugar for instance — it leads to inflammation and damages the blood vessels in our gums. This allows the bacteria to escape into our blood and get carried to distant parts of our body — hence the link to heart disease and Alzheimer's.'

'But as soon as bacteria enter our bloodstream, our immune system should kick in and make antibodies to destroy them,' I interrupted.

'Unfortunately *P. gingivalis* seems to be able to hide inside the white blood cells of our immune system so it escapes detection. And it can also enter the cells that line our artery walls and lie dormant for a long time.'

'So that's what makes it difficult for antibiotics to reach the bacteria,' I postulated.

'Yes, that's right. The best thing is to avoid gum disease in the first place.'

'What exactly constitutes gum disease? What do I need to look out for?' I wanted to know for myself and Dad, as well as for my patients.

'The mildest form of gum disease is called gingivitis. When you have plaque on your teeth, bacteria can accumulate inside the plaque and cause bleeding, receding, sore and swollen gums. Basically the tissues around your teeth become inflamed. If you don't do anything about it, gingivitis can progress to more severe gum disease called periodontitis. This is where your gums pull away from your teeth and they become loose and prone to decay. You might also develop an abscess or bad breath. Eventually the affected teeth can fall out.'

'Can I prevent gum disease by brushing and flossing every day?'

'Brushing and flossing twice daily — especially after eating carbohydrates and before going to bed — are certainly important. Plaque forms on our teeth while we sleep, as well as throughout the day as we eat and drink — it's that colourless fuzzy coating you feel when you run your tongue over your teeth on waking. The technical term for plaque is "biofilm" because it consists of bacteria surrounded by a sticky coating. The coating helps micro-organisms attach to our teeth and grow into thriving communities. The biofilm also makes it hard for antibiotics to get through. If you don't remove the plaque on a regular basis by brushing and flossing, it can collect minerals from your saliva and harden into what's known as tartar or calculus. Tartar feels rough and looks pale yellow or off-white. It provides the ideal surface for build-up of more plaque and soon you'll have a self-perpetuating process of increasing plaque and tartar formation. If this continues unchecked, gum disease is inevitable.'

'Other than brushing and flossing, is there anything else I can do to stop this from happening?'

'Make sure you use a soft toothbrush and don't brush too vigorously because over-brushing can also damage your gums and allow bacteria to enter your bloodstream. Other than that, **the best thing you can do to protect your gums is not smoke**. Tobacco helps harmful bacteria invade your gums.'

'We've known for a long time that cigarette smoking is associated with Alzheimer's,' I confirmed. More pieces of the Alzheimer's puzzle were falling into place.

'Yes — increasing the risk of gingivitis is one of the reasons that smoking is bad news for our brain. Even passive smoking is damaging, especially to baby teeth. A study of 3500 children between the ages of four and 11 years found that if one or both parents smoked, their children had double the risk of tooth decay. The researchers also measured children's blood levels of a metabolite of nicotine called cotinine. The more cotinine, the more caries.'

'Dad used to smoke and I had a lot of fillings when I was a child,' I reflected.

Dr Elizabeth nodded purposefully. 'Research has also shown that people who drink a lot of alcohol tend to have more *P. gingivalis* and more gum disease. And it goes without saying that diet plays a major role in oral health. The fewer vegetables and the more soft drinks and junk food you consume, the worse the state of your teeth and gums.'

'That means this doesn't affect me. I don't need to eat vegetables anymore!' Dad rejoiced. 'Eating sweets can't be bad for my teeth if I don't have any!'

'I'm sorry to disappoint you, but eating sweets can still give you type 2 diabetes (T2D) which is a harbinger for gingivitis,' Dr Elizabeth responded sympathetically. '**Diabetes worsens gum disease and gum disease worsens diabetes.** It's a dangerous two-way street because *P. gingivalis* can make its way to your liver and pancreas and increase insulin resistance. Treating gum disease helps regulate blood sugar levels.'

'That's extraordinary!' I gasped. 'What about using mouthwash? Do you recommend it?'

Dr Elizabeth deliberated before answering. 'Mouthwash turns out to be another interesting story. Regular use of mouthwash that contains the disinfectant chlorhexidine can lead to higher blood pressure.'

'How on earth does that happen?' I was intrigued.

'Antiseptic mouthwash blocks the first step in the production of nitric oxide. The bacteria that live on our tongue convert dietary nitrates — found in beetroot and dark leafy greens — into nitrites. The nitrites are then absorbed into our bloodstream where they're made into nitric oxide. Nitric oxide causes our blood vessels to widen by relaxing the inner muscles of our blood vessel walls.

More relaxed blood vessels mean lower blood pressure. Antiseptic mouthwash stops your tongue bacteria from producing nitrites so you can't make nitric oxide. That's not to say I never recommend mouthwash. In some cases of gingivitis, it can be helpful. But just like any other medication, mouthwash has potential side effects and I don't advise people to use it unless there's a specific reason to do so.'

How does mouthwash raise blood pressure?	
Step 1	Dietary nitrates (e.g. dark leafy greens, beetroot, radish) + tongue bacteria → **nitrites**
Step 2	**Nitrites** enter our bloodstream where they are made into **nitric oxide**
Step 3	**Nitric oxide** relaxes blood vessel walls which lowers blood pressure
However	Mouthwash blocks Step 1: Mouthwash + tongue bacteria ≠ nitrites

'I expect that after a person stops using mouthwash, their tongue bacteria resume making nitrites and their blood pressure drops back down?' I verified.

'Yes, that's correct.'

'From now on, I'll be asking all my patients with high blood pressure if they use mouthwash on a regular basis.'

Our conversation was brought to a halt as she started cleaning my teeth. When I was done, I gave Dad my brightest smile and swiftly traded places with him. To my great relief, his dentures only needed minor adjusting to alleviate the clicking and clattering. He had no pressure sores in his mouth and there were no chips or cracks in the dentures themselves.

'I told you there was nothing wrong,' he relished telling me as we walked to the car. 'You always make such a fuss about everything.'

As soon as we arrived home, I began trawling through online medical and dental journals looking for research linking gum disease to Alzheimer's. The evidence was compelling. Most thrilling of all, the first trial of a gingipain-blocking drug called COR388 (atuzaginstat) showed that it was safe and improved memory in people with Alzheimer's. The pharmaceutical company Cortexyme was now conducting a much larger trial involving 500 participants across the

US and Europe. I scanned the web pages to see how I could enrol Dad, but Australia was not involved in the study. Called the GAIN Trial, it stands for GingipAIN Inhibitor for Treatment of Alzheimer's. The objective of the trial was to evaluate whether COR388 could slow or stop the progression of Alzheimer's. For more details about the trial, visit <u>clinicaltrials.gov/ct2/show/NCT03823404.</u> I'm crossing my fingers very tightly as I wait for the results.

Meanwhile, Australia is by no means out of the picture. In 2016, scientists at the University of Melbourne developed the world's first vaccine against *P. gingivalis*. The vaccine neutralised gingipains and prevented periodontitis. Clinical trials in people with periodontitis are in the planning stages.

CHAPTER 73

Go with your gut

*Our great business in life is not to see what lies dimly
at a distance, but to do what lies clearly at hand.*

THOMAS CARLYLE (1795–1881)

Is your gut sensitive, irritable, leaky or inflamed? Are you into prebiotics, probiotics, synbiotics or psychobiotics? Why does it matter? (Definitions to follow.)

It matters because our body is home to trillions of microorganisms with a combined total weight of over 2 kg (4.4 pounds). That's more than the weight of our brain, which is about 1.4 kg (3.1 pounds). And our microorganisms — or microbes for short — have evolved to play essential roles in almost every aspect of our health. For instance, they:

- help us digest food
- control how many calories we absorb
- activate vitamins by producing enzymes that we can't make ourselves
- affect our mood and mental health
- modulate our immune system
- influence our susceptibility to allergies, asthma, autoimmune diseases, autism, diabetes, depression, **dementia,** Parkinson's, heart disease, stroke, cancer, and the list goes on
- tinker with our genes
- affect our response to medications.

The more we discover about our gut microbes, the more we realise they meddle with everything — especially our brain. Gut microbes and their metabolites (the chemicals they produce) influence brain development, brain cell communication, activation of the brain's immune system and the integrity of the blood-brain barrier (BBB). When scientists took stool samples (a rich source of gut microbes) from people with Alzheimer's and transferred them into the gut of rats, the animals began producing pro-inflammatory molecules, decreased their rate of new brain cell formation and performed worse in memory tests. **Our gut bugs carry a lot of clout when it comes to brain function.** Most of our resident microbes are bacteria, but we also house viruses, fungi and organisms known as archaea.

The gut is often described as our second brain because it has 100 million nerve cells lining its walls from oesophagus to rectum. That's about the same number of neurons as the brain of a cat. Imagine that — you have a cat brain in your gut. And these neurons enable our gut bacteria to communicate with our brain via a long, large nerve called the vagus. Do you want to know what they're saying? That's what this chapter is about: a whirlwind tour of our internal ecosystem and an insight into how **faecal transplants might stave off Alzheimer's.** Holy crapsule!

When we talk about 'gut health' we're talking about a system with three inseparable components:

1. the gut cells (called enterocytes in the small intestine and colonocytes in the large intestine) that make up the gastrointestinal tract from our mouth to our anus
2. the nerves and nerve cells (neurons) that are interwoven with our gut cells — known as the enteric nervous system (ENS)
3. trillions of microorganisms that live in every nook and cranny of the gut.

Together, these three entities — our gut cells, enteric nerve cells and microbial residents — form an incredibly complex information exchange system called the **gut-brain-microbiome axis.** This axis enables constant three-way communication between our brain, gut and microbes via nerves, hormones and immune cells. Hormones and immune cells are transported between our gut and our brain in our blood.

Thirty years ago, when I was in medical school, I was taught that the gut was nothing more than a hollow tube that broke down and absorbed food and eliminated what we didn't need — with the help of a few friendly colonic bacteria. Today we know that microbes make up more than 90% of the cells in our body and contribute more than 99% of the genes in our body. One could argue that our microbes don't exist to help *us* survive, *we* exist to enable *them* to survive. We are their planet and they live on the resources we provide for them. In return, they try and look after their planet (our body), just as we try (rather unsuccessfully) to look after our planet earth.

It's estimated that there are more bugs in our gut than there are stars in the Milky Way. One gram of faeces contains more bacteria than people on earth — and the citizens of different countries carry different microbial species. In other words, if you live in Japan, the microbes in your body are different to those of people who live in Australia or North America. In fact, no two people in the world — not even identical twins — have the same microorganisms living in their bodies. Everyone has a unique microbial identity, just as we have a unique fingerprint. Because of this, crime scene investigators are starting to use bacterial DNA in addition to fingerprints and human DNA to track down criminals. Your bacterial inhabitants are distinctively yours.

We don't only have microbes in our gut; we have bugs on every exposed surface of our body: skin, nose, ears, mouth, teeth, lungs and vagina. It's all potential real estate for microorganisms and it's all about location, location, location. Just as humans are fussy about where we live, so are microbes. Some require the intense acidity of our stomach, others the salty moisture of our armpits. The most densely populated region of our body is the colon or large intestine.

Before we continue, there are three important terms you need to understand: microbiome, microbiota and metabolites. Microbiome and microbiota tend to be used interchangeably, but to be precise:

- **Microbiome** refers to all the genes of all the microorganisms that reside in an environmental niche. Our gut microbiome is the genes of the microbes that live in our gut. Our skin microbiome is the genes of the microbes that live on our skin.
- **Microbiota** refers to the microorganisms themselves — also called microbes, commensals or flora — e.g. gut flora, skin flora and

vaginal flora. Thus, microbiota are the organisms and microbiome denotes their genes.

- **Metabolites** are the chemical byproducts of microbial activity. These metabolites are critical to our health and are influenced by not only what we eat but by all the lifestyle factors discussed throughout this book: sleep, stress, exercise and social relationships. Let me repeat that because it's fundamental to understanding the impact of gut health on brain health. **Our microbiota and the metabolites they produce are influenced by food, exercise, sleep, stress, pollution and even our social interactions.** If a person has gut problems, it may not be enough to change their diet. They may also need to improve their sleep, manage their stress, enrich their relationships, get more exercise and spend more time in nature. Do these recommendations sound familiar? Despite the explosion of new information relating to gut health, the advice about how to be healthy remains the same: **stress less, sleep more, sit less, move more, snack less, cook more, argue less, love more, and swap screen time for green time.**

Questions that researchers are currently trying to answer include the following:

- What constitutes a healthy microbiota? Is there a particular mix of species that produces optimal health? Given the enormous number and diversity of microbes that inhabit our bodies, it's unlikely there is one specific microbial signature that signifies optimal health. To date, the most consistent finding is that **the greater the diversity of microbes in our gut, the healthier we tend to be.** For instance, people with Alzheimer's have fewer distinct species than people of the same age without cognitive impairment. Therefore, our first goal is to encourage the growth of a wide variety of gut microbial species by avoiding ultra-processed food (which is toxic to microbes) and consuming a range of different vegetables, fruits and fermented foods.

- Are there key species of microbes that have a bigger impact on our brain than others? Probably, but we are yet to tease them out. A study involving bumblebees found that a type of gut bacteria called *Lactobacillus apis* improved long-term memory.

Lactobacillus apis increases circulating glycero-phospholipids (GPL), which are important constituents of neural membranes. When elderly people were given GPL supplements for several years, they demonstrated improvements in cognition. Thus, studying our gut microbiota could yield important clues to preserving brain function. Understanding what our microbes do could enable scientists to come up with pills that provide the same chemicals that our bugs produce, without having to repopulate the bacteria themselves.

- Is the absence of specific bacterial species linked to specific diseases? In relation to Alzheimer's, the answer appears to be yes. **In addition to reduced microbial diversity, people with Alzheimer's carry distinctly different gut microbial species compared to people of the same age who do not have Alzheimer's.** Unsurprisingly, the microbial mix in Alzheimer's is associated with increased inflammation and damage to our gut wall integrity.

- What comes first? Given that communication between the brain and gut is bidirectional, do changes in our brain lead to changes in gut microbes, or do changes in gut microbes produce changes in our brain? Both. Traumatic brain injury (TBI) and stroke lead to changes in the composition of our gut microbiota and subsequent gastrointestinal symptoms. Meanwhile, intestinal inflammation and constipation precede the brain changes seen in Parkinson's by several decades.

- If there is an imbalance (known as **dysbiosis**) in the ratio of essential species, what can we do to rectify the imbalance? This is where probiotics enter the scene. Patients aged 60 to 90 years with severe Alzheimer's improved their scores in the Mini-Mental State Exam (MMSE) after 12 weeks of taking a probiotic comprising *Lactobacilli* (universally recognised as good gut bugs) and *Bifidobacteria* (which are under-represented in people with Alzheimer's). Similarly, patients with severe TBI who received probiotics that contained *Lactobacilli* spent less time in intensive care and suffered fewer gastrointestinal problems as a consequence of their injury.

- Does this mean we should all be popping pre- and probiotics? If so, which ones?

Companies that offer **direct-to-consumer microbiome testing** (i.e. send us a sample of your poo and we'll tell you which foods and supplements will help you cultivate a healthy melange of microbes) claim that we have the answers to the preceding questions. We don't. One day we probably will but, at the moment, commercial services are ahead of the science.

On the other hand, there is strong evidence for the health benefits of consuming *natural* pre- and probiotics such as unpeeled vegetables, fruits and fermented foods. **Prebiotics** are non-digestible fibres in plant foods that encourage the growth of healthy bacteria in our colon. Particularly powerful prebiotics include garlic, onion, leek, asparagus, endive, chicory and Jerusalem artichoke because they contain a potent prebiotic called inulin. If you need to increase your intake of prebiotics, start low and go slow — or your gut will literally explode. However, for prebiotics to be effective, we need to have bacteria in our gut that can make use of them.

Probiotics are live microorganisms believed to provide health benefits when we eat them in sufficient amounts. The most common probiotic food is yoghurt — but make certain it is completely natural, contains live cultures and doesn't have any added sugar. Probiotics also include fermented foods such as sauerkraut, kimchi, kefir, kombucha, miso and tempeh. Every culture in the world has a range of fermented dishes from sourdough to pickled gherkins to fermented cheeses. Unfortunately, commercially made versions of these products sometimes use vinegar instead of fermentation so always check the label to ensure the product contains live cultures. Even if live bacteria have been used, the finished product is often heated to kill the bacteria because of fears around food safety. Hence, many people are learning to ferment their own foods or visiting local farmers' markets.

As for probiotics in a pill, the research is less clear. For one thing, the effects of probiotics are strain-specific. *Strain* means the subtype of *Lactobacillus* or *Bifidobacteria* — the two most common bacteria found in commercial probiotics.

Although we know that different strains perform different functions, we are far from knowing which strains are appropriate for which person. Notwithstanding the probiotic successes in Alzheimer's and TBI, research has not reached the point where we can make definitive recommendations to take specific bacterial supplements for specific ailments. Yes, you will find thousands of claims that probiotics improve symptoms of depression, diabetes, allergies, gut problems, brain fog and any other disease you care to look up. But it's still a lucky dip. In part, it depends on what's living in our gut in the first place. You might hit on a formulation that works for you and improves your condition, or you might be a 'resister' — a person who eliminates the contents of probiotics in their stool. Some probiotics can even make some people feel worse — possibly by upsetting the balance of their own resident microbiota. **Always heed your gut instinct.** Do NOT take probiotics after a course of antibiotics to try and speed up repopulation of your gut. Probiotics have been found to slow down re-establishment of a person's natural microbiota. A healthy diet (as per my previous chapters) is still the best-known way to support a healthy population of gut microbes.

Synbiotics are foods or supplements that contain a combination of pre- and probiotics. The purpose of synbiotics is to mix a probiotic (the bacteria) with a specific prebiotic (its preferred food) so that the prebiotic enhances the survival and proliferation of the probiotic.

Psychobiotics are probiotics that purportedly reduce depressive symptoms and confer mental health benefits. Research to date has yielded mixed results.

In summary:
- Prebiotics are food for probiotics.
- Synbiotics are prebiotics combined with probiotics.
- Psychobiotics are probiotics that mess with our mind.

Pre-, pro-, syn- and psychobiotics show promise in treating a wide range of conditions including Alzheimer's. However, there are many questions still to be answered.
- How can we accurately diagnose dysbiosis?
- Which probiotic is best for which condition?
- How can we predict whether someone is a responder or resister?

- How long does a person need to trial probiotics to know if they're working?
- How long do we need to keep taking probiotics when our health is restored?

Another potential approach to treating Alzheimer's is Faecal Microbial Transplantation (FMT), also known as:
- Microbiota Replacement Therapy (MRT)
- Live bio-therapeutics
- Human Probiotic Infusions (HPI)
- Bacteriotherapy
- Brugs (short for Bugs as drugs)
- Crapsules — not very popular because people don't like swallowing something that came out of someone else's bottom
- TransPOOsion
- POObiotics.

Okay, I admit I made up the last two terms, but I think there's a chance they might catch on.

FMT is not a new idea. Cattle farmers have been using what they call faecal transfer for centuries. When cows change their diet they frequently experience indigestion. Farmers treat this by sucking the fluid out of the stomach of a healthy cow and feeding it to the sick cow.

In the 1950s, shortly before antibiotics became widely available, people often died from a disease called Pseudomembranous colitis, so named because the colon becomes inflamed and develops abnormal membranes along its inner walls. Symptoms include fever, abdominal pain, diarrhoea and, in many cases, death. Doctors at the time surmised that the disease was caused by perturbations in a person's gut bacteria but they didn't have the technology to identify the culprit microorganisms. To test their theory, they infused the colon of a sick person with faeces obtained from a healthy person. The procedure was a resounding success and became known as re-setting. Seventy years later, FMT is making a comeback.

To date, I'm aware of only one clinic in Australia that treats people suffering from a variety of gastrointestinal disorders (but not

Alzheimer's) using FMT. It's called The Centre for Digestive Diseases in the suburb of Five Dock in Sydney. Apparently there's a high demand for donors because it's hard work. (Or soft for some.) In fact, it's more difficult to become a poo donor than it is to become a blood donor because the criteria are very stringent. For example:

- you can't have taken antibiotics, antacids or a range of other medications in the last two years
- you can't have any bowel issues yourself
- you can't have an autoimmune disease
- you can't have travelled to a third world country in the previous two years
- and many other criteria — the list goes on for several pages.

Felix keeps telling me I should become a donor because I'm full of it. But I'm too scared to offer my poo because I don't want to be told my shit's not good enough. If you do make the cut, you get paid very well because it's demanding work. You must deliver a fresh specimen to the clinic every morning and it's used the same day. When it becomes mainstream, I wonder what the slogan will be? Perhaps alongside a poster urging us to 'Give blood' there will be another placard imploring us to 'Give a shit'.

FMT has also recently come to the attention of brain researchers. In 2017, German scientists gave old turquoise killifish (the shortest-living vertebrates bred in captivity) antibiotics to wipe out their gut microbiota. When the old fish were then administered faeces from young killifish, they displayed more youthful behaviour and lived 37% longer than usual. In 2021, researchers from University College Cork in Ireland transplanted faeces from young mice into old mice and saw rejuvenation of their hippocampus (the brain's learning and memory centre). This was accompanied by improvements in learning and long-term spatial memory when the old mice were subjected to a maze test.

I was tempted to approach a gastroenterologist with the idea of giving my father FMT but, after my experience with the haematologist, I thought better of it. Fortunately, Chinese scientists appear to have come up with a more palatable option. In November 2019, Shanghai Green Valley Pharmaceuticals announced that China's

National Medical Products Administration approved a new drug called sodium oligomannate (GV-971) for the treatment of mild to moderate Alzheimer's.

Sodium oligomannate is obtained from a type of seaweed called brown algae. Scientists propose that the algae modulate the gut microbiome and correct dysbiosis to reduce neuroinflammation. When it was trialled against a placebo in 818 patients from 34 Chinese hospitals for 36 weeks, those taking GV-971 orally once a day scored significantly higher in cognitive tests from the fourth week until the end of the trial. So as not to bias the results, neither doctors nor patients knew who was receiving GV-971 or who was receiving the placebo.

Keen to verify the results, the US and Europe (Czech Republic, France, Netherlands and Poland) began their own trial of GV-971 in October 2020 in 50- to 85-year-old men and women with mild to moderate Alzheimer's. The trial is named the Green Memory Study and is estimated to finish in October 2026. Rigorous trials exploring efficacy, safety and side effects of medications for chronic diseases often take many years to yield meaningful results. Details of the US and European trials can be found at: clinicaltrials.gov/ct2/show/NCT04520412 and www.alzheimer-europe.org/research/clinical-trials/green-memory.

You can also download a PDF explaining the Green Memory Study at outwittingalzheimers.com/resources.

Regardless of the outcome of the Green Memory Study, it's evident the state of our gut plays a significant role in the health of our brain. Although we don't yet know exactly how this relationship plays out, we need to do everything we can to cultivate a diverse and friendly population of microbes in our gut. Eat a rich and varied array of prebiotic plants and probiotic fermented foods and consider trying a probiotic supplement under the guidance of a qualified health professional. Although it's too early to confidently assess the usefulness of probiotics, some people swear by them.

CHAPTER 74

In search of keys (again)

You realise that all along there was something tremendous within you, and you did not know it.

Paramahansa Yogananda (1893–1952)

E bor is a small town in northern NSW with a population of 166 people. It has one café, one hotel and one waterfall. I stopped there for lunch to break the five-hour drive home from Armidale, where I had given two presentations.

I ordered a vegetable lasagne and salad from Fusspots Café and asked to use their bathroom.

'I'm sorry it's out of order,' replied the friendly woman serving me. 'You'll have to drive two blocks west to the public toilet.'

'No problem,' I replied, 'I'll run the two blocks to get some exercise. By then you'll have heated my lasagne to the perfect temperature.'

After running more than two blocks, I still couldn't find the public toilet so I made my way to the hotel. As I approached, I saw a large sign on the front door. It read: *NO, you cannot use our toilets unless you are a guest of this hotel.* I opened the door nonetheless and poked my head in.

'I was going to ask if I could use your restroom but I've just read the answer,' I greeted the woman behind the counter.

She responded with a broad smile, 'I didn't write the sign so, as far as I'm concerned, you're welcome to use the restroom.'

I thanked her, completed my business and ran back to the café.

Before entering, I went to my car to retrieve my water bottle so I could refill it for the remainder of my journey. I reached into the side pocket of my handbag where I always kept my car keys and … my car keys were not there. How odd. I was sure I'd put them there as usual. Actually, I wasn't sure because I do it without thinking. But why would I not have put the car keys where I always kept them? Maybe I'd accidentally placed them in another compartment in my handbag? I had a flashback to the car key incident at the radiology clinic several years ago. This time I knew for certain the keys were not locked in the boot. Nor were they hidden in one of Dad's pockets.

I went to my table in the café, tipped my handbag upside down and sorted through every item. No car keys. I went to the woman who had taken my order and asked if she'd noticed a set of keys on the counter. No. She made an announcement to all the other café patrons that I was missing my car keys. Had anyone seen them? No.

Maybe I still had them in my hand when I'd gone to the restroom and they were lying by the washbasin at the hotel? My appetite had evaporated so I asked that my lasagne be kept warm while I ran back to the hotel to find my keys. After searching every corner of the ladies' room, and after a similar 'lost keys' announcement had been made to all the hotel patrons, my keys were still nowhere to be found. I launched into box breathing again. This time I was hoping the technique would sharpen my mind. Maybe I'd placed the keys in the pocket of my pants and they'd slipped out while I was running? I slowly retraced my steps back to Fusspots. No keys.

By this stage, everyone in town was searching for my keys, both inside and outside the café. The waitress brought out my lasagne. 'I can't keep heating this up. Why don't you have something to eat? When you stop thinking about the keys, something might occur to you.'

I reluctantly agreed.

Eating mindfully while my mind was racing was an insurmountable challenge. How could this have happened? How could I have been so careless? Was I developing Alzheimer's? How was I going to get home? Felix had been looking after Dad while I was away, but

I could sense that Dad was starting to fret. I had a spare set of car keys in a designated drawer at home but I couldn't ask Felix to drive four hours to bring them to me. It would be a huge imposition and he would have to bring Dad with him — all the while fielding question after question about where they were going and why I wasn't with them. I felt ill.

'Are you sure you checked your handbag properly? Handbags can be a bottomless pit,' the waitress interrupted my unavailing rumination.

'I tipped everything out.'

'Tip everything out again.'

I did as she suggested. No keys. As I picked up my handbag to put everything back inside, I accidentally dropped the bag. I heard the distinct clink of keys hitting the ground. Huh? I peered inside the bag but couldn't see any keys. I plunged my hand into its depths and ran my fingers along the lining. I felt the shape of my keys! But I couldn't get at them because they were underneath the lining. I examined the side compartment. Sure enough, there was a hole just large enough for my keys to slip through and disappear between the lining and the leather. Eureka!

I pulled out my keys and everyone cheered.

During the four-hour drive home, I reflected on my mini drama. I had never really lost the keys. They were in my possession the whole time — I just couldn't see them because they were hidden under a layer of lining. Likewise, **we have within our grasp the keys to a long, happy, healthy life. They're simply hidden under layers of busyness and needless complexity**.

What gives me the greatest joy? Moments of meaningful connection — with other people, animals or nature. Moments of total absorption — while walking, swimming, reading, writing, cooking, eating, working, tidying, creating or innovating. What is the underpinning of true happiness? Being immersed in whatever we're doing, wherever we are, with whomever we're doing it. **Happiness arises when we allow ourselves to experience something unfolding, rather than rushing to attain the end result**. Why do we look for answers outside ourselves when the answers lie within? If we approached everything we did as an end in itself — rather than a means to an end — we would never need to rush.

I settled into an unhurried drive home, past verdant farmland and contented cows. I had never seen so many different shades of glossy green.

CHAPTER 75

Something's in the air

If there were nothing wrong in the world, there wouldn't be anything for us to do.

GEORGE BERNARD SHAW (1856–1950)

Air pollution is one of the top 12 risk factors so far identified for Alzheimer's.

Can you recall the other 11 factors listed in Chapter 4 'Why this book?'

Test yourself before going back to check.

Air pollution also contributes to stroke, high blood pressure, heart, lung and kidney disease, Parkinson's, type 2 diabetes, depression and anxiety, all of which further promote the development of dementia. One illness compounds another. It has also been shown that people with Alzheimer's who live in areas with high levels of air pollution decline more rapidly, require more frequent hospital admissions and die sooner. Even healthy adults and children score worse on tests of cognition and memory when exposed to high levels of air pollution in the hours, days or weeks prior to testing. Take your child bushwalking the day before their next school exam. None of us are immune to the negative impacts of inhaled pollutants.

Reducing Dad's exposure to air pollution was one of the reasons we moved from traffic-choked Sydney to a quiet lakeside suburb on the Gold Coast. **Living near ducks is healthier than living near trucks.** It was a fitting topic of discussion for a Zoom meeting with Jasmin while we were both in COVID lockdown — a time that saw significant worldwide reductions in air pollution due to fewer vehicles on the road and fewer planes, boats, trains and industries operating.

'What exactly do you mean by air pollution?' Jasmin opened our exchange. 'Are you talking about bushfires, diesel fumes or industrial emissions?'

'All of the above. Air pollution comprises a diverse mixture of particles, gases, organic compounds and metals that cause harm to humans and other living organisms. It arises from fuel combustion, power stations, industry, transport and natural disasters such as fires, earthquakes, volcanic eruptions and sandstorms. But by far the greatest contribution to air pollution is human activity, not natural occurrences.'

'What is the magnitude of the harm? Has it been quantified?' Jasmin questioned.

'It's been calculated that, as at 2021, air pollution leads to over 3000 premature deaths in Australia every year — almost triple our road toll of 1100 deaths per year. Look at these figures for other parts of the world.'

Premature deaths attributable to air pollution

Country	Annual deaths attributable to air pollution
Australia	3000
United Kingdom	40 000
France	67 000
USA	200 000
European Union	500 000
Worldwide	7 million

'I've never seen "air pollution" listed as the cause of death on someone's death certificate,' Jasmin commented.

'As a matter of fact, in December 2020, a London mother, Rosalind Kissi-Debrah, made legal history in the UK when a court ruled in her favour that air pollution was a cause in her nine-year-old daughter Ella's death. The family lived 25 metres from a busy road in south-east London where levels of nitrogen dioxide (NO_2) from traffic were consistently higher than the annual legal limit.'

'How did Ella die?' Jasmin was dismayed.

'Ella had chronic and severe asthma attacks that were triggered by spikes in air pollution every winter. Eventually one of the asthma attacks led to her lungs collapsing and she died of acute respiratory failure.'

'Wasn't there anything anyone could do for Ella?'

'The family didn't know that air pollution was the problem until after Ella died. Her mother states that, if they'd known, they would have moved to another suburb. Air pollution isn't always visible to the naked eye. Rosalind has launched a charity called the Ella Roberta Family Foundation to campaign for cleaner air and raise awareness about the deadly link between air pollution and asthma. You can read about their work at ellaroberta.org. The case has prompted the British Parliament to debate a new target for air pollution in line with World Health Organisation (WHO) guidelines.'

'It goes to show that one dedicated person can make a big difference to an entire community,' Jasmin stated with resolve.

'The previous year — in 2019 — there was a similar landmark court ruling in France. A 52-year-old woman and her 16-year-old daughter sued the French government for failing to limit traffic-related air pollution in the vicinity of a ring-road in Saint-Ouen, Paris. The woman and her daughter suffered respiratory infections and bronchitis for many years before they were sent to a lung specialist who advised that their health problems were linked to air pollution. When they moved to Orléans, their symptoms resolved. In the verdict, the state was deemed at fault for taking insufficient measures to reduce concentrations of polluting gases that exceeded established limits. Never be afraid to stand up for what's right. It's not just about helping yourself but protecting others.'

'Which of the components of air pollution cause the greatest harm? Is it the particles, gases, organic compounds or metals? Can we find a way to filter out the offending component or is the whole mixture the problem? Does it help to wear a face mask for instance?' Jasmin proposed.

'Great questions. The various components of air pollution exert differential effects on our brain and body. Scientists are still unravelling all the details because each component comprises a variety of substances and we don't yet know exactly how each specific substance causes damage. Face masks protect us from some, but not all, constituents of air pollution.' I showed Jasmin another table. 'You can see the complexity of studying the relative contribution of so many diverse substances.'

Constituents of air pollution

Particulate matter (PM)	Gases	Organic compounds	Metals
• coarse particles • fine particles • submicron particles • ultrafine particles	• ground level ozone • carbon monoxide • nitrogen oxides • sulphur oxides	• polycyclic aromatic hydrocarbons • endotoxins (bacterial toxins) e.g. lipopolysaccharide (LPS)	• iron (produced by fossil fuel combustion) • manganese • vanadium • nickel • copper • zinc • cadmium • cobalt • chromium • mercury • lead

'What do you mean by particulate matter?' she asked as she pored over the list.

'Particulate matter (PM) is a combination of solid particles and liquid droplets suspended in air. PM is made up of the other three constituents. Gases, organic compounds and metals can also occur separately. **PM is classified as a neurotoxin and has been linked to brain shrinkage and build-up of amyloid β (Aβ).** The degree to which PM is toxic depends on:
• the size and chemical properties of the PM — the smaller the particle, the more readily it can enter the brain
• the surface area — the greater the surface area of the particle the greater the number of toxic substances that can stick to the particle and the more damage it can inflict

- the amount of PM a person has been exposed to
- the length of time a person has been exposed — even relatively low concentrations of air pollution contribute to chronic disease if a person has had years of ongoing exposure
- individual susceptibility to disease, based on age, sex, genetics, physical and mental health and stress levels at the time of exposure. Children — especially in utero — and the elderly are particularly vulnerable to the neurological effects of air pollution.'

'Are people with an APOE4 gene more vulnerable to the brain-damaging effect of air pollution?' Jasmin surmised.

'Yes, they are. The other nasty thing about PM is that it can give rise to secondary toxic particles from photochemical reactions and physical processes in the atmosphere. Here's a table that describes some of the differences between the three categories of PM.'

Types of particulate matter

Name	Diameter in micrometres (μm)	Examples of sources
Coarse particles (PM_{10})	2.5 to 10	• road & agricultural dust • tyre and brake wear & tear • construction & demolition works • mining operations • wood combustion
Fine particles ($PM_{2.5}$)	Less than 2.5 (30 times thinner than a human hair)	• fossil fuel combustion • industrial activities • road traffic • coalesced PM_1 or $PM_{0.1}$
Submicron particles (PM_1)	Less than 1.0	• as for $PM_{2.5}$ • biomass burning (natural lightning-induced fires or burning of vegetation for land clearing)
Ultrafine particles ($PM_{0.1}$ or UFPM)	Less than 0.1	• as for PM_1 • tobacco smoke and e-cigarettes • metal fumes produced by welding • toner pigments (desktop printers and photocopiers) • burning anti-mosquito coils

'PM is pervasive because it can stay in the air for a long time, travel hundreds of kilometres and easily enter buildings. This is particularly the case with $PM_{2.5}$ and smaller.'

'How do air pollutants enter our brain? Don't we naturally resist pollution by coughing and sneezing?' Jasmin posited.

'Yes, we do. Also, the mucous that lines our nose and upper airways traps and removes a lot of PM_{10}. However, smaller PM and gases can bypass our physical defences and penetrate deeper into our lungs. From there, pollutants can enter our bloodstream and be distributed throughout our body to any of our organs, including our brain. That's why air pollution can give rise to so many different diseases — it depends where in our body the particles end up. With respect to our brain, some particles don't even need to be transported in our blood. They can enter the brain directly through the cells and nerves in our nose, eyes and mouth. Our nose is a primary target for air pollution, which may be a reason that loss of smell is an early feature of both Alzheimer's and Parkinson's. A third route by which air pollution travels to the brain is via our gut. Air pollution changes the composition of our gut bacteria, induces chronic inflammation and damages our gut lining so that it becomes more permeable (leaky). This provides another escape route for pollutants to enter our blood or get carried to the brain along a nerve called the vagus.'

'I never realised that air pollution assaulted us on so many levels. When pollutants enter the brain, how do they cause harm?' Jasmin was keen to know all the details.

'Toxins anywhere in the body activate our immune system in an attempt to neutralise them. Exposure to large doses of toxins over a long period of time causes collateral damage in the form of oxidative stress, chronic inflammation, mitochondrial dysfunction and impaired brain energy metabolism. You'll recall from our earlier discussions that all these mechanisms underlie the development of Alzheimer's. In addition, **there's a direct correlation between levels of air pollution and brain Aβ plaques.** Epidemiological research also consistently shows that exposure to air pollution at any stage of life negatively impacts brain function. The closer people live to busy roads, power stations or industry, the worse their cognition, memory and performance on neuropsychological tests. In children this manifests as diminished vocabulary, poorer memory, lower academic performance, impaired co-ordination and ADHD. In the elderly, it increases the risk of mild cognitive impairment (MCI), Alzheimer's and Parkinson's, and produces more rapid decline in those who already have the disease. It's also postulated that early childhood exposure to air pollution can make a person more vulnerable to Alzheimer's in later life. Pregnant women living in densely polluted cities (especially within 50 metres of heavy traffic) are more likely to have miscarriages, low birth weight babies and deep vein thrombosis (DVT), not to mention all the other chronic illnesses that are triggered or exacerbated by air pollution. It has even been linked to elevated stress hormone levels (such as cortisol) and reduced fertility. It's a major global public health issue.'

'My grandmother has lived in Mascot — close to Sydney airport — for most of her life. Do you think this has increased her exposure to air pollution?' Jasmin reflected.

'Yes. Not only do aeroplanes release harmful emissions, there's a lot of traffic carrying freight and passengers to and from airports.'

'Is there a blood test that reveals how much air pollution a person has been exposed to?' Jasmin asked hopefully.

'Not yet. Some clues that your health might be compromised by air pollution include recurrent itchy eyes, scratchy throat, sinus problems, respiratory infections and intractable asthma. These symptoms can also be due to allergies, but I would definitely stay away from pollution hotspots if I suffered from any of the above.'

'What are examples of pollution hotspots? I imagine coal-fired power stations, industrial zones and busy roads would top the list.'

'Correct. Whenever you walk somewhere, take the quietest back road you can find and avoid rush hour traffic. Diesel exhaust fumes are particularly toxic and have been classified by the WHO as a Class 1 carcinogen for lung cancer, and an overlooked cause of stroke. Compared to petrol engines, diesel-powered vehicles emit significantly higher levels of PM and nitrogen dioxide (NO_2).

Unfortunately, even concentrations of air pollution well below current quality standards is associated with adverse health effects. Another hotspot is two-minute drop-off zones outside schools, where parents leave their cars idling. Even though it's only for a short time, children are exposed to high levels of pollution twice a day, five days a week.'

'Where can a person find out about the air quality in their local area?'

'Many countries use a colour-coded tool called the Air Quality Index to inform the public of daily levels of air pollution and to provide corresponding health advice. For instance, a rating of "good" (green) encourages people to enjoy outdoor activities. A rating of "very poor" (crimson) recommends rescheduling strenuous outdoor activities for another day when air quality is better. A rating of "hazardous" (red) advises people to stay indoors. Simply type the words "air quality index" into your browser and select your location. The USA has an excellent government website airnow.com where the day's air pollution data is clearly displayed and the primary pollutants, e.g. ozone, $PM_{2.5}$, PM_{10}, nitrogen dioxide (NO_2) and carbon monoxide (CO) are listed in order of highest to lowest concentration. In Australia, I recommend downloading an app created by the Asthma Foundation called Airsmart.

'Being cooped up indoors isn't the best for our cognition either, is it?' remarked Jasmin.

'No, it's not. A recent study by the University of NSW revealed that carbon dioxide (CO_2) levels in school classrooms were often four times the limit recommended by the Australian Building Codes. High levels of CO_2 impair concentration, compromise learning and make students and teachers feel tired and drowsy. Another 2021 study by the Harvard T.H. Chan School of Public Health in Massachusetts found that high indoor $PM_{2.5}$ and CO_2 levels correlated with reduced accuracy and slower reaction times on cognitive tests. The year-long research involved 302 office workers in 40 urban commercial buildings located in six countries (China, India, Mexico, Thailand, USA and UK). Each person's workspace was fitted with a pollution sensor linked to an app on their phone. When levels of $PM_{2.5}$ and CO_2 were above or below a certain threshold, participants were notified to perform a short series of cognitive tests. The higher the indoor pollution, the worse their test scores. We need to ensure that all buildings have good ventilation and filtration. Not only will people be more alert, sharp and productive, it will boost overall brain health and reduce transmission of infections.'

'This is such a complex and far-reaching problem … where do we even begin?' Jasmin was sounding despondent.

'The first step is always raising awareness. Scientists, health professionals and governments play an important role in educating people about the hazards of air pollution and how to mitigate them. Also remember that high levels of air pollution do not mean a person is unequivocally destined to get Alzheimer's. Air pollution, like excessive alcohol consumption and high blood pressure, is another piece in the puzzle — a risk factor, not an immutable determinant. No risk factor operates in isolation. A study published in the journal *Alzheimer's & Dementia* involving 542 women found that those who reported more stressful life events and disturbed sleep were more vulnerable to the brain-damaging effects of $PM_{2.5}$. In other words, $PM_{2.5}$ is more likely to push a person towards Alzheimer's if they're also under a lot of stress and not sleeping well. **Alzheimer's is the cumulative effect of multiple interacting factors.'**

'How can we reduce our exposure to air pollution and make the air cleaner in our local community?' I could see Jasmin formulating a list.

'Why don't you give me some of *your* suggestions?' I encouraged.

'Okay … here goes:

- Don't smoke or vape.
- Replace wood heaters with clean heating sources such as split systems or heat pumps that rely on renewable energy sources. This may require lobbying government to make legislative changes.
- Use public transport or carpool to reduce the number of cars on our roads.
- Avoid idling your vehicle and turn off your engine at drop-off zones to reduce vehicle emissions.
- Offer to write an article about the issue for your local paper or child's school newsletter.

- Take quiet, scenic, back streets whenever you're walking or cycling.
- Keep track of the Air Quality Index where you live and work, and wear a face mask on days that have a poor rating. I've seen cyclists wear high tech masks but I suspect any mask is better than no mask when it comes to reducing the amount of pollution we breathe in.
- Plant tall trees around your property boundaries to act as physical barriers to pollution and to release fresh oxygen.
- Lobby your local council to improve air quality by planting more trees, protecting green spaces, creating safe cycling paths and discouraging idling.

'And I'll be taking my grandmother to more parks and gardens. All our hospitals and aged care facilities need gardens for staff and residents to spend time in,' she concluded.

'Excellent!' I beamed. 'You might also like to join Doctors for the Environment Australia (dea.org.au) whose credo is "healthy planet, healthy people" and call on the government to strengthen air pollution standards. Nothing is impossible if we fervently commit to achieving it. The UK has pledged to ban the sale of all petrol and diesel vehicles by 2030, and to ensure all new cars and vans are fully zero emission from the tailpipe by 2035. This will improve air quality and support economic growth throughout the country.

'Everyone can do something to reduce air pollution, even if it's just starting a conversation. As for your personal air pollution detox plan, try forest bathing.'

'What's forest bathing?' Jasmin brightened up.

'That's the start of another conversation.'

CHAPTER 76

Have you tried forest bathing?

When you look deep into nature, you will understand everything better.

ALBERT EINSTEIN (1879–1955). It obviously worked for him.

Since the 1980s there's been a deluge of research on the health benefits of spending time in nature. The Japanese call it Forest Bathing; the British have introduced Ecotherapy and a growing number of doctors are being certified in Forest Medicine. But does it really work? Or is it just a feel-good fad? Jasmin was ready with a line-up of questions.

'What exactly is Forest Bathing?' she began. 'I'm guessing it doesn't mean skinny dipping in a forest stream?' she grinned impishly.

'You can incorporate that into the experience if you want, but it isn't mandatory,' I returned her grin. 'Forest bathing means immersing yourself in a forest or simply spending time in nature and soaking up the environment with all your senses — more commonly referred to as Nature Therapy or Green Therapy. It originated in Japan in 1982, and the term in Japanese is *shinrin yoku*. The practice arose from a marketing campaign by the Japanese Forestry Agency to encourage people to visit Japan's magnificent forests. City dwellers soon started reporting how much better they felt physically, mentally and emotionally — even after just five minutes of wandering among trees — so doctors began testing whether there were measurable bodily changes in response to contact with nature.'

'What did they find?'

'**Nature nurtures us** on many levels. For a start, being in **nature strengthens our immune system**. Many plants emit airborne chemicals called **phytoncides** that have anti-bacterial and anti-fungal properties to help them fight microbial predators and insects. When humans breathe in phytoncides, we increase the number and activity of white blood cells known as Natural Killer (NK) cells that help us fight infections and tumours.'

'How long do the benefits for our immune system last?'

'Japanese studies have found that after a day trip to a forest park in Tokyo, during which people walked in the forest for two hours in the morning and two hours in the afternoon, NK activity remained boosted for at least seven days afterwards. The forest experience also increased blood levels of anti-cancer proteins for over a week. After three days of forest bathing, the health effects lasted up to 30 days. Researchers are now investigating whether regular forest bathing can lower the risk of cancer.'

'That would be incredible!' Jasmin exclaimed.

'That's only the beginning,' I continued. '**Exposure to natural environments also markedly decreases stress** as measured by saliva samples that reveal reductions in two hormones that are released when we're tense and anxious: cortisol and alpha-amylase. In addition, **nature lowers our heart rate and blood pressure**, and people report feeling calmer, happier and more relaxed. They also fall asleep more easily and sleep better through the night. All these factors contribute to improved brain and heart health.'

'Nature sounds like a panacea for all bodily ills!' Jasmin declared with mounting excitement.

'Not just bodily ills, but mental ones as well. Functional MRI scans of the brain confirm that spending time in **nature reduces anger, depression, rumination and ADHD**. Research on children has found that the further they live from parks and green spaces — especially boys — the more likely they are to be diagnosed with ADHD and subsequently prescribed medication. In addition, a 2020 worldwide review of 186 studies confirmed that children and adolescents who spent more time in nature (green time) had better mental health, academic achievement and overall cognitive functioning than young people who engaged in more screen time (social media, video games and computer-based activities). On the other hand, if you're tired or mentally drained, nature will re-energise you and improve your concentration and creativity. This is referred to as Attention Restoration Theory. In contrast to the demands of our concrete-bound lives, nature holds our attention without straining us, and thus replenishes our exhausted mental faculties. It also provides a sense of "getting away from it all" and we heave an unconscious sigh of relief. Many people report that when they step into nature, their anxiety automatically dissipates. Performance in mentally challenging tasks improves after exposure to nature and gets worse after spending time in urban environments. This holds for children and adults alike. When grandparents take their grandchildren for a walk in a park or forest, it brings enormous health benefits for both generations. **Start swapping screen time for green time.**'

'What about the beach?'

'A stroll along the beach likewise reduces stress and improves mental health, but you're probably inhaling fewer phytoncides.'

'Maybe you're inhaling chemicals or microbes related to the ocean that have a similar effect?' Jasmin suggested.

'Quite likely. There hasn't been as much research focusing on the salutogenic (health-generating) effects of blue spaces (oceans, rivers, lakes and streams) compared to green spaces, but this is being addressed through the BlueHealth Project (bluehealth2020.eu).'

'What's the BlueHealth Project?' Jasmin asked.

'The BlueHealth Project is the biggest ever study across Europe exploring the relationship between blue spaces and human health. Unsurprisingly, the researchers found that **blue spaces wash away the blues**. One study involving 20 000 people in the UK used a smartphone app that sent participants a brief questionnaire about how they were feeling at random moments. The participants' locations were determined by GPS, and they had to submit their answers immediately. The researchers collected over one million responses and found that people felt substantially happier when they were in natural versus urban environments, and especially when they were in the vicinity of water. As a corollary of the findings, scientists are now recommending policies and tools to enable more people to experience blue environments regardless of where they live.

'The overarching message is to enjoy whatever natural environment is accessible to you because nature in all its forms is healing. Simply **living in coastal regions or greener towns is associated with fewer hospitalisations** and a longer lifespan due to less heart disease, stroke, obesity, type 2 diabetes, asthma and mental distress. Children are also less likely to be short-sighted. The best scenario of all appears to be living where green and blue spaces meet.'

'I find that being in nature also prompts people to be more physically active, which means you're getting two brain-boosters for the price of one.' Jasmin looked pleased with her appraisal.

'Blue and green spaces are also often associated with positive social interactions: a family picnic, camping, bushwalking, playing in the sand, swimming, paddling, surfing, snorkelling, diving or sailing. The other wonderful thing about nature is that it induces effortless mindfulness — it captivates us and quiets our mind chatter — which is yet another brain-boosting corollary. In fact, brain scans demonstrate that meditation and nature have similar effects on our prefrontal cortex — the part of our brain responsible for higher order thinking and decision making.'

'How much time do we need to spend in nature to start seeing benefits?'

'Great question. A study of over 19 000 adults living in various parts of England revealed that **we need at least two hours in nature per week to boost our physical and mental health** and the benefits peak between 200 and 300 minutes a week.'

'Is it better to do an hour-long walk in the park twice a week or 18 minutes every day?' Jasmin quickly calculated.

'We don't have all the answers yet, but it doesn't seem to matter how you divide your time in nature — just try to get out there as often and for as long as you can,' I encouraged. 'Quality is more important than quantity.'

'What do you mean by quality?'

'The more we engage with nature and the more connected we feel to it, the greater the benefits to our mental wellbeing. That means turn off your phone and focus on experiencing your surroundings with all your senses. Try to let go of troubling thoughts and simply take in the present moment.'

'What about gardening?' Jasmin asked eagerly.

'Gardening is a great brain-booster and antidepressant, thanks also to a species of bacteria called *Mycobacterium vaccae* that we inhale from the soil. *M. vaccae* increases our levels of serotonin (as does Prozac), and is found to reduce anxiety and improve mental processing. Mice fed live *M. vaccae* navigate mazes twice as fast and with less angst than regular mice. Researchers are currently looking into developing medications containing *M. vaccae* to treat depression, asthma, cancer and skin conditions such as psoriasis and eczema.'

'Is there any research exploring a direct relationship between exposure to nature and Alzheimer's?'

'Yes. A Chinese study of over 38 000 elderly people found that those who lived in greener suburbs had better cognition than those surrounded by concrete. Meanwhile, in the UK **green dementia care** has been found to improve mood, motivation and social interaction among aged care residents.'

'What does green dementia care entail?'

'It simply means incorporating outdoor and indoor nature-based activities into people's daily routine. For example, tending to a pot plant or kitchen garden, arranging flowers in a vase, visiting public parks, gardens and lakes, going on a picnic, participating in community revegetation projects, even just opening a window and looking at a tree or listening to birds. It depends on a person's mobility and access to green spaces.'

'Does looking at nature from a window really make much difference?' Jasmin looked dubious.

'Yes, it does. **Surgical patients recover more quickly and require fewer painkillers if they're in a hospital room that has a view of nature.** If that's not possible, flowers in the room will help them. And whenever you're studying or working at your desk, do the same. Periodically switching your gaze from a screen or book to a pot plant or flower relieves what is known as Directed Attention Fatigue. You'll feel less mentally drained and you'll focus better on the task at hand.'

'What about employing virtual reality (VR) to deliver the experience of nature? Sadly, there are people who simply don't have access to the natural world,' reflected Jasmin.

'More than 200 studies examining the health effects of still images, videos and simulations of nature have demonstrated that in terms of reducing stress, restoring concentration and improving mood, VR can be very effective. Obviously you don't get to sniff phytoncides, but virtual nature is better than no nature,' I affirmed.

'Someone will try to bottle phytoncides before long,' Jasmin commented astutely.

'Someone already has! Scientist Qing Li from Nippon Medical School in Tokyo vaporised essential oils from Japanese cypress trees and infused the scent into an urban hotel. He tested and confirmed the presence of phytoncides in hotel room air and then asked 12 healthy men aged 37 to 60 to stay at the hotel for three nights from 7 pm to 8 am. Blood and urine samples were taken before and after the three-night stay. The effect of the phytoncides was a significant increase in NK cells and cancer-fighting proteins in blood, and a reduction in stress hormones in urine.'

'Okay then, my take home from this conversation is that all hospitals and aged care homes need to:
- include accessible gardens for patients and staff to enjoy
- create kitchen gardens for residents to tend
- instal living green walls
- have pot plants in every room
- vaporise cypress or cedar tree oils with a humidifier each night
- display pictures of nature

- screen nature videos
- and provide VR nature experiences.'

'Sounds wonderful!' I endorsed.

'And I'll be giving all my patients a green prescription to spend at least 18 minutes a day in nature without their mobile phone,' Jasmin concluded.

'Go easy on giving "nature prescriptions",' I cautioned. 'Research has shown that if people feel pressured to spend time in nature, it becomes a chore and they don't find it as enjoyable as when it's their choice. By all means, encourage people to seek out green and blue spaces, but don't insist on it.'

'Noted,' Jasmin nodded.

'You might also like to have **sounds of nature** playing in the background. A study from Carleton University in Canada analysed sound recordings from 251 sites at North American national parks and found that exposure to natural versus artificial sounds was associated with more positive mood states, better health and higher mental performance, along with lower levels of stress, pain and annoyance. Some scientists are even recommending different sounds for different conditions. Water sounds are more effective for improving mood and general health, while bird sounds are better at reducing stress and irritation.'

'We really need to connect all our senses to nature, don't we?'

'Absolutely. It's the most natural thing in the world.'

CHAPTER 77

Heads up!

Nothing will ever be attempted if all possible objections must first be overcome.

SAMUEL JOHNSON (1709–1784)

I f you knew that doing something you loved — I mean *really* loved — could give you dementia, would you still do it?

What if that thing was playing your favourite sport? For instance, boxing, ice hockey, American football (gridiron or NFL), soccer (association football), Australian Football (AFL), rugby league (NRL) or rugby union (RU)?

Would you let your children participate in these sports if you knew that it raised their risk of developing dementia later in life?

What happens when sport clashes head on with medicine?

Boxing

In 1928, New Jersey pathologist Dr Harrison Martland noticed that a high percentage of professional boxers developed neurological problems after they retired. They suffered from confusion, loss of co-ordination, headaches, shaking, behavioural changes, speech deficits and other symptoms resembling dementia. He originally called the condition 'punch drunk syndrome' but it was later renamed *dementia pugilistica* from the Latin *pugil* meaning 'boxer'.

In 1949, British neurologist Dr MacDonald Critchley changed the name again to more accurately describe what was occurring in the brain. He coined the term chronic traumatic encephalopathy, which now goes by its acronym CTE. Over the ensuing half century, one in five professional boxers were struck with CTE — today recognised as a unique type of dementia.

In 1969, researchers from the Royal College of Physicians in the UK identified a subset of boxers who were more likely to acquire the disease. The boxers tended to have longer careers, more fights and more knockouts. They were also inclined to have a sparring style of fighting in which they sustained multiple light blows that dazed them but didn't bring them down. Their tactic was to wear out their opponent through endurance. It was only decades later that neurologists realised these **sub-concussive hits could cause cumulative brain damage**.

Our brain is a squishy, mushy, wrinkled lump of fatty tissue that deforms with the slightest pressure. If you held a brain in your hand, your fingers would leave indentation marks. It has the consistency of soft tofu and floats freely inside our hard bony skull. Surrounding our brain is cerebrospinal fluid (CSF), which acts like a cushion and protects our brain from banging against our skull. It's akin to jelly suspended in a jar of water.

Now imagine shaking the jar. What happens to the jelly? Every time a boxer receives a blow to the head, his brain gets shaken and knocks against his skull. Even if the punch isn't hard enough to make the brain strike the skull, every punch produces vibrations that bounce from the skull onto the brain. Vibrations through our brain disrupt normal cell functioning, stretch and tear nerve fibres and cause multiple tiny haemorrhages. If this happens often enough, the brain may never recover and continues to deteriorate for the rest of a person's life. On average, symptoms start appearing 16 years after a fighter retires but, in some cases, symptoms have emerged sooner.

In 1984, three years after retiring from boxing, Muhammad Ali was diagnosed with Parkinson's disease. He was 42 years old. Did boxing lead to his disease? The question is still being debated but the majority of doctors believe yes. *Pugilistic parkinsonism* has been listed as an official disease. Five years earlier, in 1989, Ali's idol, Sugar Ray Robinson, died at age 67 with a diagnosis of Alzheimer's.

Robinson's professional boxing career spanned 25 years from 1940 to 1965. Every decade, dementia ravages the brains of more and more boxers: Wilfred Benitez, Riddick Bowe, Bobby Chacon, Billy Conn, Jimmy Ellis, Peter Flanagan, Joe Frazier, Emile Griffith, Thomas Hearns, Floyd Patterson, Willie Pep, Jerry Quarry, Mike Quarry, Freddie Roach, Meldrick Taylor, Jimmy Young and Fritzie Zivic.

Boxing is as big a risk for dementia as smoking is for lung cancer.

American football

In 2005, CTE claimed another casualty: American football.

Michael Lewis Webster, known as Iron Mike, was one of the greatest centres in NFL history. He played for the Pittsburgh Steelers and Kansas City Chiefs from 1974 to 1990 and died in 2002 at the age of 50. Throughout his career, he played through multiple concussions that damaged the frontal lobes of his brain and led to depression, paranoia and excruciating headaches. The pain was so intense he used a stun gun to shock himself unconscious so he could get some relief. At autopsy, neuropathologist Dr Bennet Omalu examined Mike's brain under a microscope and found distinctive patterns of tau tangles — the same proteins that are seen in a brain with Alzheimer's but with no other evidence of Alzheimer's.

This sparked a string of autopsies in boxers and football players that kept revealing the same brain lesions. In 2014, Dr Ann McKee, together with seven other neuropathologists from around the world, described the unique characteristics that now define CTE: multiple phosphorylated tau tangles clustered around blood vessels deep in the folds (sulci) of the outermost region of the brain (the cortex). CTE is distinct from Alzheimer's even though both diseases share the presence of tau. CTE is a specific type of dementia that results from multiple blows to the head over a period of several years. How many blows and how forceful the blows need to be is currently under investigation. A few studies suggest that carrying the APOE4 gene increases the likelihood that a person will develop CTE in response to head trauma.

Another feature of CTE is that it can present in different ways. If it occurs at a younger age, the main features appear to be mood and behavioural problems. If it develops later in life, memory and thinking are more likely to be affected. Researchers currently describe the disease as having four stages.

In stage one, a person experiences headaches and dizziness with episodes of confusion and disorientation. The mean age of onset is 28 years but this can vary by 13 years in either direction. Stage two involves impulsive behaviour, poor judgement and personality changes. It tends to occur between the ages of 30 and 50. Stage three usually starts after age 50 and stage four after age 65. Stages three and four encompass progressive unravelling of thinking, memory, speech and movement.

A disturbing study published in the *Journal of the American Medical Association* (JAMA) in 2017 reported that CTE was found postmortem in 99% of brains donated by NFL players, 91% of brains from college footballers and 21% of brains from high school players. Even though the results are skewed by the fact that players with symptoms are more likely to donate their brains to science, the findings reveal that a shocking number of footballers at all levels suffer brain damage that leads to dementia.

Like boxers, what seems to be driving CTE in American football players is the number of years they played the game. In October 2019, analyses published in the *Annals of Neurology* found that after 15 years of professional football, almost everyone ended up with CTE. The odds of having CTE went up by 30% for every year of play. Each additional three years of football doubled a player's chances of developing CTE.

To date, the American National Football League has paid out more than US$629 million (A$895 million) to compensate brain-impaired footballers. The US National Hockey League is also facing ongoing class action from CTE-affected players.

Soccer

Jeff Astle was a professional English soccer player who scored more than 200 goals. He was an exceptional header of the ball in the days when footballs were made of leather with an internal pig skin bladder and thus became markedly heavier in the rain. Today's balls are made of material that is impervious to water so they don't gain weight when wet. However, the dry weight of the ball is the same. In his early fifties, Astle developed symptoms of Alzheimer's, which led to death by choking in 2002 at the age of 59. Almost a decade earlier, in December 1993, another soccer player, Danny Blanchflower, died of bronchopneumonia as a consequence of both Alzheimer's and Parkinson's. The two players were subsequently found to have CTE attributed to years of heading the ball.

In 2015, Astle's family launched The Jeff Astle Foundation to raise awareness of CTE and to offer support to those who were affected. The Foundation has so far listed more than 300 ex-soccer players diagnosed with dementia, many of which are likely to be due to CTE. One of them is Sue Lopez, who won 22 caps for England and occasionally suffered concussions after heading the ball. She was awarded an MBE for services to women's football and now advocates that headers be abolished in children's soccer. Her pleas are well founded. In 2016, a frightening study by the University of Stirling found that heading a soccer ball causes immediate impairments in brain function and memory for 24 hours after routine practice. In addition to recording biochemical and electrical changes in the brain, memory was reduced by up to 67%. I wonder how this affects schoolwork and exam results? Week after week, what is this doing to a child's brain capacity?

In 2019, researchers from the University of Glasgow compared death certificates from 7676 Scottish professional soccer players to 23 028 members of the general public. They found that despite having less heart disease, soccer players were five times more likely to have been diagnosed with Alzheimer's and three times more likely to have motor neuron disease (MND) or Parkinson's. The players had not been examined for CTE so it's not known whether this was also part of the diagnosis. The fact remains that **professional soccer**

players are more likely to develop a neurodegenerative disease than are non-players.

In response to these findings, heading the ball will no longer be taught to children under the age of 11 in the US and under 12 in England, Scotland and Northern Ireland. As children get older, headers will be gradually introduced and carefully monitored. Other countries are still debating the guidelines. Science dictates that more stringent protective measures are required.

Australian rugby

In 2014, the first Australian case of CTE was diagnosed in Manly Rugby Union player Barry 'Tizza' Taylor who developed symptoms of dementia in his fifties. After his death at age 77, his widow Enid agreed to have his brain sent to the Global Brain Bank at Boston University where CTE was confirmed. Once again, the defining pattern of tau tangles was seen under the microscope. It was one of the worst cases they had ever encountered.

In June 2019, a further two cases of CTE were reported in Australian professional sportsmen by Royal Prince Alfred Hospital's Associate Professor Michael Buckland in the journal *Acta Neuropathologica Communications* — this time in rugby league players. The two men had both played more than 150 first-grade NRL games over many years and died in middle age.

Not long after, 25 retired NRL players came forward with symptoms of poor mental health and declining brain function. In October 2019, a program called *Insight* on Australian SBS television interviewed half a dozen ex-NRL players along with their families and treating doctors. From their fifties onwards, they had started having bouts of depression, anger, aggression, agitation, explosive outbursts, impaired judgement, memory loss and difficulties with comprehension. The inability to control their behaviour wreaked havoc on their relationships and was tearing apart their families and friendships. Partners and children described them as having a complete change of character. The players themselves talked about being a shell of their former selves. Previously compassionate and judicious, many of them had become unpredictable and irrational. This is the classic picture of CTE.

The interviewer closed the broadcast by asking each of the players the same question: 'Thirty years ago if you'd known you would end up with dementia, would you still have become a professional rugby player?' A heavy silence swept through the audience as several of the players nodded. The thrill of the game, belonging to the team, roaring fans and adrenalin-filled days were worth the price of CTE. They were part of a cause bigger than themselves — their lives had mattered. The camera then swung to capture the responses of their partners. All of them looked devastated.

Tragically, in February 2020, Barry Taylor's son Steven died at age 56 after falling and hitting his head. Steven had also started showing signs of cognitive impairment, despite giving up rugby at the age of 16. Why had he stopped playing so young? He'd sustained five serious concussions and determined that enough was enough. When his brain was examined postmortem, it turned out that enough was in fact too much. Steven was also found to have CTE. His case corroborates the findings of a study on American high school and college football players published in the *Journal of Neurotrauma* in March 2016. Using sensors in helmets, the researchers revealed that cumulative exposure to head impact — including hits the players hardly noticed — predicted later-life depression and apathy as well as diminished reasoning, judgement, planning and problem-solving. There was a clear dose-dependent relationship between the number of hits and long-term sequelae. Frequency of hits appeared to be more damaging than severity of hits. What is most worrying is that **hits to the head don't have to cause severe pain to disrupt brain function**.

Australian football

CTE was also diagnosed posthumously in two legendary AFL players: Graham 'Polly' Farmer and Danny Frawley. Danny had been a passionate advocate for mental health issues, having suffered from depression for many years.

What now?

CTE poses more questions than it answers. Is it more likely to occur after a few severe head injuries, a lot of mild knocks or a combination of both? Would better management of concussions — such as longer rest time — reduce the likelihood of CTE later? Would players rebel against not being allowed to return to the field if they felt subjectively well? Are some people more susceptible to developing CTE because of their genes, microbiome or other unknown factors? What percentage of Alzheimer's cases are actually CTE? At this stage, unless we examine the brain under a microscope after death, we are unable to definitively diagnose CTE.

In June 2007, Dr Chris Nowinski and Dr Robert Cantu established **The Concussion Legacy Foundation (CLF)** in Boston, USA to work towards answering these questions. The overall mission of the Foundation is to end CTE through prevention, research, education and collaboration. In 2018, Associate Professor Buckland partnered with Dr Nowinski to establish the **Australian Sports Brain Bank (ASBB)**. Both organisations study posthumous brains donated by the public. Brain banks need donations from people in all walks of life, not just from athletes, so they can make comparisons and investigate the impact of different life situations. If you're interested in pledging your brain to the ASBB, visit brainbank.org.au for an information pack. You can change your mind at any time if you no longer wish to participate. ASBB also provides a support network for CTE-affected families, and education for doctors and patients.

In September 2022, I was privileged to attend the launch of the Concussion Legacy Foundation (CLF) in Australia. One of CLF's first initiatives is to raise awareness of an international campaign called 'Stop Hitting Kids in the Head'. The campaign aims to eliminate repetitive head injuries in children as a result of playing sport. One effective strategy is to replace tackle football with touch or flag football. In flag football, instead of tackling, the defensive team must 'deflag' or remove a flag from the player with the ball. It's a much safer sport with limited contact between players.

We live in a dangerous world. Contact and collision sports are not the only cause of **traumatic brain injury (TBI)** that can culminate in CTE. Major League Baseball player Ryan Freel, BMX biker Dave Mirra and professional bull-rider Ty Pozzobon all sustained multiple concussions and died before the age of 45. Postmortem, all were confirmed to have CTE.

Motor vehicle accidents, falls, domestic violence, shockwaves from explosions, cricket balls and extreme whiplash can all give rise to TBI. The military are another high-risk group. So how is TBI defined? What level of TBI precipitates CTE?

TBI is injury to the brain caused by an external force. It is classified as mild, moderate or severe, based on intensity of symptoms, how long they last and whether the person loses consciousness. Mild TBI is known as concussion but we're beginning to realise that 'mild' is a fallacy. Many people don't even realise they've been concussed because the symptoms can be very subtle. Some contact-sportspeople admit to being dazed so frequently they consider it a normal part of the game. They brush it off as an inconsequential ding and carry on. We now know that even feeling slightly dazed after a light blow can have serious and long-lasting effects, especially with insufficient rest. That's not to say a single concussion will lead to dementia. It's to advise that any concussion needs medical attention.

Concussion is a temporary energy deficit in the brain, characterised by a transient change in awareness or impairment of brain function, with or without loss of consciousness. Symptoms include dizziness, headaches, unsteadiness, confusion, nausea, vomiting, irritability, drowsiness and disturbance of memory. If there is loss of consciousness for longer than 30 minutes, or loss of memory for longer than one day, the condition is regarded as moderate. If a person has seizures or is unconscious for over 24 hours, the injury is regarded as severe. Under-18-year-olds are more susceptible to concussion and take longer to recover. One concussion increases the risk of further concussions and a longer recovery time. This is particularly important when assessing whether players are ready to return to the game. The best approach is **when in doubt, sit them out**.

Even if someone doesn't progress to CTE, a single concussion (with or without loss of consciousness) can lead to post-concussion syndrome (PCS) lasting from a few weeks to several years. The person experiences a range of symptoms including headaches, dizziness, noise sensitivity, restlessness, irritability, anxiety, depression and problems with concentration, memory and sleep. It's critical they receive the right education, support, rest and rehabilitation, with or without medications. If you or someone you know has had a recent concussion or is suffering from PCS, visit concussiondoc.io and check out The Concussion Fix online course. It has helped thousands of people recover from PCS.

Before the discovery of CTE, doctors were aware that TBI increased the risk of Alzheimer's and other dementias. We will never know how many of these earlier cases of Alzheimer's were actually CTE. Neurologists simply documented that more severe and frequent brain injuries were more likely to precipitate dementia, even 30 years after the event.

It's obvious we need to do everything we can to reduce the incidence of TBI in life as well as in sport. Seatbelts, airbags, random breath testing and helmets have all gone a long way to head off injuries resulting from motor vehicle and bicycle accidents. Falls are common in the elderly and often have lethal consequences. Within our home, I was always on the lookout for trip hazards. I removed loose rugs, installed shower rails and immediately dried wet floors. Improving Dad's balance and muscle strength were a high priority, as was taking him to annual eyesight testing.

Mitigating head injuries in sport is a more complex issue. Playing sport enriches our lives — physically, mentally and socially. However, if we don't set guidelines that ensure the safety of players, the harms will undo the benefits. To their credit, the AFL has amended the rules to reduce the number of dangerous tackles and high collisions. In 2019, rugby union lowered the legal tackle height worldwide and immediately saw a significant drop in concussions. Protocols for managing head injuries have also been tightened. These reforms are moving AFL and rugby in the right direction but it's only a start. Another critical issue is the culture of the game. Mental and physical bravery are carved into a player's DNA. Team members fear being seen as weak if they admit to feeling unwell. They believe it's an occupational hazard and the game must go on. No one wants to let the team down by staying off the field after a 'minor' knock. However, symptoms are sometimes delayed for several hours, and continuing to play would make the player sicker later. We need to redefine 'minor' and 'bravery'. Bravery shouldn't mean playing on after an injury. Wouldn't it be braver to talk about injuries so that sport could be made safer for everyone? To quote Samuel Johnson again 'Courage is the greatest of all virtues, because if you haven't courage, you may not have an opportunity to use any of the others.'

When the rules of soccer and contact sports were created, we were unaware of the consequences. Now that we know, we need to reconsider the rules. Science is full of research that yields answers we don't like. Life is filled with events that force us to change. COVID-19 has demonstrated that the world is capable of massive — previously unimaginable — change. Surely so is sport.

The first step is raising awareness. Your voice can make a difference. Start a conversation today.

CHAPTER 78

Biomarkers

Ideas shape the course of history.

JOHN MAYNARD KEYNES (1883–1946)

A novel blood test for Alzheimer's is on the horizon. Researchers worldwide have demonstrated that a protein called neurofilament light chain (NfL) is elevated in the blood plasma of people with Alzheimer's, at least 15 years before they develop any symptoms.

NfL is a structural protein found within the axon of neurons. An axon is the tail-like nerve fibre that carries electrical signals from one brain cell to another. When an axon becomes damaged, NfL is released into the cerebrospinal fluid (CSF) and trickles into the bloodstream. In a healthy brain, small amounts of NfL are continually released during the natural process of replacing old cells with new ones. As we age, there is increasing cell turnover and the amount of NfL in our CSF and blood gradually rises. Between the ages of 20 and 50, the amount of NfL doubles, and between 50 and 70 it doubles again. Thereafter, NfL levels remain largely stable. If a person has more NfL in their plasma than is expected for their age, it signifies ongoing brain cell damage and progressive disease.

High levels of plasma NfL (pNfL) are found not only in Alzheimer's but also in other neurodegenerative diseases such as frontotemporal dementia (FTD), Huntington's disease, multiple sclerosis (MS), cerebral vasculitis and motor neuron disease (MND). Therefore pNfL cannot be a stand-alone test. To assist in making a reliable diagnosis, pNfL needs to be administered together with assessments of memory and mental functioning, and interpreted in the context of presenting symptoms.

Some of the most useful applications of pNfL will be to determine:
- whether memory loss, confusion and apathy in an older person are due to Alzheimer's or depression (both conditions can present with similar symptoms but there is no rise in pNfL in depression)
- whether personality changes in an older person are due to FTD or a psychiatric disorder (pNfL is not elevated in psychiatric diseases)
- whether or not a treatment for Alzheimer's is working (pNfL should remain stable or go down if a treatment is effective)
- whether someone with mild cognitive impairment (MCI) will progress to Alzheimer's (MCI + high pNfL predict progression to Alzheimer's). See Chapter 7 'In search of signs' for a review of MCI.

People with MCI who do NOT have elevated levels of pNfL are much less likely to progress to dementia than people who have MCI with higher than normal levels of pNfL. Hence the test has predictive value in a person with MCI. Regardless of the prognosis, MCI is a sign that a brain needs boosting.

Plasma NfL is currently only being used in Sweden and the Netherlands as part of the assessment of people with memory and thinking problems. By employing the test to diagnose impending Alzheimer's, doctors can prescribe specific lifestyle changes to stop the disease from taking hold. Health professionals in other countries are still deliberating the usefulness of the test because it is not specific for Alzheimer's.

Meanwhile, in September 2020, a study published in the journal *Alzheimer's Research & Therapy* reported that NfL could also be detected in our eyes. Seventy-seven patients with an average age of 56 who underwent routine eye surgery, gave permission for scientists to collect samples of their vitreous humour during the operation. Vitreous humour is a transparent gelatinous fluid that lies behind the lens in our eyeball. Everyone was found to have small amounts of NfL in their vitreous humour but people with higher levels of NfL had correspondingly high amounts of Aβ and tau.

Researchers are now investigating whether NfL can be measured in more accessible eye fluids such as tear secretions. If so, an eye test would be simpler than a blood test to reveal that brain cells are degenerating.

Molecules such as pNfL are called biological markers or biomarkers for short. **Biomarkers are a measurable indicator of a specific disease** or bodily process. An example of a commonly used biomarker is prostate-specific antigen (PSA). Small amounts of PSA are secreted by the prostate gland into semen. However, if levels of PSA in a blood sample are significantly higher than normal, it *may* be a sign of prostate cancer and warrants further investigation or biopsy. Thus biomarkers do not always provide definitive answers but they can alert a doctor to imminent disease before obvious clues emerge. Biomarkers can also help narrow down a diagnosis or show that a person is responding to treatment. Depending on the disease, biomarkers can be found in blood, CSF, eyes, various body tissues or imaging scans.

Biomarkers are currently a big buzzword in Alzheimer's because there is no simple way to diagnose the disease. Identifying Alzheimer's at the earliest possible stage offers the best chance that a course of action will be effective. By the time symptoms of Alzheimer's appear, drugs to date have had little impact. In addition to NfL, dozens of proteins and auto-antibodies are being studied as potential biomarkers for Alzheimer's. However, the all-important question remains: if you discovered you were on the path to Alzheimer's, how would you live your life differently?

CHAPTER 79

Aducanumab: a drug rollercoaster

If someone is too tired to give you a smile, leave one of your own, because no one needs a smile as much as those who have none to give.

SAMSON RAPHAEL HIRSCH (1808–1888)

October 2012 marked the start of an exciting new anti-Alzheimer's drug trial. The medication was called aducanumab (pronounced *add-you-can-you-mab*) and it was effective in clearing amyloid plaques from the brains of mice. It was now time to test it on humans. The initiative was called the PRIME trial.

One hundred and sixty-five patients with mild cognitive impairment (MCI) or mild Alzheimer's confirmed by MRI and PET scans were randomly split into two groups. One group served as controls and received a placebo. The second group received the medication in varying doses. Neither the patient nor the doctor administering the drug knew who was receiving the placebo or who was receiving the real deal. This is referred to as a randomised, double-blind, placebo-controlled trial (RCT). The world waited.

Hundreds of earlier anti-amyloid drugs had been dismal failures. Why was aducanumab any more likely to succeed than its predecessors?

Firstly, modern brain scanning enables us to diagnose Alzheimer's much sooner than we could a decade ago. Aducanumab was therefore being given at an earlier stage of the disease than with previous drug trials. This could provide a chance to stave off irreversible damage.

Secondly, aducanumab is what is known as a monoclonal antibody. An antibody (also called an immunoglobulin) is a protein made by our immune system that removes or neutralises foreign substances that are potentially harmful. The foreign substance is called an antigen and can include bacteria, viruses, cancer cells or damaged proteins. The term 'monoclonal' means that aducanumab comes from a specific type of human white blood cell that binds to only one antigen, in this case, abnormally folded Aβ protein fragments. These are the amyloid fragments that clump together to create plaques. Earlier anti-amyloid drugs were not as selective in removing the amyloid fragments that aggregate into plaques. Instead, they cleared out harmless forms of amyloid. The trials on mice had shown that aducanumab was more potent than previous drugs in dismantling established Aβ plaques.

How did scientists come to make aducanumab in the first place? The aducanumab antibody was first discovered in the blood of healthy 70- to 100-year-olds who were mentally sharp and free from Alzheimer's. This made scientists wonder whether aducanumab might be protecting these people from cognitive decline. Hence, they started reproducing aducanumab in the lab.

After one year of **monthly intravenous infusions,** the patients who had received the highest doses of aducanumab were found to have almost no Aβ plaques in their brains. They were also reported to have better cognition than subjects in the placebo group. Whereas the mental abilities of the aducanumab group remained stable over the 12 months, the placebo group all exhibited significant cognitive decline. These results opened the door for two much larger studies across 300 centres in 20 countries. The two trials were called EMERGE and ENGAGE, each involving 1350 Alzheimer's patients and sponsored by the pharmaceutical company Biogen. The world rejoiced.

In mid-2018, a monitoring committee was engaged to perform a futility analysis to assess how the two trials were progressing and whether the results were heading in the right direction. The trials were not due to finish for several more years so this was an interim report.

In March 2019, Biogen delivered an unexpected and devastating blow to the Alzheimer's community. It was discontinuing its two international aducanumab trials because the monitoring committee deemed that the drug wasn't working — in other words, it was failing to provide any benefits. Yes, aducanumab was able to remove Aβ plaques from the brain but, no, it was not improving symptoms nor slowing the rate at which a person declined. The world mourned.

Enrolling in a drug trial is a huge physical, mental and emotional commitment. It requires a large investment of time and energy by not only the patient but also their family. In return, participants are offered hope, meaning and purpose; an opportunity to forward a cause that will ultimately benefit the whole of humanity. Trials enable patients to feel they are part of a greater good; that their suffering is not in vain. Even if a trial yields negative results, it still provides valuable data. Science is a cumulative process whereby unexpected outcomes can spark the next big breakthrough.

Thus, when Biogen made its disappointing announcement, many participants, their families and treating physicians were heartbroken. Although no one knew who had been receiving the drug and who had been given the placebo, many patients were convinced they were in the aducanumab group and slowing their rate of decline. Was the drug truly modifying their disease or were patients enlivened by the supportive friendships they'd formed with trial staff? Were they willing themselves to stay well because of the optimistic atmosphere and the belief that they were on the cusp of a great new discovery?

In October 2019, Biogen made an even more surprising announcement: the interim futility analysis was premature and incorrect. Further analyses of additional data had shown that the EMERGE trial had yielded positive results after all. People receiving the highest dose of aducanumab (10 mg per kilogram of body weight) for the longest period (at least 10 months) experienced 23% less cognitive decline than participants on lower doses or the placebo. Furthermore, not only did aducanumab remove Aβ plaques, it also appeared to reduce tau tangles in a subset of people in a dose-dependent manner. Symptoms of Alzheimer's are more closely related to tau tangles than to Aβ plaques, even though Aβ plays a role in the disease.

Unfortunately, only a small subset of ENGAGE trial participants — once again those on the highest doses for the longest period of time — demonstrated the same benefits. What to make of these inconclusive results? Biogen pushed on. The world held its breath.

In January 2020, Biogen commenced a third trial called EMBARK involving 2400 participants from their previous aducanumab trials. This time there would be no placebo and everyone would receive aducanumab at the highest dose of 10 mg/kg for two years. This is known as an open-label study. The main purpose of the study was to assess drug safety and tolerability at the highest recommended dose and to explore how long a person might continue to benefit from the drug. The study is projected to continue until 2023. The world then became engulfed by COVID.

In July 2020 Biogen applied to the US Food and Drug Administration (FDA) for approval of aducanumab as a viable treatment for Alzheimer's. Later that same year, they filed for approval in Canada, Japan, the European Union and Australia.

In November 2020 an FDA Advisory Committee voted against the drug's approval because there was insufficient evidence that aducanumab was effective. Of the 11 committee members, 10 voted NO and one person remained undecided. The committee recommended further trials to obtain more definitive evidence. The advice of this committee was only part of the FDA decision-making process. The FDA had yet to hear from patient advocacy groups and other concerned parties. Alzheimer's associations all over the country fervently campaigned for the drug's approval. There had been no new medications for Alzheimer's since 2003 — almost 18 years earlier — and current medications only modestly reduced symptoms for a short period of time in a fraction of patients. In contrast, aducanumab was the first therapy to potentially modify the disease. In other words, rather than simply ameliorating symptoms, it slowed the rate at which Alzheimer's progressed — assuming it worked.

As with all medications, there are potential side effects. People who take aducanumab need to have brain MRI scans at least twice a year to monitor for a condition known as ARIA, an acronym for Amyloid-Related Imaging Abnormalities.

There are two types of ARIA: ARIA-E and ARIA-H. E stands for oedema (because in the USA oedema is spelt edema) and H stands for haemorrhage.

ARIA-E results from seepage of fluid from the blood into the brain causing brain swelling. It occurred in 35% of people receiving aducanumab versus 3% of people receiving the placebo. Symptoms depended on how much and where the fluid accumulated. Most of the time, patients were unaware that anything was wrong. Some experienced headaches, confusion, nausea, vomiting, tremor, loss of balance or difficulty walking. Stopping the drug usually rectified the issue. Rare cases required steroids, assisted breathing and admission to an intensive care unit (ICU). The higher the dose, the more likely a person was to develop ARIA-E. APOE4 carriers were at increased risk of ARIA-E. Up to 55% of people with two copies of the APOE4 gene on the highest dose of aducanumab (10 mg/kg) developed ARIA-E during the trials, but only one-third of them had symptoms. All recovered with no long-term effects. Starting on a low dose of aducanumab and slowly increasing the dose over a period of months seemed to mitigate ARIA-E.

ARIA-H refers to tiny brain bleeds known as cerebral micro-haemorrhages. They were seen in 20% of people receiving aducanumab but, as with ARIA-E, most patients were unaware of any problems. In comparison, ARIA-H occurs in 6% of healthy elderly and in 50% to 80% of stroke patients. These people would be precluded from receiving aducanumab.

On 7 June 2021 — in a decision that sent shockwaves through the scientific community — the FDA approved aducanumab under an accelerated approval pathway. This means the decision-makers believed the drug showed enough likelihood of benefit to warrant its acceptance. However, Biogen was required to continue testing the drug's effectiveness and it had nine years (until 2030) to prove its case. The new medication was marketed under the name of Aduhelm. Alzheimer's patients celebrated. Three of the November FDA Advisory Committee members resigned in protest. Doctors, scientists, statisticians, ethicists and politicians are deeply divided on the issue. The debate rages on.

Later the same month, Biogen initiated a study to assess whether aducanumab could be administered via subcutaneous injection (SCI) rather than intravenous infusion (IV).

Why was the decision so controversial? Why was the advisory committee unanimous that there was insufficient evidence to warrant approval? Why did the FDA go against the recommendation of its advisors? What are the pros, cons and implications of the decision?

The aducanumab story is ongoing testament to the complexity of Alzheimer's and the potential for interpreting data in multiple ways. Those who agree with the drug's approval argue that something is better than nothing, even if the benefits are small. Patients have nothing to lose by trying the medication. As the first drug of its kind, no one should expect aducanumab to be the *best* drug of its kind. As with HIV treatments, the first drug zidovudine (AZT) paved the way for more and better drugs. The belief is that aducanumab will do the same for Alzheimer's. Effective treatment of Alzheimer's will probably require a cocktail of medications, with aducanumab being the first ingredient. Aducanumab has also given Alzheimer's patients and their families tremendous hope and optimism. **Hope and optimism contribute to healing** and motivate people to engage in behaviours that further improve their condition. Anything that raises the human spirit raises our wellbeing.

Those who vehemently oppose the drug argue that it provides no benefits and submits patients to uncomfortable, time-wasting and expensive procedures that take them away from things that actually make a difference — such as physical exercise and quality time with family and friends. At US$28 200[3] (A$40 000) per patient per year, insurance premiums will go through the roof for everyone. Many patients will still be out of pocket to the tune of thousands of dollars and these figures do not include the hospital costs of administering the drug and MRI scans to monitor for ARIA. The money would be better spent educating the entire population about

[3] The original cost of aducanumab was US$56 000 but in January 2022 Biogen cut the price by half because the pharma company believed that patients were not being offered the drug due to its expense.

Alzheimer's risk-reduction strategies and implementing brain-boosting programs. Daily physical exercise is unequivocally more effective than aducanumab in improving symptoms and slowing the rate of cognitive decline. Engaging a personal trainer for one hour a day, five days a week would be less expensive and much more beneficial. There is also a strong argument that Aβ is the wrong treatment target and aducanumab will only push research in a flawed direction. We should focus on reducing inflammation, oxidative damage, insulin resistance and tau tangles, while simultaneously raising blood ketone levels.

Can anyone in the USA with a diagnosis of Alzheimer's receive aducanumab? No. Only people with MCI or mild Alzheimer's have been approved to take the drug. People with moderate or severe Alzheimer's have not been shown to benefit and are at higher risk of ARIA. In addition, anyone receiving aducanumab must have prior confirmation of brain Aβ plaques on PET scan or abnormal levels of Aβ in CSF (via lumbar puncture). Aducanumab's supporters contend that this requirement will accelerate development of less invasive and less costly biomarker tests.

At the time of writing, the Australian Therapeutic Goods Administration (TGA) — the FDA equivalent — is deliberating whether to approve aducanumab for use in Australia. Most Australian physicians do not support its approval.

In summary:
- Everyone agrees that aducanumab removes Aβ plaques from the brain.
- Whether this translates into clinical benefit remains to be seen.
- Aducanumab is only recommended for people with MCI or mild Alzheimer's. It does not help people in later stages of the disease.
- The cost is US$28 200 per person per year plus hospital and monitoring expenses.
- More than one-third of people taking the drug experience brain swelling or micro-bleeds called ARIA. Most of the time these side effects do not cause problems but a small percentage of patients require admission to an intensive care unit (ICU).

- Physical exercise and other lifestyle measures discussed in this book are more effective in treating Alzheimer's than aducanumab. The problem is that **our current healthcare system is built around medicating, radiating or operating on patients rather than educating, encouraging and exercising patients.**

Taking all the above into consideration, I'll leave you with four questions to reflect on:

1. If you had Alzheimer's and were eligible to receive aducanumab, would you take it?
2. Would your answer be different if the person in question was not you but someone close to you?
3. If you're a doctor and your patient was eligible to receive aducanumab, would you prescribe it?
4. If you were given US$28 200 to spend on an Alzheimer's patient and their care-partner every year, what would you do for them?

CHAPTER 80

Dad's answer for everything

When an old man dies, a library burns down.

African proverb

On my father's 87th birthday, I asked him for his most important life advice. My first question was 'What's the key to a lasting happy relationship?'

He answered unwaveringly. 'Find someone you can laugh with, cry with and play with, whom you love and respect, and who loves and respects you in return.'

Then I asked, 'And what's the key to success and fulfilment in work?'

Again he answered resolutely. 'Work with people you can laugh with, complain with and play with, whom you love and respect, and who love and respect you in return.' He uttered the word 'complain' with an impish grin.

For a third time I asked, 'And what's the key to happiness and fulfilment in life as a whole?'

For a third time he answered, 'Fill your life with people you can laugh with, cry with, play with and complain with, whom you love and respect, and who love and respect you in return.'

The same conclusion was reached by Dr Robert Waldinger and his team of Harvard University researchers who'd studied the lives of over 700 men for 75 years. Due to the length of the study, several generations of researchers had been involved. The question they were looking to answer was 'What lifestyle factors have the greatest impact on health, happiness and longevity?' Unsurprisingly, regular physical exercise, eating minimally processed food, effectively managing stress and not smoking all played a role. But what was the strongest predictor of a long, happy, healthy life? The answer was the quality of a person's relationships. Not how many friends they had on Facebook but how connected they felt to the people who truly mattered to them. The recipe was simple: **good relationships lead to good health.** Good relationships also lead to greater life satisfaction than a lucrative and successful career. I laughed at the thought of a man with dementia intuitively knowing what had taken illustrious scientists three-quarters of a century to discover. You can watch Dr Waldinger's TED talk here:

www.ted.com/talks/robert_waldinger_what_makes_a_good_life_ lessons_from_the_longest_study_on_happiness?language=en

'Is there anything else I need to know to navigate my way through life?' I prompted my father.

'Don't die having wasted your heart.'

'What do you mean by that?' I asked.

'Don't waste a single opportunity to do a kind deed, say a kind word or think a kind thought.'

* * * * *

A few months later, Dad seemed to contract a urinary tract infection. I asked him to take a clean catch sample of his urine (which took considerable explanation and several attempts), made sure he drank plenty of water and started him on antibiotics. However, his urine came back without evidence of infection, he had no fever and the antibiotics made no difference to his urinary frequency and urgency. Reluctantly, I took him to our local hospital where he was admitted for scans, blood tests and catheterisation. Understandably, he found it highly distressing. I didn't want to leave him in hospital overnight but it was the sensible thing to do. I decided to stay with him and sleep in the chair beside his bed. The hospital staff urged me to go home so I could have a comfortable, undisturbed sleep. 'You need to be well rested for tomorrow so you can be fully present for your dad,' the nightshift nurse urged. I knew the hospital team were capable of looking after him but I was afraid that if Dad woke up during the night he would have no idea where he was and start to panic.

'Go home,' Dad reassured me, 'I'll be fine.'

I ended up waiting until he fell asleep and then tiptoed out of his room. 'Come back!' he called out unexpectedly.

I turned around to find him holding out his hand. 'Take my wristwatch with you.'

'Why?' His request puzzled me. 'You always sleep with your watch on. No one will steal it.'

'I want you to wear my watch so I can *watch* over you even when I'm not there,' he whispered.

His lucidity in the moment was staggering. I tearfully acquiesced. However, I was certain he'd think it was stolen if he woke up before I returned, so I asked the nurse to make a note that his daughter had taken his watch.

Every evening before falling asleep, I visualised my father cocooned in healing white light. It was a comforting ritual I'd started when we moved to the Gold Coast. That night was the first time I struggled to get a clear picture of him in my mind's eye. All I could conjure up was an indistinct silhouette. Why couldn't I get my imagination working?

I was jolted awake shortly before six o'clock the following morning. I almost fell out of bed reaching for my phone. It was Dad's doctor at Robina hospital. Oh dear, I thought, what has Dad done now?

'I'm sorry to inform you that your father passed away in his sleep during the early hours of the morning. When the nurse went to check on him, she found that his heart had stopped.'

'What? No! *No! No!!* But he was fine yesterday ...' my voice trailed off. The rest of the day was a blur. It was 6 March 2019. I had never felt such crushing, overpowering heaviness in every part of my body.

As I continue to reflect on Dad's words of advice, they reveal an even greater depth than I first realised. To be able to laugh, cry, 'complain' and play with people means to feel our feelings and allow ourselves to be vulnerable. His passing would not be so searingly painful if our relationship hadn't bestowed an equal measure of joy. Pain is the price we pay for truly connecting with each other. Our lives would be empty and meaningless if we had no one for whom to grieve when they passed away.

As for his counsel to think for myself, I'm reminded of the words of psychiatrist Theodore Isaac Rubin (1923–2019): 'Kindness is more important than wisdom, and the recognition of this is the beginning of wisdom.'

In today's world, to think for ourselves means to value kindness above competitive advantage. To value respect above reward; health above wealth; adventure above achievement. The irony is that if we filled our days with kindness, respect, healing and adventure, everything else we were striving for would naturally ensue.

If there was one word to describe my father, it would be 'kind'. As his brain started to falter, so did his motivation and energy. But four magic words worked a spell on him every time. Those words were: 'Can you help me?'

If I said to him, 'Let's go shopping,' he'd answer, 'No, I'm too old'. But if I asked, 'Can you help me do the shopping?' he would come with me and make every effort to assist. When a care-partner asked if he wanted to go for a walk, he'd reply that he was too tired. But if she asked him to help her post a letter, his tiredness would be supplanted by his desire to help.

When someone asked him how he wanted to be remembered, he answered, 'It doesn't matter if people don't remember me after I'm gone. Memories fade. *My* memories certainly have. What's important is making a positive difference to people's lives while I'm still alive. Face to face. Here and now.'

Despite Dad's physical absence, I still feel his presence. I don't believe we ever lose someone because they live on in the things they taught us and the countless ways they touched our lives. Dad had no medical training but he gave me salubrious advice: 'Kindness is the healthiest of all habits. And like any habit, you need to practise it daily to maintain it.'

CHAPTER 81

The search continues

Music is the universal language of mankind.
HENRY WORDSWORTH LONGFELLOW (1807–1882)

Three years after Dad passed away, and shortly before this book was due to be published, I came across the Numeric Language of Music ® (NLM) program conceived by Patty Carlson. Patty is a film score composer and producer, concert pianist and music educator. She taught herself to play the piano at the age of 21 by listening to music, memorising individual parts and finding the matching tones on the keyboard.

While working as a film score producer in Aspen, Colorado, USA, she began teaching children to play the piano using her unique method of 'understanding the language of music,' which was completely different from traditional piano lessons. Unexpectedly, her students not only learnt to play *and compose* complex and elegant music after just a few months — in some cases after only a few lessons — they also showed dramatic improvements in reading, writing and arithmetic. Even more extraordinary were the effects of her piano lessons on children with special needs and those on the autism spectrum.

Eleven-year-old Kaden was in fifth grade but performing at the level of third grade. His brother Cale had been diagnosed with Childhood Apraxia of Speech (CAS) in which the brain has difficulty co-ordinating movements of the tongue, jaws and lips. This makes the child's speech unintelligible and often leads to reduced vocabulary and difficulty with word order. In many cases, the condition persists into adulthood despite intensive speech pathology. Patty gave the family her Piano for Special Needs program and the boys were taught by their mother and grandmother following the instructions in Patty's manual. One month later, Kaden progressed to Patty's Piano Logic DVD program. Three months later, his school-teachers were astounded that he'd gone from reading at a 3.4 level to a 5.8 level and his maths had advanced more quickly than any student they'd ever seen. During the same time, Cale had a 70% improvement in his speech and was being understood by everyone around him. In the world of CAS, this was unheard of.

These and many more remarkable results compelled Patty to test her Numeric Language of Music ® (NLM) program with people who had neurodegenerative disorders (such as Alzheimer's and Parkinson's), stroke and brain injury. She approached an assisted living centre in San Luis, Colorado and began teaching three volunteers. The results were phenomenal.

One of the volunteers was a woman with advanced Alzheimer's who was struggling to eat because she had difficulty bringing a fork to her mouth. Within four weeks of Patty's piano lessons, her movements became smooth and co-ordinated and her eating improved dramatically. She also started engaging with fellow residents after years of silence.

A second volunteer had severe Parkinson's with incomprehensible speech, poor balance and loss of hand dexterity. After five months of practising the NLM program, she was no longer dropping her consonants, people could follow her speech, and her movements were deft and flowing. A third volunteer had suffered a stroke 10 years previously. Once again, the NLM program produced reversal of symptoms.

As yet, scientists can only theorise how NLM might exert its ostensibly miraculous effects. Firstly, music is multidimensional and links seemingly disparate regions of the brain. By activating one region, an associated dormant region could fire into action. Music is also a universal emotional language that triggers the brain's reward and memory systems. These systems are intricately tied to motivation and movement. In human evolution, music appears to pre-date language and served as a means of bonding and communication. By helping humans operate as a cohesive group, music enhanced our survival and is associated with the most primal functioning of our brain.

Sound is one of the first external stimuli we experience in utero. Children respond to music before they can speak, and a baby's emotional reaction to music is similar to that of an adult. Brain imaging studies show that newborns notice if music is jarring or misses a beat and, by five months of age, we are able to move our bodies in time with music. The better a baby can do this, the more they smile. These are innate skills that we retain into old age. When we listen to music, our brain is one step ahead of the rhythm and tries to predict the next beat. When study participants were played 100 pieces of unfamiliar music composed for the experiment in question, both young and old were able to identify if the music ended in an expected or unexpected way.

Could it be that Patty's unique method of musical education operated like computer code that reprogrammed the brain to regain lost functions?

Patty does not claim to have a cure for dementia or any other brain disease. Instead, she invites people with advanced Alzheimer's and their care-partners to try her NLM program FREE of charge and to report on their results. Her website offers an instructional video that is very easy to follow and can be taught to anyone at any stage of Alzheimer's. It simply involves playing specific keys, with specific fingers, in a specific order. If Dad were still with me, I wouldn't hesitate in trying the program with him. If you or someone you know has Alzheimer's, I encourage you to join Patty's quest to learn about the potential of her program to reverse the symptoms of Alzheimer's.

On her dementia website (alzheimersresearchproject.com) she writes:

Watch the 20-minute NLM instructional video and repeat the steps without deviation. The parameters of our research project are basic. Played twice a week for one to three months, let us know if and when the symptoms of Alzheimer's disease begin to reverse. Let's find out together.

You can learn more about Patty Carlson, her method of piano teaching and her results with children at <u>pattycarlsononline.com.</u> She is an incredibly humble, generous and loving human being with a genuine desire to help people heal.

CHAPTER 82

Closing thoughts

As long as you live, keep learning how to live.

SENECA (4 BCE–65 CE)

Dementia is currently the second most common cause of death in Australia after heart disease and the number one cause of death in women. Globally, as at September 2022, dementia is the seventh most common cause of death and a major driver of disability and loss of independence. But it doesn't have to be this way.

A major reason for writing this book is to overturn the notion that a diagnosis of dementia means 'get your affairs in order because there's nothing we can do about it'. Sadly, many doctors — and therefore their patients — still believe this to be the case despite overwhelming evidence to the contrary.

Allow me to present the FINGER trial — an acronym for Finnish Geriatric Intervention Study to Prevent Cognitive Impairment and Disability. Between September 2009 and November 2011, 1260 men and women aged 60 to 77 years with established risk factors for heart disease and dementia were randomly divided into two groups. One group participated in a comprehensive anti-Alzheimer's program that involved cognitive training, physical exercise, dietary advice and assiduous management of their heart disease. The second group received only general health advice. All participants underwent comprehensive neuropsychological testing at the start and end of the two years. The results made scientific headlines around the world: those who participated in the multi-pronged anti-Alzheimer's program improved their cognitive functioning compared to the group who were not proactive about their brain health. The most encouraging finding was that carriers of the APOE4 gene benefited just as much as non-carriers. Our genes do NOT seal our fate.

A decade later, in 2021, a disturbing US study of almost 150 000 older adults (97% male, 86% non-Hispanic white and an average age of 75) found that a recent diagnosis of dementia (within the preceding two years) increased the risk of attempted suicide by 44%, while a diagnosis of mild cognitive impairment (MCI) raised the number of suicide attempts by 73%. This strongly suggests that cognitive decline and dementia continue to be viewed through the lens of despair and hopelessness. This is a needless tragedy because dementia — particularly in the early stages — is not only potentially reversible, it can be a stimulus for life-enhancing personal and global transformation.

All the factors that lower our risk for Alzheimer's and curb its progression are synonymous with a joyful, meaningful, socially connected life. One of my patients poignantly admitted that a diagnosis of Alzheimer's finally gave her an 'excuse' to prioritise her health and pursue her long-buried passions. Why do we need an 'excuse' to follow our heart? Start following your heart *now* — and watch how it can bring about healing.

Don't let perfection get in the way of progress. Whatever small steps you can take towards better brain health for yourself and your family, take them. Don't worry if you can't implement everything. Any shift in the right direction will push dementia further away. Alzheimer's is not the result of one causal agent; it's due to many factors coming together to slowly erode brain function over several decades. **There are many pieces to the puzzle of Alzheimer's.** This gives us multiple opportunities to do something to prevent, halt or — at the very least — slow progression of the disease. The sooner we start the better, but even starting late is better than not starting at all. There is always something we can do to improve a situation.

From my observations, the biggest obstacle to better health is living in a world that doesn't value health. We pay lip service to the adage 'If you don't have your health, you don't have anything' but how many of us genuinely put health at the top of our priorities? Instead of squeezing healthy choices into a busy life, wouldn't it make more sense to create a fulfilling life around healthy choices? This is not a personal failing. It's a modern Western cultural phenomenon. Workplaces continue to demand more of us and if we fail to toe the line, we risk demotion or loss of our job. Humanity is under the illusion that the only way to succeed in life is to do more, consume more and have more. Have more what? And how are we defining success? Being materially wealthy but physically and emotionally unhealthy? As philanthropist and peace advocate Andrew Carnegie (1835–1919) acutely observed, 'There is little success where there is little laughter.'

I believe humanity is at a pivotal point in our evolution. We can continue as we are — sacrificing our health and our planet for short-term gain — or we can pause, reflect on our soaring rates of chronic diseases and environmental devastation and re-evaluate what *really* matters. It's never too late to create. To quote Seneca once again: 'A gem cannot be polished without friction, nor a man perfected without trials.'

Alzheimer's is not merely a personal or medical challenge. It's bigger than a family or community challenge. It's a global challenge that affects every facet of our lives: physical, psychological, emotional, social and economic. Even if you don't personally know someone with Alzheimer's, your life is, or will be, affected by it — from the taxes you pay to provide care and resources for patients and their families, to increasing numbers of the workforce being funnelled into caring roles. In 2019 the estimated global cost of dementia was US$1.3 trillion. If we don't start implementing effective public health policies, we will bankrupt every healthcare system in the world.

Fortunately, we already have the solution. We don't need to wait for new whiz-bang dementia drugs. We simply need to understand what constitutes TRUE MEDICINES.

TRUE MEDICINES is an acronym for what it takes to create long-term health and healing.

Acronym	Explanation
Take	
Responsibility	**T**ake **R**esponsibility for your own health.
Understand	**U**nderstand that modern medicine is not a path to healing. **The role of modern medicine is to keep us alive long enough to allow us to heal.**
Educate	**E**ducate yourself about your disease and the support that is available through multiple channels: books, podcasts, forums, chat rooms and advocacy groups. Then incorporate the following into your life.
Mindfulness and **M**editation	See the chapters 'Stillness' and 'Meditation' in my prequel *In Search of My Father*.
Exercise	See Part 3 'Let movement be your medicine'.
Diet	See Part 4 'Let food be your medicine'.
Intermittent fasting	See Chapter 50 'Fast to last'.
Connection and **C**ommunity	See Chapter 70 'Friends for life'.
Intention	Get clear on what truly matters to you and what you want to achieve; **give your brain and body compelling reasons to continue working at their best** — see Chapter 68 'Education prevents stagnation'.
Nature	See Chapter 76 'Have you tried forest bathing?'
Enthusiasm and **E**xcitement	**E**nthusiasm for life and **E**xcitement about what each new day will bring. See Chapter 24 'In search of meaning'.
Sleep	See Chapter 17 'Snore no more', Chapter 18 'Blow it off' and Chapter 19 'Let sleep be your medicine'.

If we maintain an open and inquiring mind, **dementia can be a doorway** to positive social change and a better way of life. **Dementia can inspire us to discover** our true values and deepen our relationships — whether we're the person with the diagnosis, their care-partner, family member, friend, colleague, employer or health service provider.

The nature of Alzheimer's actually shows us the meaning of life: to live fully in each moment. What could be more effective in teaching us the power of the present moment than someone with a disease that erodes everything other than the present moment? In the words of Scottish essayist, Thomas Carlyle (1826–1866), 'Every man is my superior in that I may learn from him.'

To close, as I started, with a poem.

> Draw stick figures
> Sing out of tune
> Dance out of step
> Gaze at the moon.
>
> Write silly poems
> Splash as you swim
> Laugh at yourself
> Go out on a limb.
>
> Dress with flamboyance
> Run at your pace
> Learn something new
> Life's not a race.
>
> It's great to be
> a lifelong beginner
> Giving things a go
> is what makes you a winner.

Songs

A Spoonful of **Mustard**

Adapted from *A Spoonful of Sugar* sung by Mary Poppins.

See Chapter 36 'Broccoli just got even better' for context.

*In every **meal that we must eat***
*There **needs to be a healthy treat***
You find the fun and snap!
*The **meal's** a game*
*And every **vegetable** you **chew***
*Becomes a **part** of **you***
Your brain! Your knee! Your fine anatomy – and

*A spoonful of **mustard** helps the broccoli go down*
*The **broccoli** go down-wown*
*The **broccoli** go down*
*Just a spoonful of **mustard** helps the **broccoli** go down*
In a most delightful way

Our brain needs lots of leafy greens
As well as cabbage, kale and beans
And Brussels sprouts and cauliflower too
They are delicious raw or cooked
The taste and crunch will get you hooked
The more you chew the healthier for you

*A spoonful of **mustard** helps the **broccoli** go down*
*The **broccoli** go down-wown*
*The **broccoli** go down*
*Just a spoonful of **mustard** helps the **broccoli** go down*
In a most delightful way

*The **mustard powder or the seeds***
*Are **what your cauliflower needs***
To keep you fit and strong and flourishing
*If you just take a little **bite***
*From every **vegetable in sight***

*And **chew** (And **chew**)*
*You'll find (**You'll find**)*
***Great health** is not a grind.*
Ah-h-h-h-h-h-h-h-h-h ah!

*A spoonful of **mustard** helps the **broccoli** go down*
*The **broccoli** go down-wown*
*The **broccoli** go down*
*Just a spoonful of **mustard** helps the **broccoli** go down*
In a most delightful way

Songwriters: Richard Sherman, Robert Sherman

A Spoonful of Mustard lyrics © Dr Helena Popovic MBBS

What's **Food** Got to Do With it?

Adapted from *What's Love Got to Do With it?* sung by Tina Turner.

See Chapter 39 'The Noxious List' for context.

*You must understand, though the **taste** of your **snack***
*Makes **your brain** react*
*That it's only the thrill **of a quick sugar hit***
And our brain's been hacked
It's physical
Only logical
We** must try to ignore **all the slick tempting ads

*Oh-oh, what's **food** got to do, got to do with it?*
*What's **food** but **the fuel for all our brain power?***
*What's **food** got to do, got to do with it?*
*Who needs **to eat junk** when **junk causes brain fog?***

*It may seem to you that I'm **being too strict***
Saying no soft drinks
Having water instead clears our skin and our head
Research shows the links
There's a name for it:
Being smart and fit
*But whatever the reason, **fresh food helps us think***

*Oh-oh, what's **food** got to do, got to do with it?*
*What's **food** but **the fuel for all our brain power?***
*What's **food** got to do, got to do with it?*
*Who needs **fast food** when **fast food slows** our **brain down?***

Oh-ohhhh

I've been taking on a new direction
But I have to say
*I've been thinking about my **brain's** protection*
*It **thrills** me to feel this way*

*Oh-oh, what's **food** got to do, got to do with it?*
*What's **food** but a **plate of home-cooked veggies?***
*What's **food** got to do, got to do with it?*
Let's eat green veg 'cause green veg boost our brain cells!

*Oh-oh, what's **food** got to do, got to do with it?*
*What's **food** but **the fuel for all our brain power?***
*What's **food** got to do, got to do with it?*
*Who needs to **eat junk** when **junk causes brain fog?***

*Oh-oh, what's **food** got to do, got to do with it?*
*What's **food** but **the fuel for all our brain power?***
*What's **food** got to do, got to do with it?*
*Who needs **fast food** when **fast food slows** our **brain down?***

*Oh-oh, what's **food** got to do, got to do with it?*
*What's **food** but a **plate of home-cooked veggies?***
*What's **food** got to do, got to do with it?*
Let's eat green veg 'cause green veg boost our brain cells!

Songwriters: Terry Britten, Graham Lyle

What's Food Got to Do with It lyrics © Dr Helena Popovic MBBS

*How Do You Solve a Problem Like **Dementia?***

Adapted from *How Do You Solve a Problem Like Maria?* sung by the nuns in the movie *The Sound of Music.*

See Chapter 67 'Let music be your medicine' for context.

Dementia makes me feel perplexed
About what's going on
I don't remember people's names
And when I do, they're gone
*And underneath **my friendly smile***
I feel that life's a con
*I even **wonder what's the date tomorrow?***

I'm often lost and muddled
I do not know what is real
I don't remember how to plan
Or cook a healthy meal
I hate to have to say it
But I very firmly feel
My brain is** not an asset to **my body

*I'd like to say a word **on my** behalf*
***Poems** make me laugh*

*How do you solve a problem like **dementia?***
*How do you catch a **thought** and pin it down?*
*How do you find a word that means **dementia?***
A memory glitch! A brain under siege! A dare!

*Many a thing **I** know **I'd** like to tell **you***
*Many a thing **I** ought to understand*
*But how do **I concentrate***
When I am in this state?
My brain no longer follows my command

*Oh, how do you solve a problem like **dementia**?*
*How do you hold a **memory** in your hand?*

*When **I shop I get** confused*
Out of focus and bemused
And I never know exactly where I am
Unpredictable as weather
***The disease is like** a feather*
It's annoying! It's frustrating! It's a jam!

There are many different types
Many causes of my gripes
Is it Alzheimer's or vascular or both?
Is it fronto-temp-oral?
Or a Lewy body curl?
Is it trauma or a tumour
What a whirl!

*How do you solve a problem like **dementia**?*
*How do you catch a **thought** and pin it down?*
*How do you find a word that means **dementia**?*
A memory glitch! A brain under siege! A dare!

*Many a thing **I** know **I'd** like to tell **you***
*Many a thing **I** ought to understand*
*But how do **I concentrate***
When I am in this state?
My brain no longer follows my command

*Oh, how do you solve a problem like **dementia**?*
*How do you hold a **memory** in your hand?*

Songwriters: Richard Rodgers, Oscar Hammerstein II

How Do You Solve a Problem Like Dementia?
lyrics © Dr Helena Popovic MBBS

APPENDIX 1

TYPES OF DEMENTIA

This list provides a brief overview of the most common dementias. It is by no means an exhaustive catalogue.

LATE-ONSET DEMENTIAS (LOD)

These constitute the vast majority (90–95%) of dementias. Symptoms can start as early as 65 years but are more common after the age of 70. Most are NOT inherited.

1. **Alzheimer's dementia (AD)** — this is the most common type of dementia in Western countries. It accounts for 60–70% of all dementias and is twice as common in women as in men. The recommendations in this book are aimed at preventing this type of dementia.
2. **Vascular dementia (VD)** — this is the second most common type of dementia. It accounts for 15–20% of all dementias. The recommendations in this book will also reduce your risk of vascular dementia. There are several subtypes. The two most common are:
   (a) Multi-infarct dementia (MID) — this is caused by multiple strokes (interruptions to brain blood flow from clots or bleeds). Strokes can be large (causing a variety of symptoms depending on which areas of the brain are affected) or silent (with no apparent symptoms but which add up over time to cause cognitive deficits). MID is more common in men than women.
   (b) Binswanger's disease — also called subcortical VD or subcortical leukoencephalopathy or subcortical arteriosclerotic encephalopathy (SAE). It is caused by widespread damage to the brain's white matter that produces a characteristic pattern on CT and MRI scans.
3. **Lewy body dementia (LBD)** — also called Lewy body disorder or diffuse Lewy body disease. LBD is characterised by the accumulation of a misfolded protein in the brain called alpha-synuclein. This protein is also found in the brains of people

with Parkinson's disease (PD). Hence Parkinson's can lead to the development of LBD. It is also more common in men than women. There are two subtypes:

(a) Dementia with Lewy bodies (DLB) — no previous history of Parkinson's disease.

(b) Parkinson's disease dementia (PDD) — this is when someone with Parkinson's disease goes on to develop dementia.

4. **Wernicke-Korsakoff syndrome (WKS)** — this is due to vitamin B1 (thiamine) deficiency. Symptoms include confusion, memory loss, eye-muscle weakness, hypothermia, low blood pressure and ataxia (lack of balance and coordination). Vitamin B1 deficiency can result from consuming more than three standard alcoholic drinks per day (on average), poor diet, prolonged vomiting, chemotherapy or gastrectomy (partial or total surgical removal of the stomach). Some doctors describe WKS as occurring in two stages:

(a) Wernicke's encephalopathy — the earlier (acute) phase of the disease.

(b) Korsakoff syndrome — also called Korsakoff's amnesic syndrome — the later (chronic) phase of the disease in which memory formation and retrieval is the main problem.

5. **Normal pressure hydrocephalus** — this is due to excessive fluid in the brain. It occasionally develops after head injury, brain haemorrhage or severe meningitis but in most cases the cause is unknown. It is treated by surgically draining the excess fluid. The sooner the diagnosis is made, the greater the chance of complete recovery.

6. **HIV-associated neurocognitive disorder (HAND)** — also known as neuroAIDS. People with HIV can develop mood changes, apathy, memory problems, slowed movements and difficulty concentrating due to the virus spreading to their brain. Anti-retroviral therapy (ART) is often able to keep the symptoms in check.

7. **Syphilis-associated dementia** — also known as neurosyphilis. If the diagnosis is made early enough, a course of penicillin can reverse the symptoms.

EARLY-ONSET DEMENTIAS (EOD)

Early-onset dementias — also referred to as younger-onset dementias (YOD) — occur before the age of 65. They can start as early as 30 years of age but are more common between 50 and 65. They account for 5–10% of all dementias.

There are three broad categories of EOD:
1. **Familial** — this means the disease is due to a gene that has been inherited from a parent. 60% of EODs are familial.
2. **Specific** — this is due to a specific cause such as trauma, infection or alcohol. These dementias can be early- or late-onset depending on the age at which the person was exposed to the causative agent.
3. **Sporadic** — as yet there is no known cause.

People often confuse the terms 'early-onset dementia' and 'early stage of dementia'. Early stage of dementia refers to the first few years of late-onset dementia during which symptoms are mild and the person is still able to perform most activities of daily living. It's simpler to avoid the phrase 'early stage of dementia' and use the more precise staging system outlined in Appendix 3.

SUBTYPES OF EOD
1. **Early-onset familial Alzheimer's disease (EOFAD)** — this accounts for 30% of EODs and is due to a person inheriting a specific form of one of the following three genes from either their mother or father. The inheritance of these genes is known as **autosomal dominant,** meaning you only need to inherit one copy of the faulty gene in order to have the disease. The child of a parent with the disease has a 50% chance of inheriting the gene.
   (a) Presenilin 1 (PSEN1) gene — alterations in the PSEN1 gene are the most common mutations causing autosomal dominant familial Alzheimer's disease (FAD). More than 185 different pathogenic (disease-causing) versions of this gene have been identified.
   (b) Presenilin 2 (PSEN2) gene
   (c) Amyloid precursor protein (APP) gene
2. **Frontotemporal dementias (FTD)** — so called because they involve the frontal or temporal lobes of the brain. FTDs account for 20% of EODs and many of these (but not all of them) are

familial. They are equally common in men and women. To date, three genes have been linked to this condition: MAPT, C9orf72 and GRN. There are several subtypes including:

(a) Behavioural variant of FTD
(b) Primary progressive aphasia (impaired ability to understand or produce speech)
   (i) semantic
   (ii) non-fluent grammatical
(c) Corticobasal syndrome
(d) Progressive supranucluear palsy
(e) FTD associated with motor neuron disease (MND)
(f) Pick's disease — this was the name originally given to all FTDs but it is now reserved for one specific subtype.

3. **Posterior cortical atrophy (PCA)** — also known as **visual Alzheimer's (VA)** or **Benson's syndrome.** This involves damage to the posterior region (back) of the brain and causes visual problems such as difficulty reading and recognising faces. Memory and thinking skills are often preserved for many years and only start to decline in the later stages of the disease.

4. **Huntington's disease** — this is a familial EOD that usually begins with movement and co-ordination problems. As the disease progresses, the person experiences increasing difficulty with planning, organising, concentrating and short-term memory.

5. **Chronic traumatic encephalopathy (CTE)** — discussed in detail in Chapter 77 'Heads up'.

6. **E280A mutation** — also known as the **Paisa mutation**. Paisa refers to the race of people who carry the gene mutation and live in a small town in the Columbian state of Antioquia. It is extremely rare outside this region. The Paisa people are currently participating in trials of anti-Alzheimer's medications.

7. **Creutzfeldt-Jakob disease (CJD)** — this is caused by an abnormal protein in the brain called a prion. There are two subtypes:
(a) Sporadic — as yet we don't know where the prion came from.
(b) New variant CJD — caused by eating meat from cattle infected with bovine spongiform encephalopathy (BSE). Colloquially referred to as mad cow disease.

APPENDIX 2

Mini-Mental State Examination (MMSE)

Patient's Name: _____   Date: _____

Instructions: Score one point for each correct response within each question or activity.

Maximum Score	Patient's Score	Questions
5		"What is the year? Season? Date? Day? Month?"
5		"Where are we now? State? County? Town/city? Hospital? Floor?"
3		The examiner names three unrelated objects clearly and slowly, then the instructor asks the patient to name all three of them. The patient's response is used for scoring. The examiner repeats them until patient learns all of them, if possible.
5		"I would like you to count backward from 100 by sevens." (93, 86, 79, 72, 65, …) Alternative: "Spell WORLD backwards." (D-L-R-O-W)
3		"Earlier I told you the names of three things. Can you tell me what those were?"
2		Show the patient two simple objects, such as a wristwatch and a pencil, and ask the patient to name them.
1		"Repeat the phrase: 'No ifs, ands, or buts.'"
3		"Take the paper in your right hand, fold it in half, and put it on the floor." (The examiner gives the patient a piece of blank paper.)
1		"Please read this and do what it says." (Written instruction is "Close your eyes.")
1		"Make up and write a sentence about anything." (This sentence must contain a noun and a verb.)
1		"Please copy this picture." (The examiner gives the patient a blank piece of paper and asks him/her to draw the symbol below. All 10 angles must be present and two must intersect.)
30		TOTAL

Interpretation of the MMSE:

Method	Score	Interpretation
Single Cutoff	<24	Abnormal
Range	<21	Increased odds of dementia
	>25	Decreased odds of dementia
Education	21	Abnormal for 8th grade education
	<23	Abnormal for high school education
	<24	Abnormal for college education
Severity	24-30	No cognitive impairment
	18-23	Mild cognitive impairment
	0-17	Severe cognitive impairment

Interpretation of MMSE Scores:

Score	Degree of Impairment	Formal Psychometric Assessment	Day-to-Day Functioning
25-30	Questionably significant	If clinical signs of cognitive impairment are present, formal assessment of cognition may be valuable.	May have clinically significant but mild deficits. Likely to affect only most demanding activities of daily living.
20-25	Mild	Formal assessment may be helpful to better determine pattern and extent of deficits.	Significant effect. May require some supervision, support and assistance.
10-20	Moderate	Formal assessment may be helpful if there are specific clinical indications.	Clear impairment. May require 24-hour supervision.
0-10	Severe	Patient not likely to be testable.	Marked impairment. Likely to require 24-hour supervision and assistance with ADL.

Source:
- Folstein MF, Folstein SE, McHugh PR: "Mini-mental state: A practical method for grading the cognitive state of patients for the clinician." *J Psychiatr Res* 1975;12:189-198.

APPENDIX 3

STAGES OF ALZHEIMER'S

Different doctors classify Alzheimer's in different ways. Most geriatricians and neurologists use the seven stages proposed by Dr Barry Reisberg (geriatric psychiatrist) at New York University (NYU).

Stages 1–3 are designated as pre-dementia stages.

Stages 4–7 indicate a confirmed diagnosis of dementia.

From stage 5 onwards, an individual is unable to live without assistance.

The table on the following pages is adapted from Dr Reisberg's Global Deterioration Scale (GDS). It provides a general outline without delving into the nuances of each stage.

Stage number	Stage name	How is it defined?	How is it diagnosed?	How is it treated?
1	Preclinical or Pre-symptomatic or Asymptomatic	The person appears to be perfectly healthy. There are no symptoms of memory loss or any other problems with thinking. However, Alzheimer's-related changes have started happening in the brain. This stage begins 20 to 30 years before any outward signs of dementia.	Scientists are currently developing tests to detect changes in our eyes, blood and cerebrospinal fluid (CSF) that indicate something is amiss in the brain. These tests look for telltale proteins and other molecules called biomarkers.	This is the best time to implement the brain-boosting strategies discussed in this book. Progression to SCI, MCI and Alzheimer's can be averted in the majority of people if they adopt a healthy active lifestyle as early as possible. Since none of us know if we are in the preclinical stage of Alzheimer's, it would be prudent for everyone to live in a way that supports their optimal brain health.
2	Subjective Cognitive Impairment (SCI)	The person feels that something is not quite right but those around them cannot notice anything different. People describe what they are experiencing as 'brain fog', 'memory glitches' or 'I'm not as sharp as I used to be'.	As above. Scores on the MMSE (see Appendix 2) and other tests of cognition are normal.	This is the second-best time to implement the brain-boosting strategies outlined in this book. Progression to MCI and Alzheimer's can still be averted in most people.
3	Mild Cognitive Impairment (MCI) or Mild Neurocognitive Disorder See Chapter 7 'In search of signs'.	The person starts to experience mild decline in memory and thinking skills. This becomes apparent to the people around them. However, they are still able to look after themselves and go about their usual activities.	A doctor makes a clinical judgement based on the changes described by the patient and their family. Treatable conditions such as hypothyroidism, vitamin deficiencies and OSA (obstructive sleep apnoea) need to be excluded.	There is still time to make lifestyle changes to improve brain function. Many people can avoid progression to Stage 4 Alzheimer's if they become highly proactive about boosting their brain.

Stage number	Stage name	How is it defined?	How is it diagnosed?	How is it treated?
4	Mild Alzheimer's	Memory and cognition decline to the extent that a person experiences difficulties looking after themselves. The main difference between Stages 3 and 4 is the need for help with complex activities of daily living (ADLs) such as managing finances, planning trips or preparing meals. Judgement is also impaired.	• Physical examination • Neuropsychological assessment • Odour identification • Blood tests • Brain scan, e.g. CT, MRI or PET	It is still vitally important to engage in physical exercise, social activities and pleasurable hobbies. A regular daily routine needs to be balanced with novelty and appropriate levels of mental stimulation. Many people with mild Alzheimer's derive great meaning from advocacy work. This is the stage when a type of medicine classed as a cholinesterase inhibitor (e.g. rivastigmine, donepezil, galantamine) may be helpful.
5	Moderate Alzheimer's	The person is still able to eat, dress, shower and engage in conversation but they have difficulty making decisions, recalling names and remembering recent events. They require assistance with most activities of daily living. Personality changes may also start to emerge.	Transition from mild to severe Alzheimer's does not occur in a distinct, stepwise fashion. Instead, functioning can go up and down from one day to the next until a new baseline of lower functioning becomes the norm.	As above + this is the stage when a type of medicine classed as a glutamate receptor antagonist (memantine) may be helpful.
6	Moderately severe Alzheimer's	The person has trouble recognising family and friends and struggles to recall aspects of their past. They may lose control of their bowel and bladder and are frequently disoriented with respect to time and place. Personality and emotional changes become more evident.	Decline from the previous stage	Ongoing stimulation especially through music

Stage number	Stage name	How is it defined?	How is it diagnosed?	How is it treated?
7	Severe Alzheimer's	The person can no longer care for themselves in any capacity. They may even forget how to walk or swallow. They appear to be unable to communicate or respond to their environment, but they are still alive inside and able to appreciate kindness and compassion.	Decline from the previous stage	Love

APPENDIX 4
FAT BIOCHEMISTRY BASICS

Fats are made up of **fatty acids** (FAs) just as carbohydrates are made up of sugars. A fatty acid is a chain of carbon atoms with an acid (carboxyl) group at one end. The other end of the molecule is called the methyl or omega end.

The length of a FA chain can be:
- short (called short chain fatty acids and abbreviated SCFAs or SFAs) — five or fewer carbon atoms
- medium (MCFAs) — six to 12 carbon atoms
- long (LCFAs) — 13 to 21 carbon atoms
- very long (VLCFAs) — 22 or more carbon atoms.

Each carbon atom can link (bond) to four other atoms. Think of a carbon atom as having two arms and two legs. Each limb can bond to another atom. Most of the carbon atoms in a fatty acid are bonded to two other carbon atoms and two hydrogen atoms. Imagine 10 people standing in a line holding hands. Each person's body represents a carbon atom and their arms represent the bonds linking one carbon atom to the next. Meanwhile, each of their legs has a hydrogen atom attached to it. In this scenario, both our arms and legs are bonded to something and we have no free limbs to bond to anything else. A fatty acid with no free bonds is described as **saturated**. It is not able to bond to any other atoms and is described as chemically stable.

If one of the limbs is not attached to a hydrogen atom, it forms a double bond with the carbon atom next to it. A double bond has the potential to release its neighbour and grab a passing oxygen atom. This chemical reaction is known as **oxidation** and it leads to **rancidity**. Rancid oils have a bitter taste and unpleasant odour. More importantly, they are damaging to our health. Heat and light also promote oxidation hence FAs with double bonds need to be kept in dark airtight bottles or metal containers and stored in a cool dark place.

FAs with at least one double bond are classified as **unsaturated**. Unsaturated FAs are further subdivided on the basis of how many double bonds they contain. The more double bonds, the more prone to oxidation and the more carefully the FAs need to be stored. In summary:

1. **Saturated** fatty acids (SFAs) have NO double bonds.
2. **Monounsaturated** fatty acids (MUFAs) have ONE double bond.
3. **Polyunsaturated** fatty acids (PUFAs) have TWO OR MORE double bonds.

Unsaturated fatty acids are also sub-classified according to where their double bonds are located. I discussed double bonds in Chapter 45 'The fat is in the fire' but here is a recap for completeness.

If the first double bond occurs between the third and fourth carbon atoms from the omega end of the molecule, it is called an **omega-3** fatty acid and is written as n-3 or ω-3. Examples of omega-3 fatty acids are alpha-linolenic acid (ALA), eicosa-pentaenoic acid (EPA), and docosa-hexaenoic acid (DHA). ALA is found mainly in plant foods such as flaxseeds (linseeds), hemp seeds, chia seeds, walnuts, soy beans, edamame, tofu, tempeh and dark leafy greens. EPA and DHA are found in seaweed, fatty fish, oysters, mussels, shrimp and prawns. **There is no debate about the health benefits and anti-inflammatory properties of omega-3 fatty acids. Everyone gives them a big tick, especially in relation to brain and heart health.**

If the first double bond occurs between the sixth and seventh carbon atoms from the omega end, it is called an **omega-6** fatty acid and is written as n-6 or ω-6. The predominant omega-6 fatty acid in the human diet is linoleic acid (LA). It is found in most nuts and seeds (including those that also contain n-3), peanuts, soybeans, margarine and vegetable (seed) oils. Natural sources of omega-6 fatty acids are healthy. Industrially made vegetable (seed) oils containing high amounts of omega-6 FAs are toxic.

If the first double bond occurs between the ninth and tenth carbon atoms, it is called an omega-9 fatty acid and is written as n-9 or ω-9. The most common omega-9 fatty acid in our diet is oleic acid. It is found in olives, macadamia nuts, avocados, almonds, hazelnuts, pecans, peanuts, cashews, pistachios, eggs, cheese, tallow and lard.

As with omega-3 fatty acids, everyone agrees that oleic acid is anti-inflammatory and improves brain and heart health.

Omega-3 (ALA, EPA and DHA) and omega-6 (LA) are the predominant PUFAs in the human diet. Omega-9 (oleic acid) is the predominant MUFA in the human diet.

One more distinguishing feature of unsaturated fatty acids is whether the hydrogen atoms at a double bond lie in the same or different planes.

Unsaturated fatty acids in real foods usually have all their hydrogen atoms on the same side of the double bond. This is known as a **cis** configuration. Cis is Latin for 'on this side of'. A cis double bond causes a kink or bend in the chain of carbon atoms and prevents fatty acids from being tightly packed together. Loosely packed chains mean the fat remains liquid at room temperature and is called an oil.

Unsaturated fatty acids created in laboratories for use in processed foods have a significant proportion of their hydrogen atoms in opposite planes. This is known as a **trans** configuration. Trans is Latin for 'on the other side of'. Trans double bonds enable the carbon chain to remain straight. Straight chains can be tightly packed together which allows the fat to stay solid at room temperature. Imagine having two piles of solid metal rods. One set of rods are straight (trans) and the other set have bends (cis). If you had to pack them into a rigid box, which shape allows the rods to be more tightly packed inside the box? The straight rods.

Why does all this biochemistry matter? The chemical structure of a fatty acid determines how it behaves in our body. In other words, the health effects of different fatty acids depend on:
* the length of the carbon chain
* the number of double bonds (saturated, monounsaturated or polyunsaturated)
* the location of the double bonds (omega-3, omega-6 or omega-9)
* the orientation of the hydrogen atoms (cis or trans).

How are fatty acids held together to make a fat molecule?

A fat molecule consists of three fatty acids attached to a compound called glycerol. Glycerol is a type of alcohol that contains three carbon atoms. Glycerol serves as the backbone of the fat molecule because each of its three carbon atoms attaches to one fatty acid chain. You can visualise this arrangement as the letter E. The chemical name for a fat molecule is triglyceride (TG) or more precisely tri-acyl-glyceride (TAG). The term 'acyl' denotes the specific way the fatty acids are attached to the glycerol. Triglycerides are the form in which fatty acids occur in our food and are stored in our bodies. Triglycerides also travel around in our blood attached to transport proteins called lipoproteins. These are the same lipoproteins that carry cholesterol.

Short (SCFAs), medium (MCFAs) and long chain fatty acids (LCFAs)

SCFAs are generated from the fermentation of dietary fibre by bacteria in our colon. The three most common SCFAs are acetate, butyrate and propionate. They provide energy to cells lining the colon and play a role in vitamin production. This makes them critical to good gut health. They also increase satiety and help to lower blood pressure.

MCFAs are found in palm kernel oil, coconut oil and in much smaller amounts in cow, goat and sheep's milk — approximately 10–20% of the fatty acids in milk are MCFAs. They are more easily absorbed than LCFAs and do not require bile acids so they are not a problem for people who have had their gallbladder removed (cholecystectomy).

LCFAs (frequently called free fatty acids or non-esterified fatty acids) can be saturated, monounsaturated or polyunsaturated and are found in all foods that contain fats: dairy, meat, fish, nuts, avocado, coconut oil, palm kernel oil and vegetable oils. The longer the FA chain, the more steps it takes to digest and absorb. This is not unlike the situation with carbohydrates. The more carbon atoms and branches, the longer it takes for the glucose and fructose to reach our bloodstream, i.e. the lower the glycemic index. The only harmful LCFAs are those in vegetable (seed) oils.

The length and saturation of a FA chain affect the properties of the cell membrane in which the FA occurs. Shorter chains with more double bonds are more fluid and flexible (less stiff) than longer saturated chains. This influences the traffic of molecules into and out of a cell and has important consequences for how the cell functions.

Another reason why too much dietary omega-6 damages cells in blood vessel walls

When we consume a diet high in omega-6 FAs, they start to replace saturated FAs in cell membranes. This makes the cell membrane less stable because n-6 FAs have two potentially reactive double bonds while saturated FAs have none. Just as oxidation of unsaturated FAs can occur outside the body and cause rancidity, it can also occur inside the body, causing what is known as **lipid peroxidation.** Lipid peroxidation occurs when free radicals (molecules with unpaired electrons) steal electrons from unsaturated fatty acids in cell membranes producing fatty acid radicals (a FA with a missing electron). The FA radical immediately seeks to replace the stolen electron by grabbing it from oxygen and creating a peroxyl-FA radical. This sets off a chain reaction of ever-increasing FA radical production and ever-increasing cell membrane damage. The chemical products of lipid oxidation are collectively known as lipid peroxides or lipid oxidation products (LOPs). The chain reaction of LOP production can be stopped by:

- two radicals (rather than a radical and a non-radical) reacting with each other or
- antioxidants getting in on the action.

Unfortunately, by this time, considerable cell membrane damage has already occurred.

APPENDIX 5

WHAT ARE PHYTOCHEMICALS?

Phytochemicals are compounds produced by plants that are believed to play a role in human health. The prefix phyto- comes from the Greek *phyton* meaning 'plant'. All plants produce phytochemicals of different types to protect them from bacteria, viruses and fungi and to stop insects and other animals from eating them. For humans, however, it's a case of what doesn't kill us makes us stronger. At least that's the current theory.

More than 100 000 phytochemicals have so far been discovered and they're being intensively studied because we're still trying to understand exactly what they do. Regulatory food labelling agencies throughout the world do not support food companies making health claims about phytochemicals because we simply don't have all the answers yet.

There are currently two exceptions. In 2014, the European Food Safety Authority (EFSA) approved health claims for the following phytochemicals (both of which are polyphenols — see the table):

1. Flavanols (also called flavan-3-ols) in cacao — believed to contribute to the health of our blood vessel walls

2. Hydroxytyrosol in olives and olive oil — believed to protect blood lipids from oxidative damage.

Phytochemicals can either be phytonutrients (good for our health) or phytotoxins (damaging to our health). In fact, some phytotoxins have historically been used as poisons. Thus, phytonutrients and phytotoxins are subsets of phytochemicals with divergent effects.

There are many classes and subclasses of phytochemicals. Some are found in all plant foods while others are specific to a particular plant. Two major classes of phytochemicals are carotenoids (found in yellow, orange and red fruits and vegetables) and polyphenols. Polyphenols are further subdivided into flavonoids, phenolic acids, stilbenes, and lignans. Each of these categories is further and further subdivided.

The following table provides a simplified overview of phytochemicals in relation to cacao.

PHYTOCHEMICALS		
Polyphenols		Carotenoids
Flavonoids are the most common polyphenols in the human diet.	The main types of flavonoids are: 1. **Flavanols** 2. Flavonols 3. Flavones 4. Isoflavones 5. Flavaones 6. Anthocy	Carotenoids are a group of >750 pigments made by plants, algae and bacteria. Humans consume about 50 of these carotenoids through eating yellow, orange and red fruits and vegetables.
Phenolic acids		
Stilbenes		
Lignans		

Confusing as it looks, both flavanols and flavonols are subclasses of flavonoids. I have to wonder why scientists would use two such similar names for different, albeit related, compounds.

Examples of foods that contain flavonoids are cacao, parsley, kale, onions, berries, apples, citrus fruits, bananas and black and green tea.

Flavanols are further classified as catechins, epicatechins and proanthocyanins. One particular epicatechin called (-)-epicatechin (pronounced minus epicatechin) is credited with many of the purported health benefits of cacao. Unfortunately, a lot of flavanols in cacao are removed during chocolate-making because of their bitter and astringent taste.

There is currently no evidence that taking supplements containing phytonutrients benefit our health. Maybe in the future?